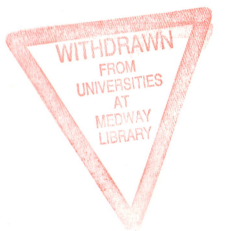

Advanced
Scanning Electron
Microscopy and
X-Ray Microanalysis

Advanced Scanning Electron Microscopy and X-Ray Microanalysis

Dale E. Newbury
National Bureau of Standards
Gaithersburg, Maryland

David C. Joy
AT & T Bell Laboratories
Murray Hill, New Jersey

Patrick Echlin
University of Cambridge
Cambridge, England

Charles E. Fiori
National Institutes of Health
Bethesda, Maryland

and

Joseph I. Goldstein
Lehigh University
Bethlehem, Pennsylvania

PLENUM PRESS • NEW YORK AND LONDON

Library of Congress Cataloging in Publication Data

Main entry under title:

Advanced scanning electron microscopy and X-ray microanalysis.

Includes bibliographies and index.
1. Scanning electron microscope. 2. X-ray microanalysis. I. Newbury, D. E. [DNLM:
1. Electron Probe Microanalysis. 2.Microscopy, Electron, Scanning. QH 212.S3 A244]
QH212.S3A38   1986   502.'8'25   85-28261
ISBN 0-306-42140-2

© 1986 Plenum Press, New York
A Division of Plenum Publishing Corporation
233 Spring Street, New York, N.Y. 10013

Printed in the United States of America

Preface

This book has its origins in the intensive short courses on scanning electron microscopy and x-ray microanalysis which have been taught annually at Lehigh University since 1972. In order to provide a textbook containing the materials presented in the original course, the lecturers collaborated to write the book *Practical Scanning Electron Microscopy (PSEM),* which was published by Plenum Press in 1975. The course continued to evolve and expand in the ensuing years, until the volume of material to be covered necessitated the development of separate introductory and advanced courses. In 1981 the lecturers undertook the project of rewriting the original textbook, producing the volume *Scanning Electron Microscopy and X-Ray Microanalysis (SEMXM).* This volume contained substantial expansions of the treatment of such basic material as electron optics, image formation, energy-dispersive x-ray spectrometry, and qualitative and quantitative analysis. At the same time, a number of chapters, which had been included in the *PSEM* volume, including those on magnetic contrast and electron channeling contrast, had to be dropped for reasons of space. Moreover, these topics had naturally evolved into the basis of the advanced course. In addition, the evolution of the SEM and microanalysis fields had resulted in the development of new topics, such as digital image processing, which by their nature became topics in the advanced course.

Thus, following this progression of development, the lecturers of the advanced course have collaborated to produce a book containing the principal topics covered in that course. In comparison to the introductory *SEMXM* volume, the topics covered in this book are undergoing rapid development. Our current efforts represent a snapshot of the field at this point in time. We fully expect these areas to develop quite substantially, and we hope that our efforts to assemble these chapters may be of aid to our readers in making their own contributions to a most exciting field of work.

Dale E. Newbury
David C. Joy
Patrick Echlin
Charles E. Fiori
Joseph I. Goldstein

Contents

Advanced Scanning Electron Microscopy and X-Ray Microanalysis

Modeling Electron Beam–Specimen Interactions

1.1. Introduction

In order to interpret features in SEM images or to develop microanalytical procedures, it is often necessary to formulate a model of the interaction of the electron beam with the specimen. Such models can provide a quantitative description of one or more of the measurable products of the beam–specimen interaction: backscattered electrons, secondary electrons, characteristic and bremsstrahlung x-rays, absorbed current, and so on. There are at least four distinct approaches to modeling these interactions: (1) simple analytic equations based on scattering cross sections; (2) Monte Carlo electron trajectory simulation; (3) electron transport calculations; and (4) dynamical diffraction theory. A detailed description of the various approaches to modeling could easily fill an entire volume. In our discussion, consideration will be limited to a description of analytic forms and Monte Carlo techniques, which are the most flexible of the modeling techniques and the most easily understood. Readers interested in electron transport methods should refer to the detailed review by Fathers and Rez (1979); dynamical diffraction theory, which is applicable to crystalline materials, particularly in the form of thin foils imaged in the transmission electron microscope (TEM) or scanning transmission electron microscope (STEM), is described in detail by Hirsch *et al.* (1965).

1.2. Cross Sections for Scattering Processes

1.2.1. General Properties

The starting point for most modeling is a mathematical description of the scattering processes of interest as expressed in terms of a cross section. A cross section, Q, is a measure of the probability that a scattering process will occur and is given in terms of the effective size of the scattering center:

$$Q = N/n_t n_i \tag{1.1}$$

where N is the number of events per unit volume (events/cm³), n_t is the number of target sites per unit volume (atoms/cm³), and n_i is the number of incident particles per unit area (e^-/cm²). The complete dimensions of Q (also commonly denoted as σ) are thus events/e^- per (atom/cm²) or cm², when the "dimensionless" quantities (events, electrons, and atoms) are not considered. It is important to be aware of the complete dimensions of the cross section, because dimensional arguments can be used in constructing the simplest analytical models, as will be illustrated below.

The cross section forms the basis for the derivation of two other parameters that can be used to describe the scattering situation: (1) the mean free path and (2) the probability of scattering. (1) The mean free path, λ, is the average distance the beam electron must travel through the specimen to undergo an average of one event of a particular type. The cross section can be converted into a mean free path by means of a dimensional argument:

$$Q \text{ [events/}e^- \text{ per (atom/cm}^2)] \times N_0 \text{ (atoms/mol)} \times 1/A \text{ (mol/g)}$$
$$\times \rho \text{ (g/cm}^3) = 1/\lambda \qquad \text{events/cm} \tag{1.2}$$

or

$$\lambda = A/QN_0\rho \qquad \text{cm/event} \tag{1.3}$$

where N_0 is Avogadro's number, A is the atomic weight, and ρ is the density.

The mean free path for a given type of event i is obtained by substituting the appropriate cross section Q_i into equation (1.3). Thus, mean free paths can be separately calculated for elastic scattering, inner shell ionization, plasmon scattering, and so on. If several different scattering processes can occur, the total mean free path, λ_T, which considers all of the processes, can be calculated as

$$1/\lambda_T = \sum_i 1/\lambda_i \tag{1.4}$$

(2) The probability of scattering, p (events/e^-), gives the number of scattering events per electron as it travels through a specimen of thickness t,

and from the arguments given above, the probability is given by

$$p = QN_0\rho t/A \tag{1.5}$$

Scattering events fall into two general categories: (1) elastic scattering, in which the direction of flight of the electron is altered but the energy remains the same, and (2) inelastic scattering, in which both the direction of flight and the energy of the beam electron are altered. Inelastic scattering is responsible for the transfer to the specimen of energy which subsequently can result in the emission of secondary radiation, including secondary electrons, characteristic x-rays and Auger electrons, bremsstrahlung x-rays, and so on. Cross sections are generally functions of the energy of the incident electron, E, the scattering angle θ by which the electron is deviated from its incident path, the element of solid angle into which the electron is scattered, $d\Omega$, and the energy of the secondary product, which can be created in an inelastic interaction. A cross section is termed a "differential cross section" if it can be expressed in terms of a derivative function, for example:

$$dQ/d\theta = f(\theta) \tag{1.6}$$

A total cross section (with respect to one or more variables) is found by integration over the complete range of the variable(s).

1.2.2. Elastic Scattering

Elastic scattering results from the deflection of the beam electron by the positive charge of the nucleus of the atom, as screened or reduced in value by the orbital electrons. The Rutherford differential cross section for elastic scattering as a function of the scattering angle θ for a constant value of the electron energy E is given by

$$dQ(\theta) = \frac{e^4 Z^2}{16(4\pi\epsilon_0 E)^2} \frac{d\Omega}{[\sin^2(\theta/2) + (\theta_0^2/4)]^2} \tag{1.7}$$

where $d\Omega = 2\pi \sin \theta \, d\theta$ is the element of solid angle into which the electron of energy E is scattered at an angle θ from its incident direction, e is the electronic charge, Z is the atomic number of the scattering atom, ϵ_0 is the dielectric constant, and $\theta_0^2/4$ is the screening parameter δ and is numerically equal to

$$\delta = \theta_0^2/4 = 3.4 \times 10^{-3} Z^{2/3}/E \quad (E \text{ in keV}) \tag{1.8}$$

A full derivation of equation (1.8) from first principles has been given by Henoc and Maurice (1976).

Equation (1.8) can be integrated over all possible scattering angles from 0 to 180° to give a total elastic scattering cross section:

$$Q = \frac{e^4 Z^2}{4E^2} \frac{\pi}{\delta(1 + \delta)} \tag{1.9}$$

The total elastic scattering cross section for copper is shown in Figure 1.1. Up to energies of approximately 50 keV, relativistic effects of the electron velocity can be safely ignored, representing a correction of only 1% to the cross section at 10 keV. Above this energy, a relativistic correction should be applied. Equation (1.8) can be corrected for relativistic effects by first substituting the Bohr radius, a_0, where

$$a_0 = \frac{\epsilon_0 h^2}{\pi m_0 e^2} = 5.29 \times 10^{-9} \text{ cm} \tag{1.10a}$$

where h is Planck's constant and m_0 is the electron rest mass. The electron wavelength λ is also substituted in equation (1.7), where

$$\lambda = h/(2m_0 E)^{1/2} \tag{1.10b}$$

The transformed equation is thus

$$dQ(\theta) = \frac{Z^2 \lambda^4}{64\pi^4 a_0} \frac{d\Omega}{[\sin^2(\theta/2) + (\theta_0^2/4)]^2} \tag{1.11}$$

The relativistic correction is then made by substituting the relativistically corrected wavelength λ_r into equation (1.11), where

$$\lambda_r = h/[2m_0 E(1 + E/2m_0 c^2)]^{1/2} \tag{1.12}$$
$$= 3.87 \times 10^{-9}/E^{1/2}(1 + 9.79 \times 10^{-4} E)^{1/2} \text{ (cm)}$$

The probability for elastic scattering into an angular range from 0 to a given angle θ_1 can be found by integrating the cross section differential in scattering angle as normalized by the total elastic scattering cross section:

$$P(\theta) = \int_\Omega [Q(\theta)/Q] \, d\Omega = \int_0^{\theta_1} [2\pi \sin \theta Q(\theta)/Q] \, d\theta \tag{1.13}$$
$$P(\theta) = (1 + \delta)[(1 - 2\delta)/(1 - \cos \theta + 2\delta)]$$

where $\delta = 3.4 \times 10^{-3} Z^{2/3}/E$.

The Rutherford elastic scattering cross section has been found to be reasonably accurate for intermediate beam energies, e.g., 20–50 keV, and for targets of low to intermediate atomic number, e.g., Cu. It has been demonstrated that the exact quantum mechanical formulation of the elastic scattering cross section should be employed at low beam energies and for high-atomic-number targets (Reimer and Krefting, 1976). Unfortunately, the exact elastic cross section (see Mott and Massey, 1965) cannot be expressed in a simple analytic form such as equation (1.7) for the Rutherford cross section. Reimer and Krefting (1976) have provided graphical comparisons of the Rutherford and Mott cross sections, and Figure 1.2, which shows the comparison for Ge and Au, is taken from their work.

Elastic scattering of the beam electrons gives rise to the interaction volume in a solid target and to the phenomenon of electron backscattering, which yields a useful signal for imaging the sample. Strictly speaking, backscattering results from a single scattering event which causes the electron path to deviate by more than 90° from the incident direction. After such a scattering event, the electron propagates back into the unit hemisphere of solid angle from which it entered. In the sense in which the term is used in scanning electron microscopy, backscattering includes beam electrons which undergo multiple elastic and inelastic scattering events before emerging from the surface of the specimen.

1.2.3. Inelastic Scattering

Inelastic scattering occurs through a variety of interactions of the beam electron with the electrons and atoms of the sample. The type of interaction and the amount of energy loss depend on whether the specimen electrons are excited singly or collectively and on the binding energy of the electron to the atom. The excitation of the specimen electrons leads to the generation of secondary products which can be used to image or analyze the sample. Separate cross sections can be described for the processes of low-energy ("slow") and high-energy ("fast") secondary electrons, inner shell ionization, which leads to the emission of characteristic x-rays and Auger electrons, bremsstrahlung x-rays, plasmon scattering, and thermal diffuse scattering.

1.2.3.1. Single Electron Excitations

1.2.3.1.1. Low-Energy Secondary Electrons. Secondary electrons are generated by scattering of the beam electron by the loosely bound conduction-band electrons of the solid. The energy transferred to the conduction-band electron is relatively small and in the range of 1–50 eV.

Because of the low energy of the secondary electrons, their range in the solid is only of the order of 5 nm. Although secondary electrons are generated along the entire trajectory of the beam electron within the target, only those secondaries generated when the beam electron is near the surface of the solid have a significant probability of escape.

The differential cross section with respect to secondary electron energy is given by (Streitwolf, 1959)

$$Q_{SE}(E_{SE}) = n_C e^4 k_F^3 A / 3\pi E \rho N_0 (E_{SE} - E_F)^2 \qquad (1.14)$$

where the cross section is expressed in terms of secondary electrons per unit energy interval per incident electron per (atom/cm²). In equation (1.14), n_C is the number of conduction-band electrons per atom, A is the atomic weight, k_F is the magnitude of the wave vector ($k_F = 1/\lambda_F$), which corresponds to the Fermi energy E_F, E_{SE} is the secondary electron energy, and E is the beam energy, with all energies in keV. A total cross section can be obtained by integrating equation (1.14) over the practical range of secondary electron energies. Since the cross section in equation (1.14) is undefined at $E_{SE} = E_F$, the lower limit of integration can be arbitrarily set at $E_{SE} = E_F + 1$ eV. The upper limit of integration is also set arbitrarily at a value of 50 eV, which defines an energy range covering the practical extent of secondary electron energies:

$$Q_{SE} = e^4 k_F^3 A n_C [1/(E_F - 0.050 \text{ keV}) - 1/(0.001 \text{ keV})]/3\pi E \rho N_0 \qquad (1.15)$$

Values of the constant in equation (1.15) for several metals are listed in Table 1.1, as well as calculated values of the total cross section for a beam energy of 20 keV.

1.2.3.1.2. Fast Secondary Electrons. Although the most numerous secondary electrons are those of low energy, $E_{SE} \leq 50$ eV, it is possible for the beam electron to interact with more tightly bound electrons and transfer larger amounts of energy, creating the so-called "fast secondary

Table 1.1. Production of Secondary Electrons in Various Metals

Element	E_F (eV)	k_F (1/cm)	n_C (e^-/atom)	Q (E = 20 keV) [secondaries/e^- per (atom/cm²)]
Cu	7.0	1.35×10^8	1	3.2×10^{-18}
Au	5.5	1.20×10^8	1	3.1×10^{-18}
Li	4.7	1.10×10^8	1	3.1×10^{-18}
Na	3.1	9.00×10^7	1	3.1×10^{-18}
Ag	5.5	1.19×10^8	1	3.1×10^{-18}

electrons." Fast secondary electrons are of interest because their range is greater than that of low-energy secondaries and their angle of emission is nearly at right angles to the beam electron trajectory. Murata *et al.* (1981) have demonstrated that fast secondary electrons play a significant role in the degradation of lateral spatial resolution in the exposure of the electron beam resists.

Fast secondary electrons can be generated with energies up to that of the incident electron. Since the primary and secondary electrons cannot be distinguished after the collision, the cross sections for the two electrons are added, and the maximum possible energy loss is restricted to $\Delta E <$ $0.5E$. The cross section differential in secondary electron energy has been given by Moller (1931) as

$$Q(E_{FSE}) = \pi e^4 Z_i [(1/\epsilon)^2 + 1/(1 - \epsilon)^2]/E^2 \qquad (1.16)$$

where ϵ is the energy transferred to the fast secondary electron normalized by the beam electron energy, $\epsilon = E_{FSE}/E$, and Z_i is the number of atomic electrons. This equation can be integrated over the range of fast secondary electron energies, with the lower limit of integration set at $E_{FSE} =$ 0.050 keV and the upper limit set at $E_{FSE} = 0.5E$. The result is given by

$$Q_{FSE} = \pi e^4 Z_i \{(1/\epsilon_{min}) - [1/(1 - \epsilon_{min})]\} \qquad (1.17)$$

The scattering angle of the primary electron after the collision relative to its incident direction is given by

$$\sin^2 \theta = 2\epsilon/(2 + E' - E'\epsilon) \qquad (1.18)$$

where $E' = E/511$ keV. The scattering angle of the fast secondary electron relative to the incident primary is given by

$$\sin^2 \phi = 2(1 - \epsilon)/(2 + E'\epsilon) \qquad (1.19)$$

For a beam electron energy of 20 keV and a fast secondary electron energy of 1 keV, the fast secondary electron is scattered at an angle of 77° from the incident beam electron trajectory.

1.2.3.1.3. Inner Shell Ionization. Inner shell ionization occurs when the beam electron transfers sufficient energy to a tightly bound inner shell electron to eject it from the atom. The atom is left in an excited state and subsequently undergoes deexcitation by means of electron transitions from outer shells. The energy released during these transitions can manifest itself as either a characteristic x-ray or an Auger electron. The fraction of ionizations which leads to x-ray emission is given by the fluorescence yield, ω. The fraction of Auger electrons produced is given by $1 - \omega$. The total cross section for inner shell ionization is given by (Bethe, 1930)

$$Q_i = \pi e^4 n_s b_s \log[c_s(m_0 v^2/2)/E_c]/(m_0 v^2/2)E_c \qquad (1.20a)$$

where n_s is the number of electrons in the shell, b_s and c_s are constants appropriate to the shell, E_c is the critical excitation energy, m_0 is the rest mass of the electron, and v is the velocity. At the low beam energies appropriate to most scanning electron microscopy and x-ray microanalysis, the mass of the moving electron is very nearly that of the rest mass, so that the term $m_0 v^2/2$ can be set equal with little error to the kinetic energy of the electron, which is the energy imparted to the electron as a result of its acceleration through the potential drop V, or kinetic energy $= eV$, where e is the electronic charge:

$$\text{Low } V (< 50 \text{ kV}) \qquad m_0 v^2/2 = eV = E \qquad (1.20b)$$

With this subsitution, equation (1.20a) thus becomes

$$Q_i = \pi e^4 n_s b_s \log(c_s E/E_c)/E_c E \qquad (1.20c)$$

where E is the beam energy. Equation (1.20c) is often expressed in terms of the overvoltage, $U = E/E_c$, and also expressing the constant πe^4 for E in keV:

$$Q_i = 6.51 \times 10^{-20} n_s b_s \log(c_s U)/U E_c^2 \qquad (1.20d)$$

where the dimensions are ionizations/e^- per (atom/cm^2).

At high beam energies, $E > 50$ keV, the relativistic velocity of the electron becomes important, and the mass of the moving electron deviates significantly from the rest mass, so that the term $m_0 v^2/2$ can no longer be set equal to the kinetic energy. Bethe and Fermi (1932) and Williams (1933) have described a relativistic modification to equation (1.20a):

$$Q_i = \{\pi e^4 n_s b_s/[(m_0 v^2/2)E_c]\}\{\log[c_s(m_0 v^2/2)/E_c]$$
$$+ \log(1 - \beta^2) - \beta^2\} \qquad (1.21a)$$

where $\beta = v/c$ and c is the velocity of light. The term $m_0 v^2/2$ can be replaced by the substitution $m_0 v^2/2 = m_0 c^2 \beta^2/2 = 255.5\beta^2$ (keV units) since $m_0c^2 = 511$ keV. The value of β can be calculated from the accelerating potential V (kV units) by the relation

$$\beta = \{1 - [1 + (V/511)]^{-2}\}^{1/2} \qquad (1.21b)$$

The constants b_s and c_s depend on the shell which is excited and have been assigned a range of values by different authors. Thus, for K-shell ionization, Mott and Massey (1949) gave $b_K = 0.35$ and $c_K = 2.42$. In an extensive examination of available experimental data, Powell (1976) deduced that for the overvoltage range $4 < U < 25$, the constants have the values $b_K = 0.9$ and $c_K = 0.65$.

Note that the Powell constants should not be applied at low overvoltages, since with the choice of $c_K = 0.65$, the cross section becomes negative due to the log term below $U = 1.55$. In the analysis of solid specimens, we are frequently interested in inner shell ionization from the incident beam energy down to $E = E_c$, since a significant fraction of the electrons lose all their energy in the solid. For calculations in solid specimens, the constants given by Brown (1974) are useful:

$$c_K = 1 \qquad b_K = 0.52 + 0.0029Z \qquad (1.22a)$$
$$c_{L23} = 1 \qquad b_{L23} = 0.44 + 0.0020Z \qquad (1.22b)$$

where Z is the atomic number. With $c_K = c_{L23} = 1$, the cross section remains positive down to $U = 1$.

If the relativistic form of the ionization cross section is used, it should be noted that there is an important consequence of making the substitution $m_0v^2/2 = m_0c^2\beta^2/2$. At a kinetic energy $E = 100$ keV, the term $m_0v^2/2$ expressed in keV units is only 76.7 keV. If the constant c in the log term is taken as unity, then the log term will be negative for a significant range of electron kinetic energy above the edge. To avoid the physical unreality of this situation, it is necessary to adjust the constant c_K to reflect the change in the term $m_0v^2/2$ (Williams *et al.*, 1984).

1.2.3.2. Multiple Electron Excitations

1.2.3.2.1. Bremsstrahlung. As the beam electron passes through the coulomb field of the atom, it can undergo deceleration which decreases the magnitude of the velocity and, hence, the kinetic energy. The energy lost by the beam electron is emitted as a photon of electromagnetic radiation. This radiation is known as "bremsstrahlung" or "braking radiation" and since any deceleration is possible from no loss up to total loss of the kinetic energy of the electron, the bremsstrahlung forms a continuous spectrum from zero energy to the incident beam energy. The intensity of bremsstrahlung emission depends on the angle relative to the beam electron trajectory.

Kirkpatrick and Weidmann (1945) described algebraic equations which provided a fit to the Sommerfeld (1931) theory for bremsstrahlung production. These equations give the components of the cross section for bremsstrahlung production of energy E_b along axes x, y, z oriented such that x lies along the beam electron trajectory and y and z lie in a plane orthogonal to x. Following Statham (1976a), the units of these cross sections are given in terms of [(keV photon energy/keV energy interval per steradian per (atom/cm^2)]:

$$Q_x = 4.5 \times 10^{-25} Z^2 \{0.252 + a[(E_b/E) - 0.135] $$
$$- b[(E_b/E) - 0.135]^2\}/E \quad (1.23a)$$

$$a = 1.47B - 0.507A - 0.833$$
$$b = 1.70B - 1.09A - 0.627$$
$$A = \exp(-0.223E/0.2998Z^2) - \exp(-57E/0.2998Z^2)$$
$$B = \exp(-0.0828E/0.2998Z^2) - \exp(-84.9E/0.2998Z^2)$$

$$Q_y = Q_z = 4.5 \times 10^{-25} Z^2 (-j + \{k/[(E_b/E) + h]\}/E)$$
$$h = (-0.214y_1 + 1.21y_2 - y_3)/(1.43y_1 - 2.43y_2 + y_3)$$
$$j = (1 + 2h)y_2 - 2(1 + h)y_3$$
$$k = (1 + h)(y_3 + j) \quad (1.23b)$$
$$y_1 = 0.220[1 - 0.390 \exp(-26.9E/0.2998Z^2)]$$
$$y_2 = 0.067 + 0.023/[(E/0.2998Z^2) + 0.75]$$
$$y_3 = -0.00259 + 0.00776/[(E/0.2998Z^2) + 0.116]$$

These components resolved along the three axes of the coordinate system can be combined to give the cross section at a particular angle ψ in the x–z plane which contains the beam direction:

$$Q(\Psi) = Q_x \sin^2 \psi + Q_y + Q_z \cos^2 \psi \quad (1.24)$$

The total cross section is found by integrating over 4π steradians:

$$Q_B = 8\pi(Q_x + Q_y + Q_z)/3 \quad (1.25)$$

1.2.3.2.2. Plasmon Scattering. The coulomb field of the beam electron can perturb the free electron gas of conduction-band electrons of a metal at long range. The beam electron excites oscillations or "plasmons" in this free electron gas. The cross section differential in scattering angle per conduction-band electron per unit volume is given by (Ferrel, 1956)

$$Q_p(\phi) = \phi_p/2\pi a_0(\phi^2 + \phi_p^2) = 3 \times 10^7 \phi_p/(\phi^2 + \phi_p^2) \quad (1.26)$$

where a_0 is the Bohr radius and $\phi_p = \Delta E_p/2E$, where ΔE_p is the energy transferred to the plasmon wave. Plasmon scattering results typically in an energy transfer ΔE_p in the range 3–30 eV, depending on the atomic number. For an aluminum target, $\Delta E_p = 15$ eV, hence for a beam energy of 10 keV, the plasmon scattering angle $\phi_p = 1.5 \times 10^{-3}$ radian. Plasmon scattering is peaked so sharply forward that the total plasmon scattering cross section can be found by setting $d\Omega = 2\pi \sin \phi \, d\phi = 2\pi\phi \, d\phi$:

$$Q_p = \int_\Omega Q_p(\phi) \, d\Omega = (\phi_p/2\pi a_0) \int_0^{\phi_1} [2\pi\phi/(\phi^2 + \phi_p^2)] \, d\phi \quad (1.27)$$

Taking the upper integration limit as $\phi_1 = 0.175$ rad where $\phi \cong \sin \phi$ and incorporating the factor $n_C A/\rho N_0$ to put the cross section on the basis (atom/cm^2) gives the total cross section as

$$Q_p = n_C A \phi_p [\log(\phi_p^2 + 0.175^2) - \log(\phi_p^2)]/2N_0\rho a_0 \quad (1.28)$$

1.2.3.3. Comparison of Cross Sections

Figure 1.1 is a plot of the elastic, plasmon, slow secondary electron, fast secondary electron, L-shell ionization, and K-shell ionization cross sections for a copper target over the energy range 1–50 keV. For this element, the largest cross section is that for elastic scattering, while the largest inelastic cross section, which has a similar value, is found to be that of plasmon scattering. For lighter elements, e.g., aluminum, the elastic scattering cross section decreases relative to the inelastic cross sections so

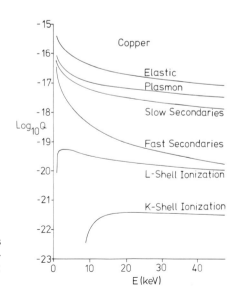

Figure 1.1. Cross sections for various scattering processes calculated for a copper target over the energy range $1 < E < 50$ keV.

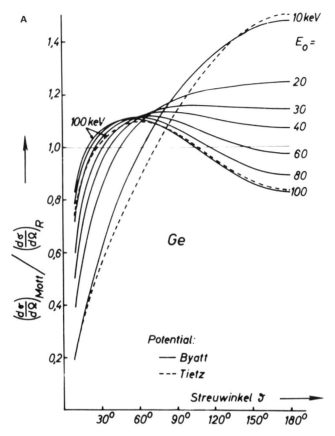

Figure 1.2. Ratio of the Mott elastic scattering cross section to the Rutherford elastic scattering cross section (Reimer and Krefting, 1976). (A) Germanium; (B) gold.

that inelastic scattering dominates. For elements of high atomic number, the elastic cross section increases relative to the inelastic cross section, so that elastic scattering dominates.

1.2.3.4. Continuous Energy Loss Approximation

The energy loss rate due to all of the inelastic scattering processes can be estimated from the continuous energy loss approximation of Bethe (1933). The energy loss dE per unit of distance dx traveled in the solid is given by

$$dE/dx = (-2\pi e^4 N_0 Z\rho/A E_m) \log(1.166 E_m/J) \tag{1.29}$$
$$= -7.85 \times 10^4 (Z\rho/A E_m) \log(1.166 E_m/J) \quad \text{(keV/cm)}$$

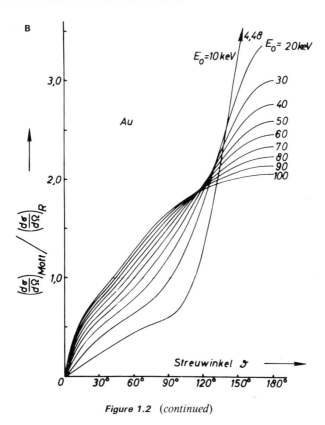

Figure 1.2 (*continued*)

where E_m is the mean energy across the distance interval dx. J is the mean ionization potential, which is the average energy loss per interaction considering all possible energy loss processes. J has been given as (Berger and Seltzer, 1964)

$$J = (9.76Z + 58.5Z^{-0.19}) \times 10^{-3} \quad \text{(keV)} \quad (1.30)$$

1.3. Analytic Modeling

An "analytic model" of electron–specimen interaction is a mathematical model which can be expressed in the form of an analytic expression, that is, an algebraic formula relating the parameters of the beam, such as energy and current, and the parameters of the specimen, such as atomic number, tilt, dimensions, shape, and so on. In order to illustrate the development of analytic models, we shall consider the calculation of x-ray generation in two types of specimens: (1) thin foils and (2) semi-infinite, flat solids.

1.3.1. X-Ray Generation in Thin Foils

A foil shall be considered "thin" if its thickness is equal to or less than the mean free path for elastic scattering. In passing through such a foil, the average electron will undergo no more than one elastic scattering event. Simultaneously with elastic scattering, the various processes of inelastic scattering can occur. In particular, the beam electron can cause inner shell ionization with the subsequent production of x-rays during deexcitation. The cross section Q_i, given by equation (1.24), has dimensions ionizations/e^- per (atom/cm^2). This crosss ection can be utilized to calculate the x-ray production along a path t by the following dimensional argument:

$$
\begin{array}{ccc}
n_x & = & Q_i \\
\text{(photons/}e^-\text{)} & & \text{[ionizations/}e^-\text{ per (atom/cm}^2\text{)]}
\end{array}
$$

$$
\begin{array}{ccc}
\times & \omega & \times & N_0 \\
 & \text{(photons/ionization)} & & \text{(atoms/mole)}
\end{array}
$$

$$
\begin{array}{cccccc}
\times & 1/A & \times & \rho & \times C_A \times & t \\
 & \text{(moles/g)} & & \text{(g/cm}^3\text{)} & & \text{(cm)}
\end{array} \tag{1.31}
$$

$$
n_x = Q_i \omega N_0 \rho C_A t / A
$$

where ω is the fluorescence yield, N_0 is Avogadro's number, A is the atomic weight, ρ is the density, and C_A is the concentration of element A.

If we examine the scattering situation closely, the electrons incident normally on the foil of thickness t actually travel a distance greater than t due to the deviation caused by elastic scattering. In order to calculate the additional path length through the sample which results from elastic scattering, it is necessary to make use of the angular distribution of the scattered electrons. Table 1.2 gives the probability for scattering into various angular ranges and the cumulative scattering probability, derived from equation (1.13), for a copper target at a beam energy of 20 keV. A cumulative probability of 0.5 is found for a scattering angle of 4.6°. Taking this angle to approximate the average scattering angle, and making the assumption that the average electron undergoes scattering at the center of the foil, the path length as modified by eleastic scattering can be calculated as

$$
t' = t/2 + (t/2)/\cos \theta_{av} \tag{1.32}
$$

This modified path length can then be substituted in equation (1.31). Strictly speaking, a further modification to equation (1.31) should be

Table 1.2. Angular Elastic Scattering Distribution for Copper Beam Energy
20 keV

Angular increment	$P(\theta)$	Cumulative probability
1	0.045	0.045
2	0.115	0.160
3	0.140	0.300
4	0.132	0.432
5	0.111	0.543
6	0.0886	0.632
7	0.0681	0.700
8	0.0532	0.753
9	0.0415	0.794
10	0.0329	0.827
15	0.0884	0.915
20	0.0360	0.951
25	0.0174	0.968
30	0.0102	0.978
40	0.0085	0.986
50	0.0067	0.9927
60	0.0025	0.9952
75	0.0021	0.9973
90	0.0011	0.9984
105	0.00066	0.9990
120	0.00047	0.99947
135	0.00026	0.99973
150	0.00015	0.99988
165	0.00009	0.99997
180	0.00003	1.0

made. The energy of the electron decreases as it passes through the foil
due to other inelastic scattering processes. Since the ionization cross section is dependent on the electron energy, the calculation should be modified to account for the change in energy. The Bethe continuous energy
loss approximation, equation (1.29), can be used to estimate this energy
loss. From equation (1.29), the energy loss rate $dE/dx = 0.0069$ keV/nm
for copper at 20 keV. Thus, in a foil with a thickness of the order of 10
nm, the energy loss would be of the order of 0.06 keV. At 20 keV, the
ionization cross section would change by 0.3% in response to this change
in energy.

1.3.2. X-Ray Generation in Thick Targets

Eventually, as the thickness of the specimen in the previous calculation is increased, the energy loss along the electron path becomes sufficiently large to cause an appreciable change in the ionization cross section. In a semi-infinite solid target, a large fraction of the beam electrons

lose all of their energy during inelastic scattering. In such a case, it is necessary to follow the change in the beam energy and ionization cross section from the incident beam energy, E_0, to the edge energy for the shell of interest, E_c. The thin foil calculation given in equation (1.31) thus becomes the basis for an integration procedure with t replaced by dx. The procedure for this integration has been described in detail by Philibert and Tixier (1968); we shall illustrate the major steps and the final result. From equation (1.31), the differential production of x-rays dn_x along an element of path dx can be written as

$$dn_x = (C_A N_0 \rho Q_i \omega / A) \, dx \qquad (1.33)$$

In order to find the total x-ray production in the solid, we must integrate equation (1.33) along the total path length from 0 to the range corresponding to the point at which the energy of the electron decreases to the edge energy of the x-ray line of interest, $E = E_c$:

$$n_x = (C_A N_0 \rho \omega / A) \int_0^R Q_i(E) \, ds \qquad (1.34)$$

In equation (1.34) the relationship between $Q(E)$ and path length can be established by means of the Bethe expression, which gives the functional dependence of $dE/ds = f(E)$:

$$n_x = (C_A N_0 \rho \omega / A) \int_{E_0}^{E_c} [Q_i(E)/(dE/ds)] \, dE \qquad (1.35)$$

When the appropriate equations are substituted in equation (1.35) for Q_i (equation 1.20) and dE/ds (equation 1.29), and the substitution $U = E/E_c$ is made, the integration becomes

$$n_{xA} = [(C_A \omega n_s b_s)/2A_A M]\{(U_0 - 1) \\ - (\log W/W)[\mathrm{li}(U_0 W) - \mathrm{li}(W)]\} \qquad (1.36)$$

where n_{xA} is the number of x-rays produced by element A, $M = \Sigma_i (C_i Z_i/A_i)$, and W is the product $\Pi_i (1.166 E_c^A/J_i)$. The term li denotes the logarithmic integral, where the logarithmic integral of a number h is given by

$$\mathrm{li}(h) = 0.5772 + \log(\log h) + \sum_{s=1}^{s=\infty} (\log h)^s/ss! \qquad (1.37)$$

Although equation (1.36) gives the x-ray production for an electron which totally expends its energy in the target, in reality a significant fraction of the electrons are backscattered from a solid target, which removes a fraction of the energy which would otherwise have gone into the production of x-rays. Thus, a further correction must be made for the loss of x-ray production due to backscattering. Duncumb and Reed (1968) provided a graphical representation of the fraction of the total possible x-ray production, denoted "R," based on experimental measurements of the backscattering coefficient η and the energy distribution of backscattered electrons. More recently, Myklebust (1984) has provided an algebraic expression for R based on Monte Carlo electron trajectory calculations:

$$R = aZ + bZ^2 + cZ[\exp(-U)] + 1 \qquad (1.38)$$

where the constants are listed in Table 1.3.

Since R represents the fraction of total possible x-ray production, the final value of n_x calculated from equation (1.36) must be multiplied by R from equation (1.38) to give the backscatter-corrected x-ray production, n_{xBS}:

$$n_{xBS} = n_x R \qquad (1.39)$$

1.4. Monte Carlo Electron Trajectory Simulation

1.4.1. Formulation

The complexities involved in obtaining analytic expressions for electron interactions in solid samples are well illustrated by the previous example. The complex dependence of the cross sections for the various elastic and inelastic scattering processes on electron energy and the complex dependence of the rate of energy loss on electron energy [$dE/ds \sim (1/E)\log E$] lead to functional expressions which are difficult to integrate. Moreover, as is the case with the R factor given in equation (1.38), it is frequently necessary to make corrections for modifications to the production of secondary radiation caused by backscattering of the primary electrons. Finally, although the development given in equations (1.33) to (1.39) produces a useful expression for the total x-ray production, it gives

TABLE 1.3. Constants for Calculation of R, the Backscatter Correction[a]

	a	b	c
K-lines	−0.00673	1.79×10^{-5}	0.008624
L-lines	−0.00779	4.038×10^{-5}	0.007415
M-lines	−0.00751	3.262×10^{-5}	−0.006415

[a]From Myklebust (1984).

no information whatever on the distribution of the x-rays produced in the sample. The distribution of the generation of x-rays with depth in the sample, designated $\phi(\rho z)$, must be known in order to provide corrections for sample self-absorption. In fact, in the development of quantitative matrix correction procedures, it was necessary to measure the $\phi(\rho z)$ distribution experimentally, since analytic expressions could not be developed from first principles.

The technique of Monte Carlo electron trajectory simulation provides a "first principles" approach for the calculation of electron beam–specimen interactions which gives detailed information on the spatial distribution of scattering events. In the Monte Carlo technique, the beam electron is considered as a discrete particle which undergoes elastic and inelastic scattering with the atoms of the sample, which is considered amorphous. The trajectory is calculated in discrete steps, an example of which is shown in Figure 1.3. The electron undergoes a scattering interaction at location P which causes it to deviate by an angle θ from its previous path. It travels a distance S along the new path, where S is the step length of the calculation, until it undergoes another scattering event at point $P+1$. The selection of the scattering angles and step lengths is made from the scattering cross sections given above. Because significant angular deviations result only from elastic scattering events, it is common practice in Monte Carlo simulations to consider only elastic scattering when calculating the scattering angle, θ. The scattering angle distribution is found from equation (1.13) reexpressed in terms of a random number:

$$\cos \theta = 1 - [2\delta R/(1 + \delta - R)] \qquad (1.40)$$

where R is a random number such that $0 \leq R \leq 1$. Selection of random numbers linearly distributed across this range produces a histogram of

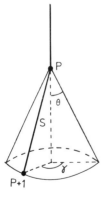

Figure 1.3. Fundamental repetitive calculation step of the Monte Carlo electron trajectory simulation technique illustrating the scattering parameters calculated for a single scattering step.

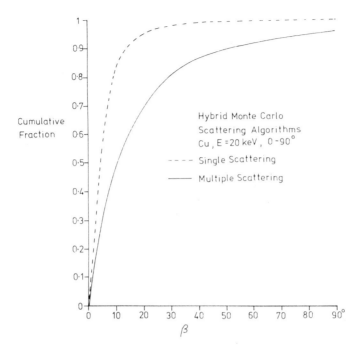

Figure 1.4. Scattering angle distributions produced by random number generator.

scattering angles, as illustrated in Figure 1.4. (The use of randomly selected numbers at several points in the calculation sequence gives the basis of the name "Monte Carlo" calculation.) The azimuthal angle γ in the base of the scattering cone shown in Figure 1.3 can take on any value in the range 0–360°, again selected by a random number.

Since only elastic scattering events are presumed to contribute to significant angular deviations, the step length between scattering events is determined from the mean free path for elastic scattering, which is found from equation (1.3) with the total elastic scattering cross section from equation (1.9). Because the mean free path is the value of the average distance between scattering events, a distribution is obtained by means of the equation

$$S = -\lambda_e \log R \qquad (1.41)$$

where λ_e is the elastic mean free path. From the scattering angles θ and γ and the step length S, the x, y, z coordinates of point $P+1$ can be calculated from the coordinates of point P.

Although inelastic scattering is neglected as far as angular deviations and the path length are concerned, energy loss due to inelastic scattering is considered by means of the Bethe continuous energy loss approximation, equation (1.29). The energy loss ΔE along a segment of path of length S is approximated as

$$\Delta E = S(dE/ds) \tag{1.42}$$

The production of secondary radiation along the electron path can be calculated from the appropriate cross section, the specimen atom species parameters (concentration, atomic number, atomic weight, and density), and the path length. Thus, for inner shell ionization, equation (1.31) is used with $S = t$. The value of electron energy appropriate to that step in the simulation is used for the calculation of the ionization cross section.

Thus, the trajectory of the electron is followed incrementally through the target, with constant knowledge of the electron coordinates, energy,

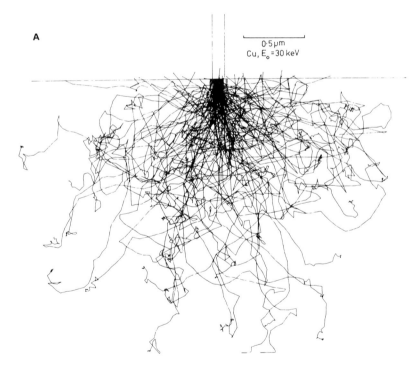

A

0·5 µm

Cu, $E_o = 30$ keV

Figure 1.5. Monte Carlo calculation for a copper target at a beam energy of 30 keV. (A) Electron trajectories; (B) sites of inner shell ionization events.

direction of flight, and production of secondary radiation. An example of electron trajectories calculated for a copper target at a beam energy of 30 keV is shown in Figure 1.5a, and the sites of possible inner shell ionization within the interaction volume are shown in Figure 1.5b. The great strength of the Monte Carlo procedure is the capability of calculating accurate spatial distributions. Of course, the accuracy of the calculation is limited by the accuracy of the cross sections used for calculation of the scattering angles and mean free path. In fact, it is usually necessary to apply a correction term to the mean free path calculated from the Rutherford elastic cross section in order to get good agreement between the Monte Carlo calculation and measured values of an interaction parameter such as the backscattering coefficient as a function of atomic number. For example, Kyser and Murata (1974) modified the Rutherford elastic mean free path with an atomic number-dependent correction of the form $\lambda'_e = \lambda_e(1 + Z/C)$ where C had a value of 300. The correspondence between the modified Monte Carlo calculation and the experimental val-

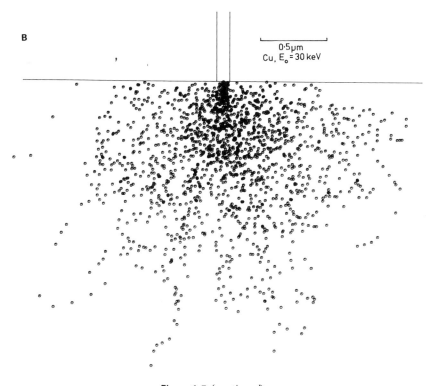

B

0·5µm
Cu, $E_o = 30\,keV$

Figure 1.5 (*continued*)

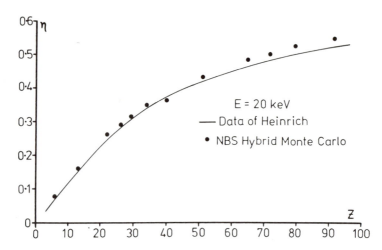

Figure 1.6. Calculation of backscattered electron coefficient from solid targets at a beam energy of 20 keV as compared to experimental data of Heinrich (1966).

ues of the backscattering coefficients is shown in Figure 1.6. The need for this empirical correction can be understood in terms of the deviation of the exact cross section from the Rutherford cross section illustrated in Figure 1.2. With this empirical adjustment to the mean free path fixed, the Monte Carlo simulation is found to be capable of calculating other experimentally measured parameters, such as the backscatter coefficient as a function of tilt, as shown in Figure 1.7, with considerable accuracy. Detailed testing of the results of Monte Carlo simulations has demonstrated their considerable utility in accurately calculating values of electron beam–specimen interaction parameters (Newbury and Myklebust, 1984).

The principal weakness of the Monte Carlo calculation is the need to calculate many trajectories in order to obtain statistical significance. Examination of the individual trajectories in Figure 1.5a reveals that each trajectory varies greatly from any of the others. The precision of a Monte Carlo calculation depends on the number of events calculated, with the standard deviation of the calculation given by

$$\sigma = \overline{n}^{1/2} \qquad (1.43)$$

where n refers to the number of trajectories which contribute to the event of interest. Thus, in a calculation of a backscattering coefficient, the precision of the calculation is not determined by the total number of elec-

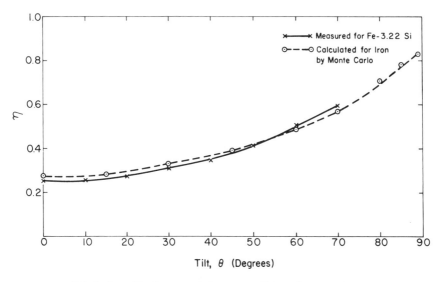

Figure 1.7. Calculation of backscattered electron coefficient from a solid iron target as a function of specimen tilt and compared to experimental data of Newbury *et al.* (1973).

trons calculated, but by the number of electrons which backscatter, so that

$$\sigma = (\eta N)^{1/2} \tag{1.44}$$

where N is the total number of trajectories calculated and η is the backscattering coefficient. In the same simulation, the calculation of characteristic x-ray production would be obtained with greater precision, since all of the incident electrons contribute to the generation of x-rays.

Because the position of the electron is continuously known, the calculation of distributions is straightforward. An example of a calculation of the depth distribution of x-ray generation is shown in Figure 1.8. An even more dramatic example of the utility of the Monte Carlo calculation for the simulation of electron interactions in complex targets is shown in Figure 1.9, where beams of various energies are shown interacting with spherical aluminum particles with a diameter of 2 μm.

The extensive development of Monte Carlo calculations has provided a major tool of great utility in the field of scanning electron microscopy and x-ray microanalysis analogous to the use of mathematical formulations of diffraction theory for the interpretation of images in the transmission electron microscopy of crystalline materials. Monte Carlo

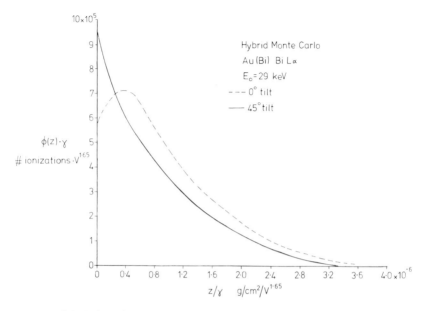

Figure 1.8. Calculation of depth distribution of inner shell ionization for gold tilted at 0 and 45°.

calculations have been applied to the study of magnetic contrast (Newbury *et al.*, 1973), x-ray emissions from particles (Yakowitz *et al.*, 1975; Newbury *et al.*, 1980), x-ray emissions from thin films (Kyser and Murata, 1974), and the resolution of signals in high-resolution images (Hembree *et al.*, 1981).

1.4.2. Applications of the Monte Carlo Method

The power of the Monte Carlo simulation for scanning electron microscopy and electron probe microanalysis lies in its adaptability to a wide range of problems. In many cases it is difficult to describe the electron interaction in a simple analytic fashion or to define the boundary conditions for solution by the transport equation. In such cases the approach of using an incremental calculation in which the electron position and velocity are followed in a stepwise fashion provides the flexibility needed to deal with difficult situations. The following examples will serve to illustrate the techniques which are used to adapt a Monte Carlo simulation to specific problems, as well as to illustrate the diversity of information which can be derived.

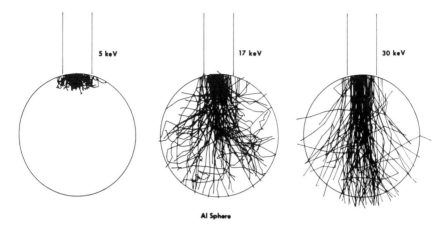

Figure 1.9. Calculation of electron interaction with aluminum spheres of diameter 2 μm at various beam energies (Newbury *et al.*, 1980).

1.4.2.1. Atomic Number Contrast

Consider a specimen which consists of regions of aluminum and gold. The specimen is flat, so that the only contrast mechanism which will operate is atomic number contrast in the backscattered electron signal. A backscattered electron detector will be employed which has an energy filter to exclude all electrons which have lost more than a defined fraction of the incident energy, E_0. We wish to calculate the contrast as a function of the fraction of the backscattered electron energy distribution which is excluded by the filter.

The information which is needed in this case is an energy histogram of the backscattered electrons. The energy of each backscattered electron is recorded when it is determined that the electron has exited through the sample surface. The backscattered electron energy distribution in increments of $0.1E_0$ is listed in Table 1.4. The atomic number contrast will be calculated by assuming that the signal is proportional to the backscattering coefficient:

$$C = \Delta S/S_{\max} = \Delta\eta/\eta_{\max} \qquad (1.45)$$

In addition to the Monte Carlo calculations of backscattering from gold and aluminum targets, Table 1.4 also contains the contrast for each energy increment as calculated by equation (1.45). From these calculations, it can be seen that the contrast increases as electrons which have lost significant amounts of energy are excluded from the signal.

Table 1.4. Energy Distribution of Backscattered Electrons[a]

Energy range	Aluminum backscatter	Gold backscatter	Contrast	ϵC^2
$E_0->0.9E_0$	0.0124	0.1614	0.923	0.1375
$E_0->0.8E_0$	0.0327	0.3072	0.894	0.2455
$E_0->0.7E_0$	0.0613	0.3904	0.843	0.2774
$E_0->0.6E_0$	0.0904	0.4388	0.794	0.2766
$E_0->0.5E_0$	0.1163	0.4674	0.751	0.2636
$E_0->0.4E_0$	0.1365	0.4861	0.719	0.2515
$E_0->0.3E_0$	0.1500	0.4960	0.698	0.2414
$E_0->0.2E_0$	0.1585	0.5011	0.684	0.2342
$E_0->0.1E_0$	0.1619	0.5035	0.679	0.2318
$E_0->0$	0.1627	0.5039	0.677	0.2310

[a]Conditions: E_0 = 20 keV. Trajectories: 20,000 on each target.

In establishing the threshold current which is necessary to ensure the visibility of a feature, it is not the contrast alone which sets the limitations, but instead the product of the efficiency of signal collection and the contrast squared. Assuming that the efficiency is proportional to the collected signal, which in turn is proportional to the backscatter coefficient, the parameter

$$\epsilon C^2 \cong \eta C^2 \tag{1.46}$$

can also be calculated, and this value is tabulated in Table 1.4. The behavior of this term as a function of energy demonstrates that the best visibility is not achieved with the maximum contrast, which occurs for the interval $E_0-0.9E_0$, but rather occurs when the filter is set to the window $E_0-0.7E_0$. A further increase in the width of the accepted energy window beyond this range produces a decrease in visibility.

With data derived from a Monte Carlo simulation such as that shown in Table 1.1, it is possible to calculate other situations of interest. For example, if a solid-state silicon backscattered electron detector is used, such a detector modifies the signal through an energy response function which increases linearly with electron energy above a threshold value. This response has the effect of producing an output signal which is weighted in favor of the high-energy fraction of backscattered electrons. Alternatively, if a secondary electron conversion detector is used, the resulting signal is skewed to favor the low-energy fraction of the backscattered electron energy distribution. It should be noted that the knowledge of the backscattered electron energy distribution gained from the Monte Carlo calculation is critical in determining the magnitude of such effects.

1.4.2.2. Modeling Type II Magnetic Contrast

The Monte Carlo simulation has been used to study the properties of type II magnetic contrast (Fathers *et al.*, 1973a,b; Newbury *et al.*, 1973). Type II magnetic contrast arises because of the deflection of the beam electrons traveling in the sample by the magnetic force experienced by a charged particle moving in a magnetic field:

$$\mathbf{F} = e\mathbf{v} \times \mathbf{B} \tag{1.47}$$

In order to produce contrast, it is necessary that the sense of the deflection in domains of opposite magnetization be such that in one case the electrons undergo a net motion toward the sample surface, which increases the backscattering coefficient, while in a domain of the opposite magnetization, the electrons are deflected away from the surface, which decreases the backscattering coefficient.

To simulate type II magnetic contrast in the Monte Carlo simulation, it is necessary to modify the fundamental scattering calculation step, which is illustrated in Figure 1.3. The calculation for each scattering step is performed twice. The conventional calculation is performed first: the electron scatters at a point $P(L)$ through a scattering angle and with a step length S to bring it to a new point $P(L + 1)$. The magnetic deflection of the electron along this path is calculated from the velocity and equation (1.47). The effect of the magnetic force is to deflect the electron slightly to bring it to the point $P'(L + 1)$ instead of $P(L + 1)$.

The point $P'(L + 1)$ is calculated by the following procedure. The electron velocity and the magnetic field are first expressed as vectors:

$$\mathbf{v} = av\mathbf{i} + bv\mathbf{j} + cv\mathbf{k} \tag{1.48a}$$
$$\mathbf{B} = B_x\mathbf{i} + B_y\mathbf{j} + B_z\mathbf{k} \tag{1.48b}$$

where v is the magnitude of the velocity and a, b, c are the direction cosines of the line $P(L) - P(L + 1)$. The magnetic force imparts an acceleration to the electron

$$m\mathbf{a} = \mathbf{F} = -e\mathbf{v} \times \mathbf{B} \tag{1.49}$$

Forming the cross product, the acceleration is given by

$$\mathbf{a} = (-e/m)\mathbf{v} \times \mathbf{B} = (-ev/m)[(bB_z - cB_y)\mathbf{i} \\ + (cB_x - aB_z)\mathbf{j} + (aB_y - bB_x)\mathbf{k}] \tag{1.50}$$

This acceleration acts for a time t which is given by $t = S/v$, where v is the magnitude of the velocity and S is the step length from $P(L)$ to $P(L + 1)$. The final deflection components are thus

$$\Delta S_i = v_i t + (1/2)a_i t^2 \tag{1.51}$$

The point $P'(L + 1)$ is found by adding the deflection increments to the position of the electron at the beginning of the scattering event, $P(L)$. The magnetic modification to the conventional scattering step is illustrated in Figure 1.10.

In developing this calculation, the key point is the idea of introducing the magnetic deflection as a small perturbation on the normal calculation. This approximation can be made because the actual magnetic deflection is of the order of 0.05% of the step length of the calculation. The actual measured value of type II magnetic contrast for iron, the element with the highest magnetic field, at a beam energy of 30 keV and an optimal specimen tilt angle, is 0.3% (Fathers *et al.,* 1973a,b). Thus, Monte Carlo simulation of the contrast between domains of opposite magnetization requires calculating a difference in the backscattering of 3 parts in 1000. That is, on average when a "bright" domain yields 1000 backscattered electrons, a "dark" domain will yield 997. In order to make a statistically valid calculation of this difference, the precision of the calculated backscatter coefficients must be considered carefully. The desired precision, P, is related to the required mean number of events of interest by the relation

$$P = \overline{n}^{1/2}/\overline{n} = \overline{n}^{-1/2} \tag{1.52}$$

Thus, the mean number of events which must be calculated is

$$\overline{n} = 1/P^2 \tag{1.53}$$

Note that n refers to the number of events of interest, in this case backscattered electrons. To find the total number of trajectories, T, required, $\overline{n}$ must be divided by the yield, Y, for that type of event, which in this case means that $Y = \eta$, the backscattering coefficient:

$$T = \overline{n}/Y = \overline{n}/\eta \tag{1.54}$$

Thus, if the desired precision is a factor of ten smaller than the contrast to be calculated, a precision of 0.03% is required in the backscattering coefficient in order to calculate contrast effects at the 0.3% level. A precision of 0.03% would require the calculation of 11 million events which in turn implies that a total of 20 million trajectories must be calculated,

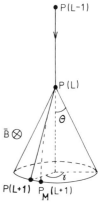

Figure 1.10. Modification of the basic Monte Carlo scattering step to incorporate magnetic deflection of the electron.

$\bar{F} = -e(\bar{v} \times \bar{B})$

since the backscattering coefficient for iron tilted to 55° is about 0.6. Moreover, an equal number of trajectories would be needed for a domain of opposite magnetic field. This is an impractically large number of trajectories. As a compromise, the magnetic field of the calculation was scaled up so as to give contrast values of approximately 5%, which allowed statistically significant results with 40,000 trajectories. In order to establish the validity of this approach, the assumed magnetic field was scaled incrementally, and the calculated contrast was found to scale linearly.

The value of the Monte Carlo simulation in studying type II magnetic contrast was realized in four ways. First, the Monte Carlo calculations were able to confirm those properties of type II magnetic contrast which were initially observed experimentally, namely the strong dependence of the contrast on the specimen tilt and the dependence of the contrast on the rotation of the magnetization vector relative to the tilt axis of the specimen. This information was important to confirm the postulated mechanism of the contrast, namely the deflection of the beam electrons by the internal magnetic field of the domains.

Second, the Monte Carlo simulation indicated that the contrast increased as the 1.4 power of the beam energy, as illustrated in Figure 1.11. The early experimental measurements of the type II magnetic contrast were limited to a maximum beam energy of 30 keV, which was insufficient to accurately measure the energy dependence. Later when SEM images were prepared in a high-voltage STEM/TEM instrument, the predicted energy dependence was confirmed.

Third, the Monte Carlo simulation was utilized to study the dependence of the contrast on the fractional energy of the backscattered elec-

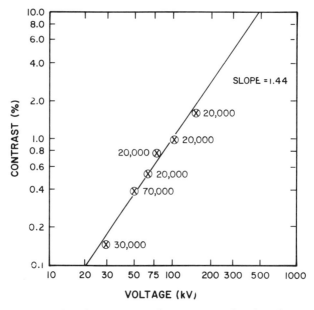

Figure 1.11. Behavior of type II magnetic contrast as a function of beam energy.

trons. As shown in the histogram of Figure 1.12, the contrast was found
to have a complex dependence on the energy of the backscattered electrons. In order to maximize the contrast, the accepted energy window had
to be extended to include electrons which had lost as much as 25% of
their incident energy. This result suggested the importance of multiple
scattering as opposed to single or plural scattering as the regime in which
type II magnetic contrast was formed. Thus, the beam electron had to
spend an adequate period traveling through the magnetic field in order
to accumulate a sufficient magnetic deflection to be sensitive to the local
magnetic character of the sample.

Fourth, experimental observations, shown in Figure 1.13, revealed
that the resolution of a domain wall depended on its orientation relative
to the tilt axis. With the domain wall perpendicular to the tilt axis, the
resolution was much sharper than when it was parallel to the tilt axis.
This difference can be understood with the aid of Monte Carlo calculations of the interaction volume. When the interaction volume is projected onto a plane normal to the tilt axis, Figure 1.14, it is seen to be
larger than when it is projected onto a plane which contains the tilt axis.
Thus, the shape of the region from which the backscattered electrons
emerge is elliptical, with the minor axis parallel to the tilt axis. When
scanning this elliptical shape across a domain wall, the best resolution is

obviously obtained when the minor axis crosses the feature. This situation is realized for domain walls which run perpendicular to the tilt axis. For domain walls which run parallel to the tilt axis, the major axis of the elliptical area crosses at right angles, which leads to poorer resolution.

1.4.2.3. Calculation of X-Ray Generation and Emission in Cylindrical Particles

The Monte Carlo simulation can be applied to study the generation and emission of x-rays in samples with unusual shape, such as particles. As an example, we shall consider x-ray calculations for cylindrical particles oriented such that the cylinder axis is at right angles to the x-ray detector axis. X-ray emission from the particle along an axis perpendicular to the beam, which is the situation encountered in many SEM–EDS systems, will be compared to x-ray emission along an axis at an acute angle to the beam, which is the typical detector axis in an electron probe microanalyzer.

To adapt the Monte Carlo calculation to this specimen shape, two

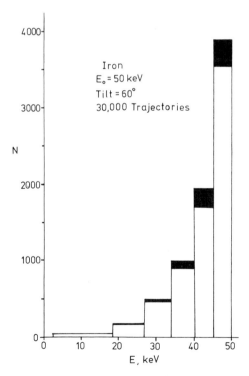

Figure 1.12. Histogram of backscattered electron energy from domains of opposite magnetization.

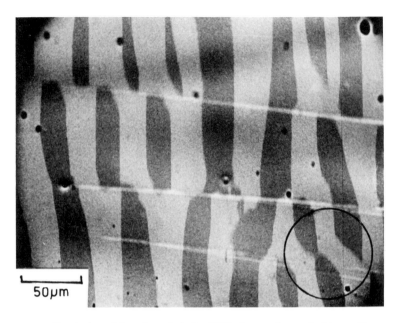

Figure 1.13. Resolution of domain walls in Fe–3%Si alloy as observed with type II magnetic contrast.

significant changes must be made to the basic simulation. For flat, bulk samples, the test for backscattering is simply penetration through the surface plane, which is described by the equation $z = 0$. Thus, whenever $z < 0$, backscattering is considered to have occurred for flat, bulk samples. However, for particle samples, backscattering is considered to have occurred whenever the beam electron passes outside of the particle boundary. For a cylindrical rod with the rod axis running parallel to the x axis (tilt axis), the test condition for backscattering requires determination when the electron passes outside the circular cross section. This circle has the equation

$$y^2 + (z - r)^2 = r^2 \tag{1.55}$$

where r is the radius of the cylindrical cross section. Backscattering therefore occurs when

$$y^2 + (z - r)^2 > r^2 \tag{1.56}$$

A further level of sophistication can be introduced in the simulation by following the trajectory of the electrons which have left the substrate to

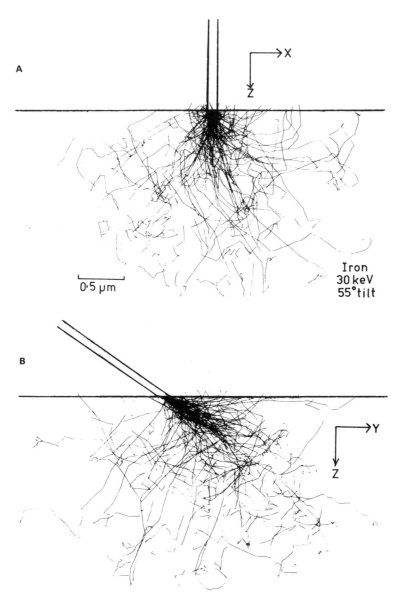

Figure 1.14. Interaction volume in iron tilted 55° as viewed (A) perpendicular and (B) parallel to the tilt axis.

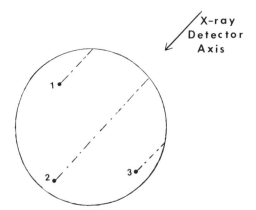

Figure 1.15. Determination of the x-ray emission path length for cylindrical particles.

determine if subsequent scattering off the sample substrate causes the electron to reenter the particle.

The second modification to the simulation which must be introduced concerns the calculation of the x-ray path length out of the particle from the sites at which x-ray generation occurs. For flat, bulk samples, a simple relation exists between the depth at which an ionization event is created, z, and the x-ray emission path length, PL, along a given detector axis, which is specified by the takeoff angle ψ (the angle of the detector axis above the horizontal):

$$PL = z \csc \psi \qquad (1.57)$$

For cylindrical particles, the emission path length depends on the y position within the particle, even at constant z coordinate, as illustrated in Figure 1.15. For a cylindrical particle, the determination of the path length along the detector axis with direction cosines AD, BD, CD requires simultaneous solution of the equation of the line and the equation of the circle:

$$\text{Circle: } y^2 + (z - r)^2 = r^2 \qquad (1.58a)$$
$$\text{Line } (y - Y_0)/\text{BD} = S = (z - Z_0)/\text{CD} \qquad (1.58b)$$

where S is the distance through the particle from the point at which the x-ray is generated (X_0, Y_0, Z_0) to the point on the circumference. To find the values of the coordinates y, z on the circumference of the circle, which can then be substituted into equation (1.58b) to solve for the x-ray path length S, substitution from equation (1.58b) into equation (1.58a) yields a quadratic equation:

$$[(BD/CD) + 1]z^2 - 2[(BD/CD)Z_0 + r]z + Z_0^2 = 0 \qquad (1.59)$$

The values of z can be found by solving the quadratic root formula,

$$z = [-b \pm (b^2 - 4ac)^{1/2}]/2a] \qquad (1.60)$$

where

$$a = (BD/CD) + 1$$
$$b = -2[(BD/CD)Z_0 + r]$$
$$c = Z_0^2$$

Note that the line defined by equation (1.58b) intersects the circle at two locations. These two separate values are generated by the $\pm$ term. In reality, only one solution is desired, the intersection in the direction of the x-ray detector. For a detector placed above the particle in negative z space,

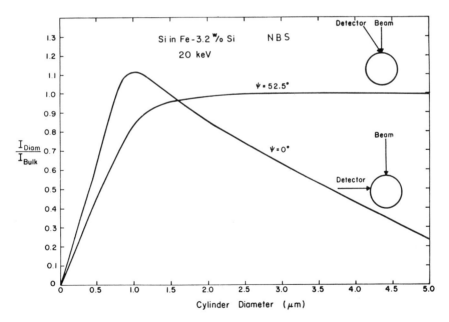

Figure 1.16. Behavior of x-ray emission from cylindrical particles for two different x-ray detector configurations.

the desired solution for *z* in equation (1.60) must be the more negative, and hence the root found with the term

$$z = [-b - (b^2 - 4ac)^{1/2}]/2a \tag{1.61}$$

is the correct value.

With these modifications to the conventional Monte Carlo simulation, the x-ray emission from cylindrical particles can be calculated. Results for two different detector axes are shown in Figure 1.16. A distinct difference is noted between a detector located at a high takeoff angle and at a low takeoff angle. As the particle diameter increases, the x-ray intensity measured with the high-takeoff-angle detector rises asymptotically to a constant value. The low-takeoff-angle detector, typical of an SEM–EDS configuration, shows an initial rise and then a sharp falloff in the emitted x-ray intensity. This behavior results from the increased mass of sample which the x-rays must pass through while traveling horizontally to reach the detector.

Appendix

Two examples of Monte Carlo electron trajectory simulations are included, together with test data, for the interested reader to utilize. These programs are written in the BASIC language for use on an APPLE II computer, but they should be readily adaptable to other types of small computers.

```
10   REM :***************************
20   REM :MONTE CARLO PROGRAM -THIN FILM
30   REM :WRITTEN BY DAVID JOY
40   REM :BASED ON NBS PROGRAM
50   HOME : LOMEM: 16384
60   REM :***************************
70   REM :SET UP STORAGE ARRAY
80   REM :***************************
90   DIM EX%(100)
100  SPEED= 140
110  VTAB 10: HTAB 10: PRINT "MONTE CARLO SIMULATION": PRINT : HTAB 14: PRINT
     "FOR THIN FILMS": PRINT
120  HTAB 16: PRINT "DCJ 6/1/84": PRINT
130  VTAB 20
140  HTAB 7
150  PRINT "-----------------------------"
160  VTAB 22: PRINT "TO RUN THIS PROGRAM..TOUCH ANY KEY": GET AN$
170  SPEED= 255
180  HOME : HTAB 9: PRINT "EXPERIMENTAL CONDITIONS"
190  HTAB 9: PRINT "-----------------------"
200  VTAB 5: INPUT "WHAT ELEMENT ?";NA$
210  FOR J = 1 TO 30
220  READ NM$
230  READ Z
240  READ AA
250  READ RH: IF NM$ = NA$ THEN GOTO 280
```

```
260   NEXT : VTAB 7: PRINT "DATA NOT STORED .. ENTER BELOW"
270   GOTO 320
280   VTAB 7: PRINT "ATOMIC NUMBER   ";Z
290   VTAB 9: PRINT "ATOMIC WEIGHT   ";AA
300   VTAB 11: PRINT "DENSITY (GM/CM3)   ";RH
310   GOTO 350
320   VTAB 9: INPUT "DENSITY OF THE FILM (GM/CM3) ?";RH
330   VTAB 11: INPUT "ATOMIC NUMBER ?";Z
340   VTAB 13: INPUT "ATOMIC WEIGHT ?";AA
350   VTAB 15: INPUT "ACCELERATING VOLTAGE (KEV) ?";EI
360   VTAB 17: INPUT "FILM THICKNESS (ANGSTROMS) ?";TH
370   REM :**************************
380   REM :CALCULATE ELASTIC MEAN FREE PATH
390   REM :**************************
400   AL = (Z ^ 0.67) * 3.4E - 3 / EI:AK = AL * (1 + AL)
410   ER = ((EI + 511) * (EI + 511) / ((EI + 1022) * (EI + 1022)))
420   SG = (Z * Z) * 12.56 * 5.21E - 21 * ER
430   SG = SG / (EI * EI * AK): REM   CROSS SECTIONS IN CM2
440   L1 = AA / (RH * SG * 6.02E23): REM   MEAN FREE PATH IN CM
450   L1 = L1 * 1.0E8 * (1 + (Z / 300)): REM   MEAN FREE PATH IN ANGSTROMS
460   ES = EI
470   JB = 9.76 * Z + (58.5 / ((Z) ^ 0.19)):JB = JB * 1.0E - 3
480   DQ = 7.85E4 * RH * Z / AA
490   REM :****************************
500   REM :GRAPHICS DISPLAY
510   REM :SET UP SCALING FOR PLOT
520   REM :INITIALISE COUNTERS
530   REM :****************************
540   HOME : HGR : HCOLOR= 3
550   ZS = 5: IF TH > 500 THEN ZS = TH / 100
560   NE = 0:BS = 0:TR = 0
570   ZZ = (20 + (TH / ZS))
580   HPLOT 1,20 TO 250,20: HPLOT 1,(ZZ) TO 250,(ZZ): HPLOT 125,1 TO 125,
      20
590   VTAB 23: HTAB 9: INVERSE : FLASH : PRINT "TO STOP TOUCH ANY KEY": FOR
      N = 1 TO 99:Q = LOG (99): NEXT : NORMAL : PRINT : PRINT : PRINT
600   VTAB 22: PRINT "TOTAL "
610   VTAB 22: HTAB 15: PRINT "BS "
620   VTAB 22: HTAB 30: PRINT "TRANS "
630   VTAB 23: CALL  - 868: PRINT "ENERGY (KEV) IS "
640   REM :**********************
650   REM :SET UP INITIAL COORDINATES
660   REM :**********************
670   X = 0:Y = 0:LAM = L1:EI = ES:RE =  RND (9):Z =  - LAM *  LOG (RE)
680   IF Z > TH THEN  HPLOT 125,20 TO 125,(ZZ + 1):XN = 0:YN = 0:Z = 0:ZN
       = TH:ST = TH: GOTO 1380
690   HPLOT 125,20 TO 125,(20 + (Z / ZS))
700   REM :**********************
710   REM :INITIAL DIRECTION COSINES
720   REM :**********************
730   CX = 0:CY = 0:CZ = 1
740   REM :**********************
750   REM :INITIAL PLOTTING POSITION
760   REM :**********************
770   Y1 = 125 - (Y / ZS):Z1 = 20 + (Z / ZS)
780   REM :**********************
790   REM :CALCULATE STEP LENGTH
800   REM :**********************
810   RL =  RND (1)
820   ST =  - LAM *  LOG (RL)
830   REM :**********************
840   REM :ELASTIC SCATTERING ANGLE PHI
850   REM :**********************
860   R1 =  RND (2)
870   CP = 1 - ((2 * AL * R1) / (1 + AL - R1))
880   SP = (1 - CP * CP) ^ 0.5
890   REM :**********************
900   REM :AZIMUTHAL SCATTERING ANGLE
910   REM :**********************
920   R2 =  RND (3):GA = 6.28 * R2
930   M =  ATN ( - CX / CZ)
940   IF CX = 0 THEN CX = 1.1E - 4
950   N =  ATN ( - CZ / CX)
960   REM :**********************
970   REM :CALCULATE NEW COORDINATES
```

```
980   REM :***************************
990   CM =  COS (M):CN =  COS (N):CG =  COS (GA):SG =  SIN (GA)
1000 CA = (CX * CP) + (CM * SP * CG) + (CY * CN * SP * SG)
1010 CB = (CY * CP) + (SP * SG * (CZ * CM - CX * CN))
1020 CC = (CZ * CP) + (SP * CN * CG) - (SP * CY * CM * SG)
1030 XN = X + ST * CA:YN = Y + ST * CB:ZN = Z + ST * CC
1040  REM :***************************
1050  REM :PLOT NEW POINT
1060  REM :***************************
1070 Y2 =  INT (125 - (YN / ZS)):Z2 =  INT (20 + (ZN / ZS))
1080  IF Y2 < 1 THEN Y2 = 1: GOTO 1100
1090  IF Y2 > 250 THEN Y2 = 250
1100  IF Z2 < 20 THEN  HPLOT Y1,Z1 TO Y2,19: GOTO 1310
1110  IF Z2 > ZZ THEN  HPLOT Y1,Z1 TO Y2,(ZZ + 1): GOTO 1380
1120  HPLOT Y1,Z1 TO Y2,Z2:Y1 = Y2:Z1 = Z2
1130  REM :***************************
1140  REM :CALCULATE DIRECTION COSINES
1150  REM :***************************
1160 CX = CA:CY = CB:CZ = CC
1170 X = XN:Y = YN:Z = ZN
1180  IF  PEEK ( - 16384) > 128 THEN  GOTO 1510
1190  REM :****************************
1200  REM :CALCULATE ENERGY LOSS
1210  REM :****************************
1220 DE = DQ *  LOG (1.166 * EI / JB):DE = DE / EI
1230 EI = EI - ST * 1.0E - 8 * DE
1240 LAM = L1 * EI / ES
1250  IF EI < 25 THEN NE = NE + 1: VTAB 22: HTAB 8: PRINT NE: GOTO 670
1260  VTAB 23: HTAB 18: PRINT ( INT (EI * 10) / 10)
1270  GOTO 810
1280  REM :***************************
1290  REM :BACKSCATTERED ELECTRON
1300  REM :***************************
1310 BS = BS + 1:NE = NE + 1
1320  VTAB 22: HTAB 8: PRINT NE
1330  VTAB 22: HTAB 20: PRINT BS
1340  GOTO 670
1350  REM :***************************
1360  REM :TRANSMITTED ELECTRON
1370  REM :***************************
1380 NE = NE + 1:TR = TR + 1
1390  VTAB 22: HTAB 8: PRINT NE
1400  VTAB 22: HTAB 37: PRINT TR
1410  REM :****************************
1420  REM :CALCULATE EXIT COORDINATES
1430  REM :****************************
1440 CX = (XN - X) / ST:CY = (YN - Y) / ST:CZ = (ZN - Z) / ST
1450 LL = (TH - Z) / CZ:XE = X + LL * CX:YE = Y + LL * CY
1460 RN = ((XE * XE) + (YE * YE)) ^ 0.5
1470 R =  INT (RN / (2 * ZS)) + 1: IF R > 100 THEN R = 100
1480 EX%(R) = EX%(R) + 1
1490  IF  PEEK ( - 16384) > 128 THEN  GOTO 1510
1500  GOTO 670
1510  POKE ( - 16368),0: HCOLOR= 0: HPLOT 1,1 TO 1,153: HPLOT 250,1 TO 2
      50,153: GET AN$: HOME : TEXT
1520 EM% = 0
1530  FOR J = 1 TO 100
1540  IF EX%(J) > EM% THEN EM% = EX%(J)
1550  NEXT
1560  FOR J = 1 TO 100:EX%(J) =  INT (EX%(J) * 150 / EM%): NEXT
1570  HGR : HCOLOR= 3: HPLOT 0,153 TO 250,153
1580  FOR J = 1 TO 50
1590  HPLOT (J * 5 - 5),153 TO (J * 5 - 5),(153 - EX%(J)) TO (J * 5),(15
      3 - EX%(J)) TO (J * 5),153
1600  NEXT
1610 SS =  INT (2 * ZS): VTAB 22: PRINT SS;" ANGSTROM BARS"
1620 WA = 0:WB = 0
1630  FOR J = 1 TO 100
1640 WB = WB + EX%(J)
1650  NEXT
1660  FOR J = 1 TO 100
1670 WA = WA + EX%(J)
1680  IF WA > (0.9 * WB) THEN  GOTO 1700
1690  NEXT
1700  VTAB 23: PRINT "90% BEAM RADIUS IS ";(J * SS);" ANGSTROMS"
```

```
1710   DATA  BE,4,9.01,1.848,B,5,10.81,2.5,C,6,12.01,2.34,NA,11,22.99,0.9
       7,MG,12,24.31,1.74
1720   DATA  AL,13,26.98,2.7,SI,14,28.09,2.34,P,15,30.97,2.2,CA,20,40,1.5
       4,TI,22,47.9,4.5,V,23,50.94,6.1,CR,24,52,7.1
1730   DATA  MN,25,54.94,7.4,FE,26,55.85,7.87,CO,27,58.93,8.9,NI,28,58.71
       ,8.9,CU,29,63.55,8.96,ZN,30,65.37,7.14
1740   DATA  GA,31,69.72,5.91,GE,32,72.59,5.32,NB,41,92.91,8.6,MO,42,95.9
       4,10.2,PD,46,106.4,12,AG,47,107.9,10.5
1750   DATA  CD,48,112.4,8.64,SN,50,118.7,7.3,W,74,183.9,19.3,PT,78,195.1
       ,21.45,AU,79,197.0,19.3,PB,82,207.2,11.34
1760   RESTORE
```

```
10   REM :****************************
20   REM :MONTE CARLO PROGRAM-BULK SAMPLE
30   HOME : LOMEM: 16384
40   REM :****************************
50   REM :SET UP STORAGE ARRAY
60   REM :****************************
70   DIM E(51),BE%(40)
80   VTAB 10: HTAB 10: PRINT "MONTE CARLO SIMULATION": PRINT : HTAB 15: PRINT
     "SOLID SAMPLES": PRINT
90   HTAB 16: PRINT "DCJ 6/01/84": PRINT
100  VTAB 20
110  HTAB 7
120  PRINT "-------------------------------"
130  VTAB 22: PRINT "TO RUN THIS PROGRAM..TOUCH ANY KEY": GET AN$
140  HOME : HTAB 9: PRINT "EXPERIMENTAL CONDITIONS"
150  HTAB 9: PRINT "-----------------------"
160  VTAB 5: INPUT "WHAT ELEMENT ?";NA$
170  FOR J = 1 TO 30
180  READ NM$
190  READ Z
200  READ AA
210  READ RH: IF NM$ = NA$ THEN  GOTO 240
220  NEXT : VTAB 7: PRINT "DATA NOT STORED .. ENTER BELOW"
230  GOTO 280
240  VTAB 7: PRINT "ATOMIC NUMBER   ";Z
250  VTAB 9: PRINT "ATOMIC WEIGHT   ";AA
260  VTAB 11: PRINT "DENSITY (GM/CM3)  ";RH
270  GOTO 310
280  VTAB 9: INPUT "DENSITY OF THE FILM (GM/CM3) ?";RH
290  VTAB 11: INPUT "ATOMIC NUMBER ?";Z
300  VTAB 13: INPUT "ATOMIC WEIGHT ?";AA
310  VTAB 15: INPUT "ACCELERATING VOLTAGE (KEV) ?";EI
320  VTAB 17: INPUT "TILT (DEGREES) ";TI
330  VTAB 19: HTAB 10: INVERSE : FLASH : PRINT "CALCULATING RANGE": NORMAL

340  ZG = Z
350  REM :BETHE ENERGY LOSS
360  DEF  FN SP(EN) = 7.85E4 * ZG * ( LOG (1.166 * EN / JB)) / (AA * EN)

370  JB = (9.76 * ZG + (58.5 / (ZG ^ 0.19))) * 1.0E - 3
380  AH = 0.263 * (ZG ^ 0.4)
390  B = 7.2E - 2 * ZG / AH
400  B = B * ((EI / 15) ^ 0.95)
410  FOR M = 1 TO 21:EN = (M - 1) * EI / 20: IF EN > = (6.34 * JB) THEN
     F = 1 /  FN SP(EN): GOTO 430
420  F = ( SQR (EN * JB)) * AA / (6.24E4 * ZG)
430  L = 2: IF M / 2 =  INT (M / 2) THEN L = 4
440  IF M = 1 OR M = 21 THEN L = 1
450  FS = FS + L * F: NEXT M:R = FS * EI / 60: REM  R IS MASSTHICKNESS/KV
460  SS = R / 50:E(1) = EI
470  FOR M = 2 TO 51: IF E(M - 1) < (6.34 * JB) THEN 520
480  A1 = SS *  FN SP(E(M - 1)): IF A1 / 2 > E(M - 1) THEN 520
490  A2 = SS *  FN SP(E(M - 1) - A1 / 2): IF A2 / 2 > E(M - 1) THEN 520
500  A3 = SS *  FN SP(E(M - 1) - A2 / 2): IF A3 > E(M - 1) THEN 520
510  A4 = SS *  FN SP(E(M - 1) - A3):E(M) = E(M - 1) - (A1 + 2 * A2 + 2 *
     A3 + A4) / 6: GOTO 530
520  EM = E(M - 1) ^ 1.5 - 9.35E4 * ZG * SS / (AA *  SQR (JB)):E(M) = 0: IF
     EM > 1E - 9 THEN E(M) = EM ^ 0.6667
530  NEXT M:E(51) = 0: FOR M = 2 TO 50:E(M) = (E(M) + E(M + 1)) / 2: NEXT
     M
```

```
540  SL = SS * 5E5 / RH: VTAB 19: CALL  - 868: VTAB 21: PRINT "RANGE (MIC
     RONS)=";SL: FOR N = 1 TO 500:FF =  LOG (999): NEXT
550  ZS =  INT (120 / SL): REM - SCREEN DIV/UM
560  HOME : HGR : HCOLOR= 3
570  ST = SL / 50: REM  STEP LENGTH IN MICRONS
580  HPLOT 1,149 TO (1 + ZS),149
590  NE = 0:BS = 0
600  HPLOT 1,20 TO 250,20: HPLOT (125 + 19 * TAN (TI / 57.4)),1 TO 125,
     20
610  VTAB 23: HTAB 9: INVERSE : FLASH : PRINT "TO STOP TOUCH ANY KEY": FOR
     N = 1 TO 99:Q =  LOG (99): NEXT : NORMAL : PRINT : PRINT : PRINT
620  VTAB 22: PRINT "TOTAL "
630  VTAB 22: HTAB 15: PRINT "BS "
640  VTAB 22: HTAB 30: INVERSE : PRINT "BULK MC": NORMAL
650  VTAB 23: CALL  - 868: VTAB 23: PRINT "ENERGY (KEV) IS "
660  REM :************************
670  REM :SET UP INITIAL COORDINATES
680  REM :************************
690  X = 0:Y = 0:Z = 0:CX = 0:CY =  SIN (TI / 57.4):CZ =  COS (TI / 57.4)
     :K = 1: HPLOT 125,20
700  FOR K = 1 TO 50
710  REM :******************
720  REM :SCATTERING ANGLES
730  REM :******************
740  NU = ( RND (1) ^ 0.5):NU = ((1 / NU) - 1):AN = NU * B / E(K)
750  SP = (AN + AN) / ((AN * AN) + 1)
760  CP = (1 - (AN * AN)) / ((AN * AN) + 1)
770  REM :************************
780  REM :AZIMUTHAL SCATTERING ANGLE
790  REM :************************
800  R2 =  RND (3):GA = 6.28 * R2
810  M =  ATN ( - CX / CZ)
820  IF CX = 0 THEN CX = 1.1E - 4
830  N =  ATN ( - CZ / CX)
840  REM :************************
850  REM :CALCULATE NEW COORDINATES
860  REM :************************
870  CM =  COS (M):CN =  COS (N):SG =  SIN (GA):CG =  COS (GA)
880  CA = (CX * CP) + (CM * SP * CG) + (CY * CN * SP * SG)
890  CB = (CY * CP) + (SP * SG * (CZ * CM - CX * CN))
900  CC = (CZ * CP) + (SP * CN * CG) - (SP * CY * CM * SG)
910  XN = X + ST * CA:YN = Y + ST * CB:ZN = Z + ST * CC
920  REM :************************
930  REM :PLOT NEW POINT
940  REM :************************
950  Y2 = (125 - (YN * ZS)):Z2 = 20 + (ZN * ZS)
960  IF Y2 < 1 THEN Y2 = 1: GOTO 980
970  IF Y2 > 250 THEN Y2 = 250
980  IF Z2 < 20 THEN Z2 = 19: HPLOT  TO Y2,Z2: GOTO 1100
990  IF Z2 > 150 THEN Z2 = 150
1000  HPLOT  TO Y2,Z2
1010  REM :************************
1020  REM :CALCULATE DIRECTION COSINES
1030  REM :************************
1040 CX = CA:CY = CB:CZ = CC
1050 X = XN:Y = YN:Z = ZN
1060  IF  PEEK ( - 16384) > 128 THEN  GOTO 1180
1070  VTAB 23: HTAB 18: CALL  - 868: VTAB 23: HTAB 18: PRINT E(K)
1080  NEXT K
1090  NE = NE + 1: VTAB 22: HTAB 8: PRINT NE: GOTO 690
1100  REM :************************
1110  REM :BACKSCATTERED ELECTRON
1120  REM :************************
1130 BS = BS + 1:NE = NE + 1
1140 J =  INT (E(K) + 0.5):BE%(J) = BE%(J) + 1
1150  VTAB 22: HTAB 8: PRINT NE
1160  VTAB 22: HTAB 20: PRINT BS
1170  GOTO 690
1180  POKE ( - 16368),0: HCOLOR= 0: HPLOT 1,1 TO 1,153: HPLOT 250,1 TO 2
     50,153: GET AN$: HOME : TEXT
1190  VTAB 1: HTAB 10: PRINT "** DATAPRINT **"
1200  VTAB 3: PRINT "TOTAL NUMBER ELECTRONS ";NE;" IN ";NA$
1210  VTAB 4: PRINT "DENSITY WAS ";RH
1220  VTAB 6: PRINT "BS COEFFICIENT ";(BS / NE)
1230 SUM = 0:AV = 0: FOR J = 1 TO EI: PRINT J,BE%(J)
```

```
1240  SUM = SUM + BE%(J):AV = AV + J * BE%(J): NEXT J
1250  PRINT "AVERAGED ENERGY = ";(AV / SUM)
1260  STOP
1270  DATA  BE,4,9.01,1.848,B,5,10.81,2.5,C,6,12.01,2.34,NA,11,22.99,0.9
      7,MG,12,24.31,1.74
1280  DATA  AL,13,26.98,2.7,SI,14,28.09,2.34,P,15,30.97,2.2,CA,20,40,1.5
      4,TI,22,47.9,4.5,V,23,50.94,6.1,CR,24,52,7.1
1290  DATA  MN,25,54.94,7.4,FE,26,55.85,7.87,CO,27,58.93,8.9,NI,28,58.71
      ,8.9,CU,29,63.55,8.96,ZN,30,65.37,7.14
1300  DATA  GA,31,69.72,5.91,GE,32,72.59,5.32,NB,41,92.91,8.6,MO,42,95.9
      4,10.2,PD,46,106.4,12,AG,47,107.9,10.5
1310  DATA  CD,48,112.4,8.64,SN,50,118.7,7.3,W,74,183.9,19.3,PT,78,195.1
      ,21.45,AU,79,197.0,19.3,PB,82,207.2,11.34
1320  RESTORE
```

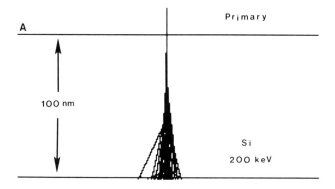

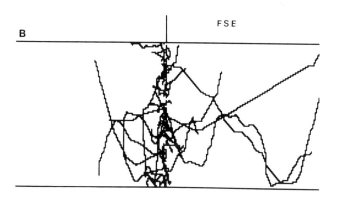

Figure 1.A1. Monte Carlo electron trajectory simulations as calculated on a personal computer. Silicon, 100 nm thick, E_0 = 100 kev. (A) Primary trajectories; (B) fast secondary electron trajectories.

2

SEM Microcharacterization of Semiconductors

2.1. Introduction

The electronics industry is now one of the principal users of the scanning electron microscope, with as many as half of all new SEMs being bought, directly or indirectly, for semiconductor applications. There are several reasons for this popularity. First, the SEM provides a variety of contrast modes which are of great value in qualitatively and quantitatively assessing the properties of semiconductor materials. Second, the SEM offers modes which allow the operation of devices such as switches, transistors, and even complete integrated circuits, to be observed under conditions which approximate those of normal use. As the size of devices has been reduced to the micrometer scale, and as devices themselves become more complex, the fact that the SEM can combine imaging and chemical microanalysis with such facilities as the ability to identify electrically active defects, or measure voltages, makes it in many cases the most versatile tool for characterization, diagnosis, and failure analysis. The major techniques in current use for semiconductor studies are discused below, but other modes of operation including electron channeling and x-ray microanalysis are also of value and the chapters dealing with these topics should be consulted as well.

2.2. Voltage Contrast

Voltage contrast is an imaging mode of the SEM in which regions of a sample which are at different potentials relative to one another appear, in the secondary electron image, to be of differing brightness. Although voltage contrast was one of the first phenomena observed in the SEM (Knoll, 1941), it remains one of the most important techniques available for the analysis of complex circuits (Gopinath *et al.,* 1978). The effect that is usually, if incorrectly, referred to as voltage contrast is the result of the mechanics of secondary electron collection in the SEM, the details of which are shown in Figure 2.1. In order to ensure efficient collection of secondaries when using an Everhart–Thornley detector, a potential of typically $+200$ V, relative to the specimen which is at ground potential, is applied to the Faraday cage which surrounds the light pipe. With the detector placed 1 cm or so from the surface, this potential results in a field of the order of 100 V/cm directed toward the detector, which is sufficient to attract toward the scintillator a high fraction of all the secondaries leaving the specimen.

Consider now the situation when a sample such as an integrated circuit, with potentials applied to its components, is observed in the SEM (Figure 2.2). In the center of an area that is negatively biased with respect to ground, there will be a higher average field from the detector, the detector efficiency will be increased, and so that region will appear to be brighter than the surrounding grounded material. An area that is positive with respect to ground will see a reduced field, the collection efficiency will be lowered, and so that region will appear darker than its surroundings. The image of such a device will therefore show signal modulations, "voltage contrast," which correspond to changes in the potentials of different regions of the surface.

The appearance of voltage contrast is often quite dramatic. Figure 2.3 compares the secondary electron images of a chip before and after

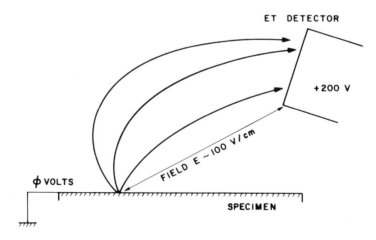

Figure 2.1. Collection fields in SEM chamber for secondary electrons.

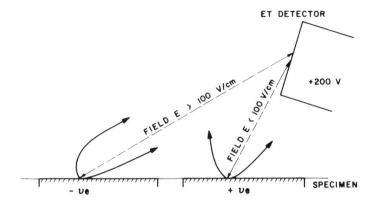

Figure 2.2. Collection fields from sample with applied potentials.

potentials are applied to it in the SEM. With all the conductors in the device grounded, the secondary electron image shows only the normal topographic detail resulting from the surface structure of the specimen. But as soon as potentials are applied to the chip (Figure 2.3B), many of the operating conductor strips can be seen in high contrast against the background level of the device. The visual impact of this kind of image, and the apparent ease with which it can be interpreted, help explain the popularity of the method.

Although a voltage contrast image of this type can give a quick visual impression of the layout of a circuit, and some indication of the magnitude and polarity of the applied potentials, a detailed quantitative interpretation is much more difficult for several reasons. First, the variation of signal level with potential is not symmetrical for the positive and negative potential cases. While raising the surface potential can significantly reduce the number of secondaries collected by reducing the detector efficiency, biasing a region negatively can usually only yield a small increase in signal because a high fraction of the secondaries is already being collected. Second, there is not a unique correlation between the signal level and the surface potential. This is illustrated in Figure 2.4 which shows the familiar sight of some dust on the surface of a sample. The particle has charged negatively, and so appears bright. However, although the region surrounding the particle is all at earth potential, the contrast is far from uniform. The strong dark ring arises because the potential difference between the particle and the surface produces a strong radial field directed toward the particle. Secondaries produced close to the particle are thus captured by this field and returned to the specimen rather than collected by the detector, and the potential contrast is modulated by the local field effect.

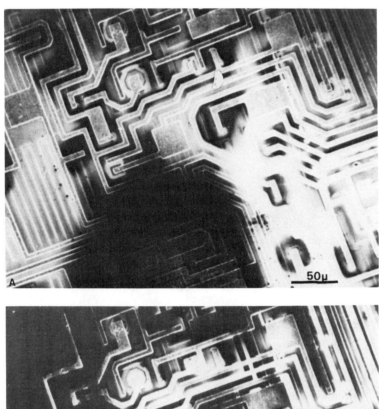

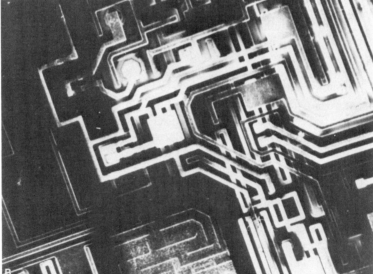

Figure 2.3. Secondary electron images of chip (A) before and (B) after application of potentials.

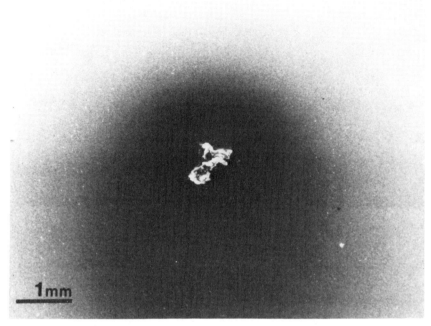

Figure 2.4. Charge ring around dust particle.

A similar situation is shown in Figure 2.5 where two conductor strips at different potentials are in close proximity on the surface of the chip. If conductor A is at +2 V with respect to ground, and conductor B is at −2 V, and the separation between A and B is 40 μm, then the field between them is 1000 V/cm, which is ten times greater than the field from the detector. An electron leaving the specimen will see the combined effect of the detector field and any local fields, and the collection efficiency and hence the signal level will thus depend not only on the potential of the region from which the secondary came, but also on the distribution of potentials around that area. In some cases the local fields might be in such a sense as to enhance collection, in other situations they will reduce the efficiency, but in all cases the result is to change the signal level from the constant value that would have been expected from the equipotential conductor. This effect can be seen by following any of the conductors visible in Figure 2.3B and noting how the contrast level changes with the proximity of another conductor, in many cases switching from bright to dark and back again within the distance of a few micrometers as it passes close to another potential. "Voltage contrast" in this mode is seen, in fact,

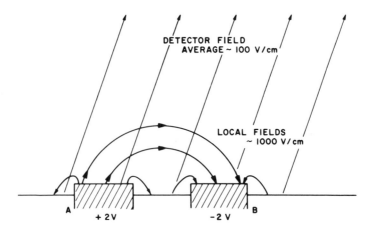

Figure 2.5. Local fields produced by conductor strips.

to be more correctly "field contrast" since the relationship between contrast and potential is indirect and many valued. It is also a pure "trajectory" effect, arising only from changes in secondary electron behavior after they leave the sample, and thus is not observable in such modes as backscattering or specimen current.

An important practical consideration when using this method is the choice of beam energy. In general, the lowest voltage should be the best choice. The observed contrast is a function of the field distribution at the specimen surface. Problems are often encountered as a result of random fields from charging. For example, insulated wires used to make contact to the device under observation can acquire a charge as the result of the impact of backscattered electrons. If this, or some other charging, occurs, then the voltage contrast image may fade after a few minutes of observation, and not reappear unless the beam is switched off for some time, or the sample is briefly removed from the vacuum. If this is seen to be happening, then lowering the beam energy will often yield a stable image, since the lower energy will give a higher secondary yield from all exposed surfaces and correspondingly less charging. The lower energy will also increase the collected secondary signal. Since many current SEMs can operate efficiently at energies as low as 1 keV, it is usually possible to find a suitable energy.

However, many integrated circuits are covered by a passivation layer of a ceramic or glass, typically 1 μm or so in thickness. While this layer can be chemically removed, in many laboratories it is considered desirable to leave it in position rather than risk the possible damage resulting from its dissolution. In such a case, it is necessary to try and observe the voltage contrast signal with the passivation in position. This can be done if the beam energy is chosen correctly. At low beam energies, the passivation layer will not charge, but since it will be an equipotential, no contrast from the underlying circuit will be visible (Figure 2.6a). At high beam energies (Figure 2.6b), the passivation layer will charge, producing local fields which will mask the contrast. At an intermediate energy (Figure 2.6c), the beam can just penetrate to the circuit. As the electrons travel through the insulating layer, they produce conductivity because of the generation of electron–hole pairs (as discussed below). This conductivity allows the potential distribution of the circuit to be transferred to the top of the passivation and thus imaged in the normal way. The energy range over which this can be successfully done is often very narrow and must be determined experimentally. In addition to keeping the beam current as low as consistent with an adequate signal/noise ratio, the scan rate

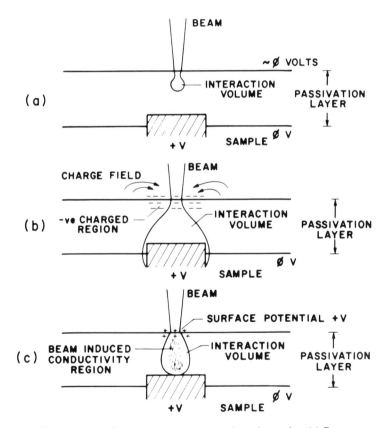

Figure 2.6. Optimization of voltage contrast on passivated samples. (a) Beam energy too low; (b) energy too high; (c) optimum energy.

used for observation can also have a pronounced effect on the stability of the image. The charge, and corresponding discharge, cycle for each point on the surface has a characteristic time which is typically of the order of seconds. When the beam is scanned slowly, the field distribution around any point is constantly changing as the result of these charging events and the voltage contrast image is very unstable. If, however, a high scan speed, such as TV rate, is used, then each point under observation is revisited so often by the beam that it cannot discharge. The surface thus reaches a temporary equilibrium condition and the image stabilizes (Welter and McKee, 1972).

2.3. Voltage Measurements

Although the qualitative voltage contrast mode described above is adequate for many purposes, there are many applications where an accurate, spatially resolved, measurement of surface potential is required. Since the mode discussed above cannot meet this need, another approach must be sought. The most common technique is based on the use of a filter to analyze the energy of the secondary electrons. The principle can be understood by reference to Figure 2.7a which shows the number $N(E)$ of electrons of energy E as a function of their energy. Ignoring the contribution from the backscattered component, which can in any event be minimized by using a low accelerating voltage so as to increase the secondary yield, the majority of the signal intensity lies within the energy range 0–100 eV. Imagine now placing a grid in front of the secondary detector and applying a potential to it. When the potential is positive or zero relative to the sample, all the secondaries will be transmitted through

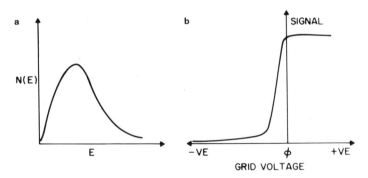

Figure 2.7. (a) Yield curve $N(E)$ versus E for secondary electrons. (b) Collected secondary signal versus detector bias—"s-curve."

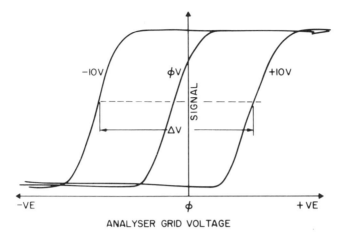

Figure 2.8. Shift of s-curves with applied potential.

to the detector. But if the grid is biased negatively, then some electrons will be prevented from passing the grid. When the magnitude of the negative potential is small, most of the signal will still get through, but as the potential is increased, more of the secondaries will have insufficient energy to pass the potential barrier and be collected so that the signal will fall. If the collected signal is plotted as a function of the grid potential, then a variation like that shown in Figure 2.7b will be obtained, the characteristic form of which is often called the "s-curve" for the retarding field energy analyzer, of which the single grid is the simplest example (Balk *et al.*, 1976; Menzel and Kubalek, 1979).

   If the potential of the sample is shifted, then the shape of the s-curve will remain the same, but it will slide along the potential axis by an amount equal to the voltage applied to the specimen, since the energy of all of the secondaries relative to the analyzing grid will have changed by the same amount. The difference in potential between two points on a surface could thus, in principle, be measured by recording "s-curves" from the two points and noting the difference in analyzer potential dV required to make the signal levels the same (Figure 2.8). Note that this is not an absolute measurement of potential unless one of the points is at ground. Although this is one way to proceed, it is not ideal, first because it would be necessary to sweep the grid potential through its whole range at each pixel in order to be able to compare the s-curves, and second because local fields due to the surface potential distribution would affect the collection efficiency of the detector just as they did in the previous example. If this occurs, then the s-curves will be distorted and an accurate potential measurement will be impossible.

These problems can be overcome by using a more elaborate form of analyzer as illustrated in Figure 2.9 and changing the way in which the measurement is made. The first modification consists of an "extractor grid" which is placed before the analyzer grid and just above the specimen surface (Fujioka *et al.*, 1981). Typically, this grid is placed 1 mm or less from the surface and is held at about 1000 V positive relative to ground, and so provides a vertical field in excess of 10^4 V/cm. This is sufficient to eliminate any effects due to surface-generated fields and so ensure a uniform collection efficiency independent of the geometry of the surface. The analyzer grid is typically placed between two grounded grids so that any potential applied to the analyzer does not change the extraction field, and to ensure that secondaries rejected by the grid flow to earth rather than cause the charge-up of a surrounding surface. Secondaries which pass the grid are deflected by an arrangement of electrodes so as to pass out through the side of the device and on to the standard secondary detector. In this way, the voltage analyzer can be inserted between the sample and the detector when quantitative measurements are required.

The analyzer grid is connected as part of a feedback loop (Balk *et al.*, 1976; Hardy *et al.*, 1975) the operation of which can be understood from Figure 2.10. For a given grid potential and sample voltage, the detector will see some fixed signal level. If the sample voltage is changed, then the signal will also change, falling if the sample voltage is increased or rising if the voltage is reduced. The change in signal will not, in general, be linear with this change except in the central portion of the "s," so the pur-

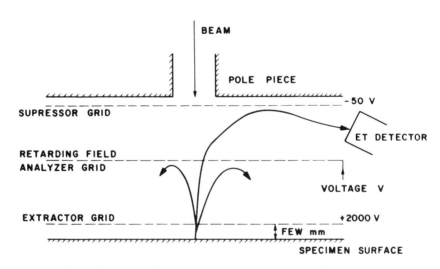

Figure 2.9. Schematic drawing of secondary electron voltage analyzer.

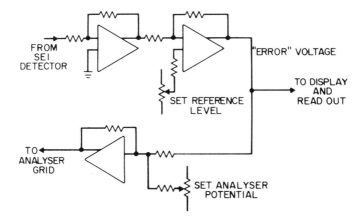

Figure 2.10. Feedback system to linearize voltage analyzer.

pose of the feedback is to linearize the response. With the sample at ground potential, the analyzer grid is adjusted (usually with a high-speed ramp and oscilloscope trace) so that for the widest range of grid potentials the signal swing is linear. The signal from the detector is passed into a comparator amplifier the output of which is adjusted to be zero at the midpoint of the "s-curve." If now the electron beam is scanned to another region of the sample where the potential is different, then the signal will change, and the output from the comparator will alter from zero to some negative value for an increase in surface voltage or a positive value for a decrease in surface voltage. This "error" voltage is passed through an amplifier, inverted, and added to the potential on the analyzer. Thus, a rise in surface potential will increase the voltage applied to the analyzer grid, and it can be seen from Figure 2.8 that the effect of this will be to cause a rise in the collected signal. With a well-designed analyzer, the change in grid potential required to bring the signal back to its original value is linearly proportional to the change in voltage at the sample. If the feedback loop is adjusted so that the signal level is held constant regardless of surface voltage, then the "error" voltage applied to the analyzer grid will track the surface potential directly and linearly over a wide range (Figure 2.11). Typically, linearity is maintained over a range of at least ± 20 V, with a resolution of 0.1 V. Provided that the feedback system has sufficient bandwidth, then the variation of the error signal as the beam scans will directly map the surface potential. With the use of a color-coded digital image recording device, the potential at every point within the field of view could be displayed quantiatively.

Alternatively, the beam can be stopped at one point of interest, and the potential followed as a function of time. In this mode the SEM is

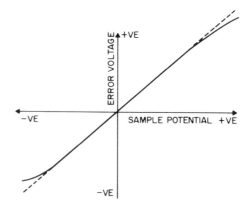

Figure 2.11. Voltage response from linearized analyzer.

behaving analogously to an oscilloscope since the waveform of a signal at any point in a circuit can be examined. Unlike an oscilloscope, however, the electron beam presents little loading to a circuit, although at most beam energies there will be some interaction with the system under test. If the beam energy is higher than that value at which the total electron yield (secondary plus backscattered) equals unity, then current will be injected into the specimen from the beam. Although the magnitude of this component is small, in many circuit topologies it is sufficient to alter the state of logic devices such as gates. If the beam energy is low enough for the yield to be greater than unity, then current leaves the sample from the point of beam impact, and the electron beam is loading the circuit. If either of these conditions is undesirable, then the beam energy must be carefully adjusted to set the specimen current to zero (Davidson, 1983).

2.4. Stroboscopic Microscopy

The techniques discussed above are applicable when the potentials under examination are changing at a rate which is slow compared to the scan speed, which means in practice that the potentials will be essentially static. However, the performance of many complex digital circuits changes considerably with the speed at which the device is being clocked; a device which runs well at a low frequency may exhibit erratic behavior, or no performance at all, at a higher driving rate. There is thus an important practical need to be able to measure potentials and extract waveforms from circuits operating at high speed. This can be done by a method which is identical to that employed in conventional photography, the technique of "stroboscopy." To obtain the stationary image of a rapidly rotating object, stroboscopy uses an intense source of light which can be controlled to give short pulses of light at a high repetition rate. If the frequency of the light pulses is made equal to the rotational rate of the object to be examined, then every time the light comes on, the object will be in the same position, and because of the phenomenon of "persistence of vision" the brain will combine these brief segments of images to give the impression of the object being stationary.

An identical approach can be used with an electron beam (Plows and Nixon, 1968) as shown in Figure 2.12. Suppose that we wish to observe a conductor carrying a potential which is varying periodically as shown in Figure 2.12a. If the electron beam is chopped on and off so that each "on" period synchronizes with the voltage variation to be observed (Fig-

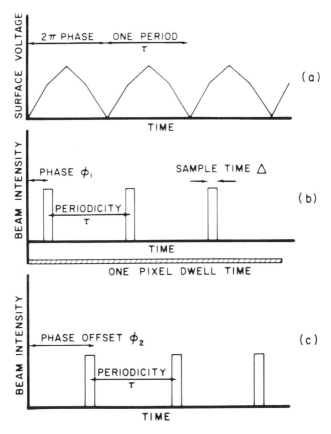

Figure 2.12. Principle of stroboscopic electron microscopy. (a) Signal variation; (b) beam intensity; (c) effect of phase shift.

ure 2.12b), then the collected voltage contrast signal will always represent the same potential value. The complete potential waveform on the conductor can be observed by leaving both frequencies constant, but altering the phase (or time offset) between them (Figure 2.12c). In the case of the SEM, there is no "persistence of vision," but provided that the signal is sampled several times at each picture point, then the image approximates that which might be expected from a continuous beam and a constant specimen voltage. This type of technique is ideally suited for the study of modern digital circuits, such as microprocessors, memory, shift registers, and so on, since the clock signal used to drive the device can also be used to control the beam (Gopinathan *et al.,* 1976; Ostrow *et al.,* 1983). Using a voltage analyzer such as that discussed above, the logical levels at different points in the circuit can be followed through the clock cycle, a facility which makes it possible to follow propagation delays through a device and compare these with those calculated during design (Wolfgang, 1983). For example, it might be found that the potential on a gate reaches the level required for switching later in the clock cycle than that assumed during design. Such a timing delay would cause the circuit to malfunction, or fail to operate at all at high clock rates, even though at low frequencies it might perform quite satisfactorily. If we are only interested in the logical state of a conductor, then the output of the voltage analyzer can be coded to give, for example, white for a "1" and black for a "0." When set up in this way, the data being transmitted along a bus can be read directly by scanning a line trace normal to the conductors in the bus and displaying the coded output directly on the SEM CRT scanned in a two-dimensional raster (Figure 2.13). Used in this way, the display can be used in much the same sort of way as the "signature" analyzers widely employed for digital diagnosis (Menzel and Kubalek, 1981; Ostrow *et al.,* 1983).

Such abilities have made stroboscopic voltage contrast an important part of device fabrication and testing laboratories. There are, however, a few important problems which must be borne in mind. In order to accurately follow the AC voltage of interest, the fraction of the time that the beam is "on" must be small compared to the time between each "on" period. This means that the effective average current striking the specimen is only a small part of the actual measured incident beam current. Typically, this "duty cycle" will be 0.1 or less. Images will therefore be noisier unless the current is increased, or the scan is slowed down so that the specimen is sampled many times at each pixel. Second, even to study quite modest frequencies, it will be necessary to be able to switch the electron beam on and off at very high speed. For clock speeds of 10 MHz, beam switching times of a nanosecond or less are required, and this level of performance must be obtained with minimal motion of the beam on

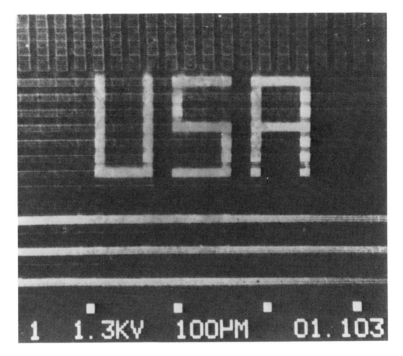

Figure 2.13. Voltage coding observation on bus lines. (From Menzel and Kubalek, 1981.)

the specimen during the switching. Most systems use electrostatic deflection, but for the very highest speeds the column has been used as a traveling wave tube to allow chopping of the beam at gigahertz rates.

2.5. Charge Collection Microscopy

The voltage contrast technique discussed above provides a way of studying in detail the behavior of a finished device. The techniques discussed in this section can also be used to study the active (junction) regions of devices but their primary application is in the characterization of semiconductor materials. The feature which distinguishes this group of techniques is that the specimen itself is used as the detector of the signal. The collective term "charge collection microscopy" covers many separate modes of operation each of which relies on the same beam interaction but provides a different type of information about the material (Leamy, 1982).

These techniques are specific to semiconductors (and some nonmetallic materials) because electron bombardment of such materials will

Table 2.1. Energy Necessary to Form
Electron-Hole Pairs in Various Materials

Material	Energy (eV) per pair
Ge	2.5
Si	3.6
GaAs	4.5
GaP	7.8
Diamond	17.0

produce a significant increase in the number of mobile charge carriers. This is because the incident electron can transfer enough energy to the sample to promote an electron from the valence band to the conduction band. Since the valence band was initially full, this action leaves behind a "hole" which acts like an electron carrying a positive charge. This hole, and its corresponding electron in the valence band, are now free to move around the lattice. Each incident electron can generate a large number of such "electron–hole" pairs because the energy required to produce each one is small (see Table 2.1), typically about three times the band-gap in the material (Sze, 1969) and thus a few electron volts, so that one 10-keV electron hitting a silicon target could produce nearly 3000 electron–hole pairs.

If left alone, the carriers diffuse randomly through the lattice until ultimately an electron and hole will come close enough to annihilate one another. However, if an electric field is applied to the specimen, then the electrons and holes will tend to move in opposite directions and the charge carried by the electrons and holes could be collected in an external circuit. The necessary field could be supplied either from an external source such as a power supply, or internally from a source such as the "built in" voltage which exists at a p–n junction or Schottky barrier. Table 2.2 lists the options and the appropriate terms (Holt, 1974).

Each of the configurations in Table 2.2 produces a distinct type of information about the sample but, confusingly, it is common practice to refer to all modes by the generic term *electron beam-induced conductivity* (EBIC). This lack of precision has also often been carried over into the

Table 2.2. Techniques for Characterization of Semiconductors

Bias source and type	Measured quantity	Mode
External constant voltage	Current	Beta conductivity
External constant current	Voltage	Beta conductivity
Internal (p–n or Schottky)	Open-circuit voltage	Electrovoltaic
Internal (p–n or Schottky)	Short-circuit current	Charge collection

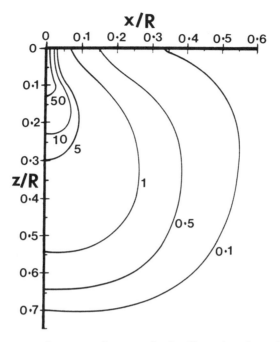

Figure 2.14. Contours of charge-carrier generation in silicon plotted as a function of electron range R. x = Horizontal distance from beam impact; z = depth.

experimental arrangements, with the result that the interpretation of image detail is made difficult. In practice, the most common mode of operation relies on the bias from p–n junctions or Schottky barriers with the current detected by amplifiers of relatively low input impedance. This mode approximates to true charge collection and in the subsequent discussion it is this technique which will be considered. Readers interested in the other modes of operation should refer to Holt (1974) for more details of the production and interpretation of these other images.

2.6. Charge Collection Images of Semiconductor Materials

The incident electron beam is scattered as it travels through the specimen, forming the familiar teardrop-shaped volume. Electron–hole pairs are produced at all points within this volume although with widely varying density (Figure 2.14). The mean rate of carrier generation is:

$$\langle g \rangle = \frac{E(1 - n)I_b}{\text{eh} \cdot q} \tag{2.1}$$

where $\langle g \rangle$ is the rate in carriers per second, I_b is the incident beam current in amperes, q is the electronic charge (1.6×10^{-19} coulomb), E is the incident beam energy (in eV), eh is the energy (in eV) required to produce one electron–hole pair, and n is the bulk backscattering coefficient. Thus, in Si a 15-keV beam of 0.1 nA generates about 3.1×10^{12} carrier pairs/s. If the excited volume were approximated as a sphere, the radius would be about 1.5 μm and so the carrier density would be about 10^{23} pairs/s per cm^3. The actual generation profile of the carriers is, of course, far from uniform (Figure 2.14) and it can be seen that the majority of the carriers are generated fairly close to the surface and within a relatively narrow radius, although the tail of the distribution extends for a considerable distance.

The carriers can, however, travel far from their generation point. If we consider the case of n-type material (i.e., one in which the majority carriers are electrons), then provided the excess electron density ΔN, introduced by the electron beam, is less than the equilibrium density N, the excess majority carriers (electrons) will follow the diffusion of the injected minority carriers (holes) so as to maintain charge neutrality. This mechanism is called drift, and the drift velocity v will depend on the local field E and the mobility ξ of the carrier:

$$v = E\xi \tag{2.2}$$

Typically, in materials such as Si, Ge, and GaAs, v saturates at a maximum value of about 100 m/s for fields of 10^6 V/cm. During this diffusion process, the electrons and holes can recombine, generally through an intermediate stage in which one species or the other is "trapped" by a defect in the crystal. The average distance traveled by a carrier before it is trapped depends inversely on the number of traps N and the probability σ of any trap capturing the carrier:

$$\lambda = 1/N\sigma \tag{2.3}$$

so the average time t that carrier travels is simply

$$t = \lambda/v \tag{2.4}$$

This quantity t is called the "lifetime" of the carrier. The lifetime of an electron–hole pair will be determined by the minority carrier lifetime, and is typically 1 ns to 1 ms. In a specimen containing a distribution of traps, and being injected with carriers from the beam, there is a balance between the generation rate g and the losses due to the recombination and diffusion. Under steady-state conditions, the minority carrier concentration p is given as

$$p = \text{const} \exp(-x/L) \tag{2.5}$$

where $L = (Dt)^{1/2}$ and D is the diffusion constant for holes. L, the "minority carrier diffusion length," is a very important parameter for semiconductor devices as it represents the average distance between the point of creation and the point of recombination for a minority carrier. This may be as large as 1 cm in very pure Si, or as low as a few micrometers for processed GaAs. Because L is such an important parameter, giving important pointers to the nature of the semiconductor material and the processing that it has received, the ability to measure L in the SEM is very useful.

On the basis of the simple outline of semiconductor physics and electron interactions given above, we can now discuss the details of charge collection imaging. The simplest case, and the one first observed experimentally (Everhart, 1958), is that shown in Figure 2.15 for a vertical p–n junction in a material. The built-in bias of the junction provides the necessary field for separating holes and electrons, so that when the generation volume of the beam overlaps the extent of the field, a current will flow in the external circuit. When the beam is moved away from the line of the junction, the current does not fall to zero, however, because some carriers will diffuse from the generation volume toward the junction and so be collected before they recombine. From equation (2.5), it can be seen that the number of carriers reaching the junction will fall exponentially, so the collected current $I(x)$ will vary with x as

$$I(x) = I(0) \exp(-x/L) \tag{2.6}$$

where L is the minority carrier diffusion length defined earlier. If the diffusion lengths on either side of the junction are different, then the resultant current profile would have the form shown in Figure 2.16. This simple experiment therefore provides a way of directly measuring L. In practice, some care must be taken to ensure that there is no surface whose distance from the beam changes with x as is the case in Figure 2.15b, because carriers will also diffuse to, and recombine on, the surface and the form of equation (2.5) must then be modified to

$$I(x) = I(0) \exp[-K(x)x/L] \tag{2.7}$$

where $K(x)$ is a variable usually of order unity (Bresse and Lafeuille, 1971). If the surface-to-beam distance is constant (as for the surface

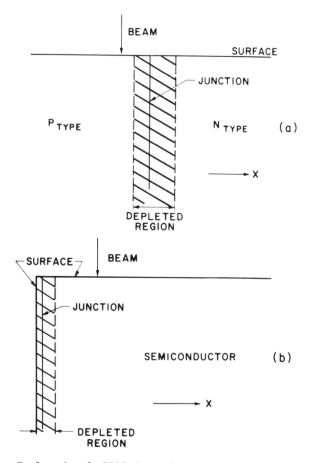

Figure 2.15. Configurations for EBIC observation. (a) p–n junction; (b) edge junction.

through which the beam enters), then the effect of surface recombination is constant and the net effect is simply to modify the observed value of L. A considerable literature exists discussing ways of extracting accurate values of L from measurements of $I(x)$ with various sample geometries.

The signal collected by a junction, or junctions, is also a common way of applying charge collection techniques to the study of devices. If the EBIC amplifier is connected across a pair of the power line rails to a device, then signals be will obtained from every junction in the device when the beam passes sufficiently close to it for collection to be possible. Figure 2.17 shows an example of this type of operation with many junction regions clearly visible. The form of the image will depend very much on the beam energy since raising this will increase both the penetration

The collected current will depend on the beam energy, the depleted depth, and the diffusion length of the material. Figure 2.20 plots the calculated gain (i.e., collected current/incident current) of a Schottky barrier on silicon at 15 keV (Joy, 1985). An increase in either the depleted depth, caused by a change in the resistivity or through the application of an external reverse bias, or the diffusion length will increase the gain up to the point where all the carriers are being collected. The gain is then about 3800 at 15 keV. Because the gain depends in a predictable way on these parameters, Schottky barriers offer an easy way to find the diffusion length L. A measurement of the gain at two different beam energies and some simple graphical analysis allow both parameters to be determined unambiguously. Unlike the methods for finding L described earlier, this approach is not significantly affected by recombination at the beam entry surface because the Schottky barrier will eliminate any flow of carriers to the surface.

Since both the diffusion length and the depletion depth change the collected current, local variations in either parameter will produce contrast. For example, in silicon slices, small changes in carbon doping impurities will change the resistivity and hence the depletion depth. The characteristic "striae" bands of contrast produced in the way are easily visible as in Figure 2.21 even though the minute differences in resistivity that they represent are very hard to measure directly (Chi and Gatos, 1978; Leamy *et al.,* 1978). However, the most important application of the Schottky technique is to study electrically active defects in semiconductor materials. If a dislocation or stacking fault is electrically active, then it can "trap" a carrier for sufficient time to allow it to recombine

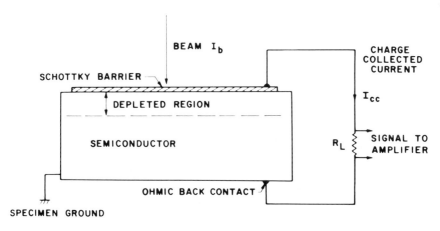

Figure 2.18. Geometry from Schottky barrier collection.

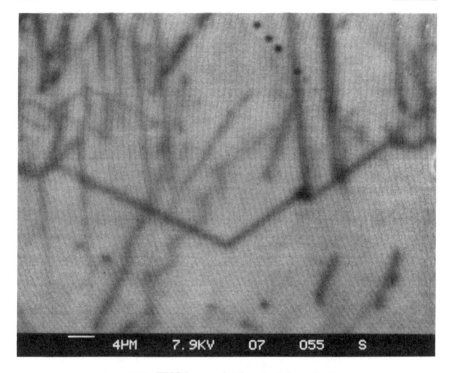

Figure 2.19. EBIC image of defects in deformed silicon.

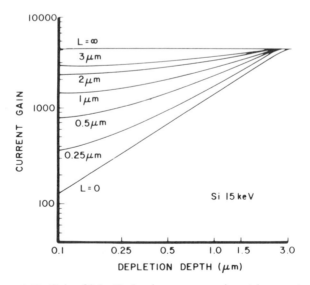

Figure 2.20. Gain of Schottky barrier versus experimental parameters.

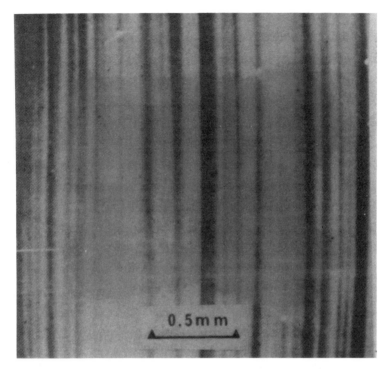

Figure 2.21. EBIC image of dopant striae in silicon. (From Leamy *et al.*, 1978.)

with a passing carrier of the other sign. Such activity occurs at such features as line or point defects, or grain boundaries and its presence can have a devastating effect on the performance of any device fabricated over top of the defect. The ability of the charge collection technique to observe these active defects is therefore an important tool for the study of materials.

If carriers are generated near an electrically active defect, then some of them will diffuse to the defect, recombine, and so not contribute to the collected charge (Lander *et al.*, 1963). The defect therefore appears as a dark line in the image (e.g., Figure 2.19). The calculation of a contrast profile is complex (Donolato, 1978) but its general shape (Figure 2.22) can be deduced straightforwardly. If we assume a line defect (i.e., a dislocation) parallel to the surface of the material and consider scanning the beam perpendicular to the defect, then clearly the signal profile as a function of the beam position will be symmetrical about the defect. The fall in signal due to carriers diffusing to the defect will depend on the number of carriers generated, the distance they have to travel to the defect, and

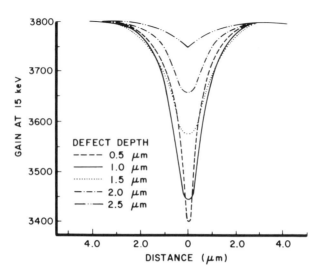

Figure 2.22. Computed line profiles across EBIC image of defect.

the diffusion length L. The simplest case is when the beam is centered over the defect: the signal loss to the defect will then mainly depend on the average number of carriers produced at the depth of the defect. As seen from Figure 2.14, this means that the contrast will be highest for a defect close to the surface; calculations show that the maximum actually occurs when the defect is at about one-third of the mean electron range. On the other hand, if the defect is at a depth greater than the electron range, then no carriers are produced in the vicinity of the defect and the only carriers recombining at the dislocation will be that small fraction which diffuse to it. Consequently, the contrast from a defect falls to zero very rapidly once the defect depth exceeds the electron range. An estimate of the dislocation depth can therefore be made by noting the beam energy at which it first becomes visible and finding the electron range R from the relation

$$R = 0.0428(E^{1.75}/\rho) \qquad (\mu\text{m}) \qquad (2.8)$$

where ρ is the density (g/cm^3) and the beam energy E is in keV. As the beam is moved away from the defect, the contrast falls because fewer carriers are being produced at the defect. The "width" of the defect image will obviously depend both on the diameter of the electron beam interaction volume at the depth of the defect, and on the diffusion length. Because the interaction volume has a teardrop shape, we can expect that the width of the image will be narrowest when it is close to the surface, or just at the end of the electron range, and greatest at about one-half the electron range. Raising or lowering the beam energy will obviously have a major effect on the defect image width since the interaction volume has a diameter varying as about $E^{1.75}$. High-resolution defect images therefore need energies that may be as low as a few kiloelectron volts. Varying the diffusion length will also change the width of the defect, but since the chance of a carrier reaching the defect falls off with distance from the dislocation as

$$(1/r) \exp(-r/L) \qquad (2.9)$$

even when L becomes very large the image width will be limited to about twice the width of the interaction volume.

The defect image is also dependent on the position of the defect relative to the depleted layer. If the defect is outside (below) the depleted region, then information about the dislocation is carried only by those carriers which diffuse back into the depleted region. Consequently, the contrast is reduced by an amount depending on the average distance that these carriers must travel, and the diffusion length. If the depleted layer is swept downwards toward the defect, by applying a reverse bias to the Schottky for example, then the contrast will rise because more carriers will be collected and the contrast will peak as the edge of the depleted layer passes through the defect line. If the bias is increased still further, then the contrast will fall because the bias field will sweep carriers away from the defect and so reduce the probability of recombination. It may also be noted here that the contrast from a defect can also be affected by other factors. Under conditions of high beam current, or low beam voltage (where the small interaction volume results in a high carrier density), the number of majority carriers injected by the beam may exceed the equilibrium density. If this happens, then the defect may become saturated with carriers and the rate of recombination will fall (Leamy *et al.,* 1976, 1978).

2.7. Quantitative Measurements in Charge Collection Microscopy

It has already been shown that the diffusion length of a semiconductor material can be measured either from charge collection profiles around a junction, or from the gain of Schottky barrier. In addition to this important parameter, other quantitative information about a semiconductor material can be obtained. The minority carrier lifetime t can be measured by rapidly switching off the electron beam and monitoring the decay of the collected current since the number of minority carriers at some time T will fall according to the formula (S. M. Davidson, 1977)

$$n(t) = n(0) \exp(-T/t) \qquad (2.10)$$

where $n(0)$ is the equilibrium number of minority carriers before the beam is switched off. Although the principle of this measurement is simple, the practical application is often difficult because the lifetime t can range from microseconds for top-quality unprocessed Si to only tens of picoseconds for heavily doped compound semiconductors. The ability to switch the beam off in a very short time is therefore essential. This can be done by electrostatically, or electromagnetically, deflecting the beam across an aperture which is usually situated between the gun and first condensor lens so as to minimize any apparent motion of the beam during switching. With care, such a system can producing switching times of the order of a few nanoseconds, although such a figure requires precise alignment and engineering. Faster switching can be obtained by pulsing the Wehnelt cylinder of the gun so as to cut off emission. This has the advantage that no beam motion occurs, but the disadvantage that significant high-voltage pulse engineering is required. Using either approach, the practical minimum lifetime measurable is of the order of 0.5 ns, the limit being set by the effect of capacitances distributed through the recording system (Possin and Kirkpatrick, 1976).

Quantitative information about the energy level of the traps giving rise to recombination can be obtained by changing the temperature of the sample. This is because the Fermi level moves from its position near a band edge at low temperatures to a position near the middle of the gap at high tempeatures, so in an n-type material the Fermi level will sweep over the top half of the band gap. As the Fermi level passes through the energy level of a defect, the electron population on the trap will fall and so the contrast will change (Kimerling *et al.,* 1977). If the temperature at which the image changes contrast is noted, then an estimate of the trap energy can be made. A practical problem with this technique is that heating the semiconductor will often produce excessive noise and leakage currents. However, in silicon the relative energies are such that lowering the temperature toward liquid nitrogen will produce the desired effect (Ourmazd and Booker, 1979) and in this case both leakage and noise will be reduced.

The two operations, beam switching and temperature variation, discussed above can be combined to produce a powerful technique known as deep-level transient spectroscopy (DLTS), which again relies on the different equilibrium occupation of a trap when it is above, or below, the

Fermi level. The DLTS technique exploits this variation to determine precisely the energy, and map the position, of the traps. The sample is connected as for normal charge collection imaging, but the beam is now pulsed on for a short time (typically 2.5 μs) and off for a longer time (typically 10 μs). In the quiescent state, each trap will have an equilibrium population of holes or electrons on it (Figure 2.23). When the beam is switched on, the local density of electron–hole pairs will be increased and this occupation level will be modified. After the beam is again switched off, the occupation of each trap will decay back to its original values as the excess electrons, or holes, are thermally excited and leave. The rate at which this occurs will depend on the energy level of the trap and the

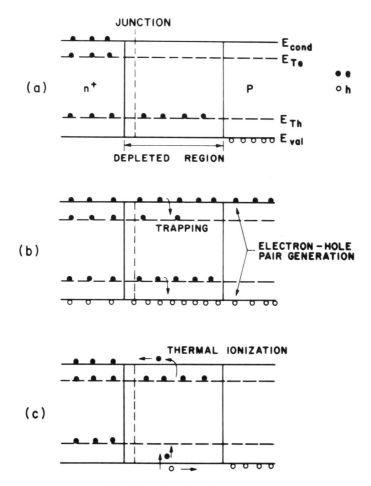

Figure 2.23. Principle of deep-level transient spectroscopy.

sample temperature. As the electrons and holes desorb from the traps, they are collected by the depletion field in the usual way and produce a transient current flow which can be measured in the external circuit. This measurement can be made by sampling the current flow at two closely spaced intervals, say 1 μs apart, and noting the difference in the readings obtained. If this quantity is plotted as a function of the sample temperature, then a spectrum is obtained which displays peaks at temperatures where traps are being emptied (Figure 2.24). The relative height and position of the peaks are characteristic of the type of traps being sampled, and such spectra can therefore be used as "fingerprints" to classify defects produced during processing. The actual energy level of a defect can be found by taking three (or more) samples of the transient current so as to measure the rate of fall of the signal. An Arrhenius plot of this against $1/T$ gives the trap energy (Petroff and Lang, 1977).

If the sample temperature is held at a value corresponding to a DLTS peak for a given trap, then the transient signal can be displayed as the beam is scanned to produce an image which will be a map of the distribution of the trap. Such an image is a convolution between the normal charge collection image (which maps the collection efficiency of the junc-

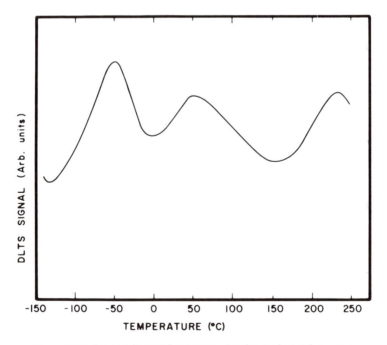

Figure 2.24. Schematic DLTS spectrum showing typical defect peaks.

tion) and the DLTS signal. A comparison between a standard charge collection image and the corresponding DLTS image is instructive because it can demonstrate that traps need not be associated with visible defects in the material. This technique is particularly effective when applied to thinned samples (Petroff *et al.*, 1978) because STEM imaging can be used to view all defects whether electrically active or not.

2.8. Practical Aspects of Charge Collection Microscopy

Before leaving the subject of charge collection microscopy, a few practical points should be made. Since, at its peak, the collected signal is typically several thousand times the incident beam current, any low-signal amplifier with low noise, good bandwidth, and a high dynamic range, can be used. However, for the image to be interpretable in a quantitative way, the collection conditions must be properly defined. If an EBIC image is desired, then the amplifier must represent, ideally, a short circuit to the specimen. The practical extent to which this is necessary will depend on the characteristics of the material being measured. Typically, the collected current is measured by allowing it to flow through a resistor of known value and sensing the voltage developed across the resistor. Figure 2.25 shows an experimental plot, for such an arrangement, of the apparent gain of a Schottky diode as a function of the load resistance R.

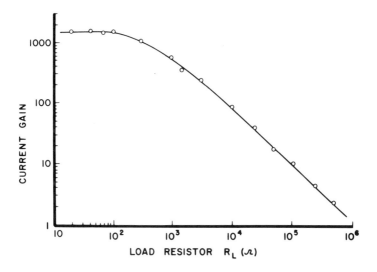

Figure 2.25. Apparent gain of Schottky barrier versus load resistance R.

When R is very high (>10 megohms), the apparent gain is small because the leakage resistance of the diode is small compared to the load resistance and so most of the current never passes through the external circuit. As R is reduced, the gain rises because less of the current is shunted through the leakage resistance, and eventually saturates at a load of about 100 ohms. On a diode with lower leakage resistance (e.g., a very large area Schottky barrier), it would be necessary to use an even lower load in order to approximate the true EBIC short-circuit condition. Even when an accurate measurment of the current gain is not required, the use of a high-input-impedance amplifier is undesirable because the ohmic drop across the input will represent a fluctuating bias applied to the sample which may result in unpredictable and unstable imaging artifacts. In addition, the combination of a high input impedance, and the inherent capacitance of a Schottky barrier or a p–n junction, acts like a low pass filter and severely limits the scan speed at which useful images can be obtained. An alternative approach to the use of a voltage amplifier and shunt resistor is the true charge-sensitive amplifier, commercial examples of which are usually specified to produce ohmic drops across their inputs of only a few millivolts. Such devices are ideal for EBIC imaging but tend to be both costly and limited in dynamic range when compared to otherwise comparable voltage amplifier systems.

In EBIV the measurement of an open-circuit voltage is required. This needs a high-input impedance amplifier, typically hundreds of megohms, such as is available from low-leakage FET devices. While the provision of such an amplifier is not usually a problem, the bandwidth limitation inherent under these conditions is, and EBIV measurements are consequently less readily performed. In either case, the connections between the sample and the external circuitry need to be arranged carefully. For example, all of the leads used for current lead-outs should exit the column through a single hole, to avoid the single-turn transformer effect in which the circulating eddy currents in the magnetic screening are coupled into the leads, and a single low-impedance earth point must be provided. Wherever possible, earth leads should be heavy-duty copper braid, and contacts should be made through screw-down terminals. Attention to details of this type can dramatically improve the noise level in images. The provision of some means of digitally recording at least line scan information is now very important, and suitable systems are available commercially in the form of modified multichannel analyzers (Russell and Herrington, 1982) or through the use of personal computers (Joy, 1982).

The other problems that routinely occur in charge collection microscopy are those associated with making contacts to the sample, and to producing good-quality Schottky barriers. The deposition of good Schottky barriers requires careful attention to detail; in particular, the surface of the specimen must be carefully cleaned by the use of a chemical etch, and the vacuum station in which the deposition is carried out must be free from any trace of hydrocarbon contamination. Table 2.3 outlines the step-by-step procedure required for the fabrication of good Schottky barriers which are typically only 200–400 Å thick since a greater thickness will result in an energy loss in the metal layer. On n-type samples, gold is usually the optimum choice, while on p-type samples, titanium seems to work best, but considerable experimentation may be required to find the correct choice of metal and etching procedure for any given situation since the chemistry of the barrier interface is very complex. The contacts to the sample must all be ohmic, a requirement that can usually be met by using a "silver dag" wire contact or a pressure-loaded probe to the metal layer. The back contact to the material can also be made in the same way, although in heavily doped specimens it may sometimes be necessary to fabricate a special region. A suitable back-contact can conveniently be made by evaporating 300–500 Å onto the material, and then heating the sample to about 560 C in an inert gas. When fabricated, the Schottky should behave like a diode when tested with an ohmmeter, and the forward to backwards resistance ratio should be 1 to 10 or better when measured at a few volts.

2.9. Cathodoluminescence Studies

In the preceding section, we examined the charge that can be collected from the production of electron–hole pairs in a semiconductor. In the context of charge collection imaging, the recombination of the electrons and holes leads to a fall in the signal, but this same recombination can result in the radiation of photons from the sample, an effect known as cathodoluminescence (CL). If these photons can be detected, then CL provides a valuable source of information about semiconductor materials and the defects that they contain (Holt and Datta, 1980; Pfefferkorn *et al.,* 1980).

Photons can be produced when the electrons and holes recombine either (a) directly from the conduction to the valence band, or (b) from a donor (n-type) impurity to the valence band. The rate R_r at which such radiative recombination events occur is given for case (b) as

$$R_r = N_r \sigma_r v \tag{2.11}$$

where N_r is the concentration of radiative recombination centers, σ_r is the probability of the donor being occupied by an electron, and v is the carrier velocity. In lightly doped material, (a) is the most probable mechanism

Table 2.3. Schottky Barriers on Si

Initial preparations

   1. Rinse several clean Teflon beakers, first in electronic-grade methanol, then trichloroethane, and finally methanol again.
   2. Obtain a clean pair of tweezers and a supply of deionized water.
   3. Bake out the evaporator basket or boat that will be used for the metal deposition.
   4. Measure charge (in grams or length of wire) for desired deposition thickness assuming uniform coverage of a sphere centered at the boat, radius equal to the distance to the specimen.

Sample preparation

   I. n-type silicon

   1. Place the Si in a Teflon beaker filled with clean methanol.
   2. Place this beaker in an ultrasonic cleaner for about 5 min.
   3. Rinse the Si in trichloroethane without letting the Si surface dry. The Si wafer must never be exposed to air, and must always be kept under the solvent surface.
   4. Rinse the Si in methanol following the same procedures as in step 3.
   5. Rinse in deionized water.
   6. Add enough hydrofluoric (HF) acid to make the Si wafer hydrophobic (i.e., so that water droplets stand on surface).
   7. Pour out the water–HF solution, checking to see that the polished surface of Si is dry. If not, the cleaning procedures 1–6 must be repeated with greater care.
   8. When removing the wafer from the beaker, use tweezers—not fingers! Only allow the tweezers to make contact with the outer edges of the wafer, as any Schottky made in a region handled by the tweezers will be defective. Also take care not to get any water–HF on the tweezers as it will react with the metal and contaminate the wafer.
   9. Place the cleaned Si wafer on a clean filter paper.
   10. Mount the wafer on the mask, Schottky side down.
   11. Place the sample in the evaporator and pump down to 10^{-7} Torr if possible, then proceed to evaporate.
   12. Keep the shutter over the basket until the charge starts to evaporate. The main function of the shutter is to keep the Si surface contaminant-free while the charge outgasses.
   13. Once the shutter is open, keep it in this position until all of the charge is evaporated, taking care not to let the Si wafer get too hot.

   II. p-type silicon

   1–5. The same as for n-type preparation.
   6. Etch the wafer in a mixture of nitric and hydrofluoric acid, adding small amounts of HF to the nitric acid. Hold the beaker at all times and swirl the solution; it should turn to a pale orange. Watch the Si surface at all times to avoid orange peeling. If the Si hazes, re-etch. The usual etching time is 1–2 min.
   7. Rinse with deionized water by gradually adding water and then pouring it out.
   Follow steps 8–13 of n-type preparation, making sure to start evaporation no later than 20 min of pumping even if a pressure of 10^{-5}Pa (10^{-7} Torr) is not reached.

---

for radiative recombination, but for most practical semiconductors, (b) is the most significant mechanism. There is, however, a third possibility (c) that recombination will occur by an intermediate deep-level trap. Such an event is nonradiative (i.e., no photons are produced in the recombination) and since events (b) and (c) will be competing for the same minority carriers, the radiated CL intensity will depend on the relative probability of these two processes. The recombination rate at the trap is

$$R_t = N_t \sigma_t v \tag{2.12}$$

where N_t is the concentration of traps and σ_t is the capture cross section. All other factors being equal, $\sigma_t \gg \sigma_r$ because the trap is farther from either the conduction or valence bands. The CL signal is thus proportional to the ratio R_r/R_t:

$$\text{CL intensity} = N_r \sigma_r / N_t \sigma_t \tag{2.13}$$

The CL spectrum will have its peak intensity at the most probable radiative transition energy, which will normally be close to the band gap energy,

$$E_{CL} = E_g - E_d - E_{ex} \tag{2.14}$$

where E_g is the band gap, E_d is the donor ionization energy (if a donor is involved), and E_{ex} is the exciton binding energy (an exciton is an electron and a hole bound loosely together).

The CL radiation therefore potentially contains a large amount of information. The fundamental problem with the technique is collecting this information. The number of photons emitted is small, and consequently the first priority is ensuring that the maximum fraction of the total available is recovered. Figure 2.26 shows a typical scheme in which

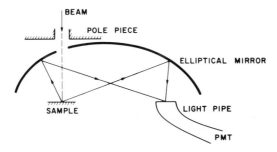

Figure 2.26. Schematic drawing of collection scheme for cathodoluminescent imaging.

the sample is placed at one focus of a parabolic mirror, the other focus being at the mouth of a light pipe which then carries the signal to a photomultiplier or other detector. Such an arrangment can collect a significant fraction of the light signal and can perform satisfactorily for most applications provided that care is taken to prevent electrons from being scattered directly onto the end of the light pipe (where they will cause low-level light production and generate a spurious background). For this same reason, the practice, occasionally found, of using the standard secondary electron detector as a CL collector after first removing the Faraday cage and scintillator should be avoided.

The material of the light pipe and window must be chosen so as to allow all the wavelengths of interest to be transmitted efficiently. For the normal visual range, many materials can be found that are suitable, but for operation in the long-wavelength regime (above 1 μm), quartz or specially formulated glasses are required. Similarly, the photomultiplier must have its sensitivity curve matched to the energy range of interest, and since the actual sensitivity of the detector can vary by more than one order of magnitude over its working range of wavelengths, the detector will require a calibration for sensitivity in quantitative applications.

The simplest approach is to use the photomultiplier to collect the whole CL signal and then amplify this signal to modulate the cathode-ray display screen in the normal way. Figure 2.27 shows the appearance of an image collected in this way from a sample of GaAs. Superimposed over the uniform contrast from the material itself, a large number of dark spots

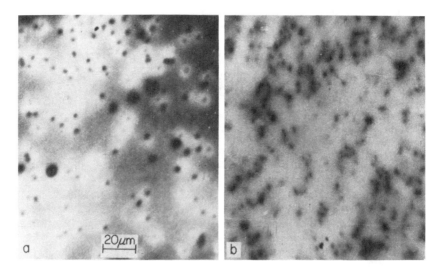

Figure 2.27. CL image of defects in GaAs. (From Davidson, 1977.)

can be seen. Each of these represents a recombination center, such as a defect. As shown by equation (2.13), this will result in a drop in the detected signal. The CL image can therefore be used in a way that is similar to charge collection microscopy to determine the number and distribution of electrically active defects. However, the CL technique has the benefit that no Schottky barrier is required. The form of the defect profile is similar to that discussed earlier for charge collection images, with a width that will depend on the beam interaction volume and the minority carrier diffusion length. The spatial resolution will not depend on the wavelength of the light produced since no imaging lenses are involved. Figure 2.28 shows another contrast mode in which changes in doping level are visible as changes in signal intensity. Although it might be expected from equation (2.13) that the intensity would vary linearly with N_r and hence with the doping level, the actual variation tends to be less than this because the trapping concentration will also vary with the doping. Relatively small changes in doping are, however, readily visible and the technique is a rapid and valuable tool for the study of devices and materials.

Although the simple CL image is useful, more information can be obtained by dispersing the photons through a spectrometer before collecting them, so that the emission spectrum of the specimen can be determined. Two kinds of analyzer are in common use, grating or prism spec-

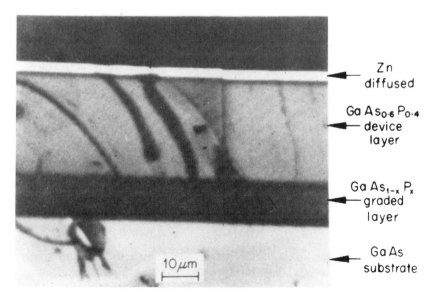

Figure 2.28. CL image showing contrast variations due to doping. (From Davidson, 1977.)

trometers in which the light is dispersed by diffraction, and Fourier transform spectrometers which rely on interference effects. Prism or grating spectrometers are available at low cost in a format ideally suited for interfacing with an SEM, but are of low efficiency. Fourier transform analyzers are not so readily available, but have a very much higher transmission factor and can therefore be used with smaller electron probes. In either case, the signal intensity after dispersion is much less than the total collected intensity, and for satisfactory results single photon counting techniques are required. Since the peak of the spectrum depends on the band gap energy (equation 2.14), a spectral analysis can be used to investigate changes in the band gap as a function of doping, for example in such devices as GaAsP LEDs or heterostructure lasers. Peaks in the spectrum may also be associated with particular types of defects as the result of decoration by an impurity, so an image formed from monochromatic radiation can be used to map such defects. Finally, it can be noted that the CL spectrum shifts with sample temperature, and thus a spectrometer attached to an SEM offers the ability to map device operating temperatures (Davidson and Vaidya, 1977).

2.10. Thermal Wave Microscopy

A final technique which deserves mention is thermal wave microscopy (Davies, 1983). This mode of operation differs from the other techniques discussed above in that it probes the thermal and mechanical, rather than the electronic, properties of the sample. However, since these are related to, or can modify, the electronic behavior, their study is important when performed in conjunction with the other techniques discussed here. The system is shown schematically in Figure 2.29 and relies on the repetitive chopping of the electron beam as it is scanned across the sample. The energy deposited in the sample by this beam causes a periodic temperature variation which will spread out as a spherical wave front from the beam point. The wavelength λ of this thermal wave will depend on the chopping frequency ω and thermal properties of the sample, and is given as

$$\lambda = (2\chi/\rho C\omega)^{1/2} \tag{2.15}$$

where χ is the thermal conductivity, C is the specific heat, and ρ is the density of the material. For common metals and a chopping frequency in the 100 kHz range, the wavelength is of the order of a few micrometers. The intensity of this temperature variation, which is typically of the order of less than 1°C, will depend on the thermal properties (density, specific

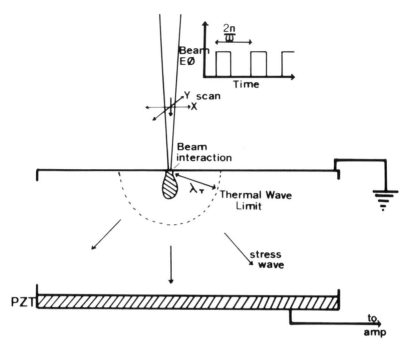

Figure 2.29. Principle of thermal wave operation.

heat, thermal conductivity) of the irradiated volume, but since the thermal wave is heavily damped it does not travel far enough from the beam impact point for it to be measured and made use of. But the temperature oscillation generates a periodic expansion and contraction of the sample which in turn causes an elastic stress wave to propagate through the sample. This elastic (acoustic) wave is at the same frequency as the thermal signal, but has a wavelength λ_a which is much longer; for example, in silicon the velocity of sound is 8945 m/s so that a 100-kHz wave has a wavelength of 8.9 cm. This wave therefore propagates freely through the sample and can be detected (Figure 2.30) by a suitable transducer bonded at a convenient point to the spectrum.

The intensity of the acoustic (elastic) signal depends on the efficiency of the conversion from thermal to mechanical energy, which in turn depends on the elastic moduli, coefficients of expansion, and so on. This efficiency is very low, usually of the order of 10^{-8}, and consequently the elastic signal is small. However, the efficiency rises linearly with the incident beam power, and with the chopping frequency, so optimum results are obtained with high beam currents (1 μA at the sample) and high-speed chopping. The detected signal depends, through the efficiency equation,

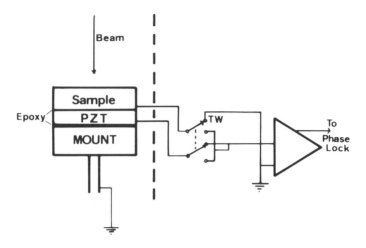

Figure 2.30. Signal detection for thermal wave operation.

in a complex way on a very large number of parameters of the sample, so that a variation in any one of these can produce contrast. Thus, changes in the density due to plastic deformation, or voids and cracks as in the example of Figure 2.31; or the thermal conductivity perhaps due to doping as illustrated in Figure 2.32; or the elastic moduli (as the orientation of the material changes from one grain to another) will all be visible. The interpretation of the images observed is thus far from straightforward, and additional imaging techniques applied to the same area are likely to be required before an unambiguous analysis can be made.

The contrast comes almost totally from the interaction volume (the "thermal wave" region) of the incident beam. This is because the wave-

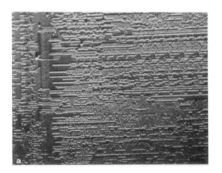
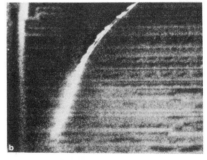

Figure 2.31. (a) SE image of chip and (b) corresponding thermal wave image showing subsurface crack. Reprinted with permission of Thermawave, Inc., Fremont, California.

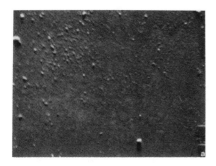 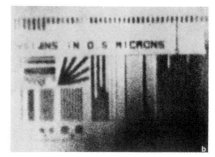

Figure 2.32. (a) SE image of silicon and (b) corresponding thermal wave image showing contrast due to ion-implanted dopants. Reprinted with permission of Thermawave, Inc., Fremont, California.

length of the acoustic wave is so large that it interacts only weakly with the specimen and thus functions mostly as a carrier for the thermal wave information. The spatial resolution of thermal wave images is then set by the quadrature sum of the beam interaction radius, the probe size, and the thermal wavelength (see Table 2.4). As seen, for common metals, at a chopping frequency of 1 MHz, it is realistic to expect resolutions of the order of only a few micrometers. To achieve higher resolutions, it is necessary to determine which is the limiting factor and reduce that. In light materials (e.g., Al, Si), the limit will be the beam interaction volume and this can only be minimized by using low beam energies. In heavier materials, the thermal wavelength is usually the limit, and this can be reduced by increasing the chopping frequency. In either case, the ultimate limit is likely to be set by the need for an adequate beam current into the sample, and for tungsten thermionic electron sources this will probably be at around the 1 μm level. However, some recent work (Balk and Kultscher, 1983) has shown that detection of harmonic signals (i.e., multiples of the

Table 2.4. Thermal Wave Imaging
Resolution in Various Materials (μm)[a]

Factor	Al	Si	Cu	Au
Probe size	1.0	1.0	1.0	1.0
Beam spread	4.8	5.5	1.4	0.7
Thermal λ	5.1	3.9	6.1	6.1
Resolution	7.1	6.8	6.3	6.2

[a]Data for 30-keV operation at 1 MHz.

original chopping frequency) produces both significantly higher resolution as well as some new types of contrast.

The lateral and depth resolution are both about three times the thermal wavelength for the chopping frequency used. The depth resolution can, however, be improved by using a phase-sensitive detection system which is referenced to the chopping of the incident beam so that both phase and amplitude information can be obtained. Because the phase of the thermal wave signal changes rapidly as a function of its depth beneath the surface, images recorded at different phase shift settings on the detector allow a depth-resolved analysis of the sample to be made, down to the maximum penetration depth.

The thermal wave technique is still new and much basic work remains to be done to generate quantitative, rather than qualitative, data. Even at this stage, however, the thermal wave mode does have promise in many areas of device quality control, as well as in studies of deformation, and even forensic science (Cargill, 1980; Rosencwaig and White, 1981).

3

Electron Channeling Contrast in the SEM

3.1. Introduction

Electron channeling is an effect of the interaction of energetic electrons with crystalline materials which can be used to detect the crystallographic properties of a sample in an SEM image. With a suitable sample and proper attention to the electron optical requirements for the detection of electron channeling contrast, it is possible in any SEM to form images of the crystallographic microstructure of a sample, including high- and low-angle grain boundaries, and it is also possible to obtain electron channeling patterns, which provide direct information on orientation relative to the incident beam, from large single crystals. With special scanning systems, electron channeling patterns can be formed from selected areas with dimensions as small as 1–5 μm in diameter. The crystallographic information available in the electron channeling pattern is analogous to that which can be obtained by x-ray diffraction of solid specimens. The advantage of electron channeling is the combination of imaging and orientation information which is available in the SEM. Electron channeling contrast has been the subject of several reviews (Booker, 1969; Newbury, 1974; Joy *et al.*, 1982).

3.2. Origin of Electron Channeling Contrast

In describing the properties of electron scattering in solids (*SEMXM,* Chapter 3), the crystallinity, or lack thereof, of a sample was ignored. To a first approximation, the measurable products of the scattering of the beam electrons, which include backscattered, secondary, and absorbed electrons, characteristic and bremsstrahlung x-rays, and low-energy photons, do not depend on the crystal structure of a bulk sample. However, when we examine the electron signals with sensitivity to changes of about 5%, crystallographic effects on the products, particularly backscattered electrons, can be detected. That is, the orientation of the beam relative to the arrangement of atoms in the crystal influences the interaction of the beam electrons with the solid and the resulting products.

The origin of these crystallographic effects is the phenomenon of electron channeling, which was first reported in the SEM by Coates (1967) and explained on a theoretical basis by Hirsch and Humphreys (1970). Electron channeling can be understood conceptually with the aid of Figure 3.1, or alternatively with a three-dimensional ball-and-stick model of a crystal lattice. As vectors representing the beam approach the crystal from various angles, or the line-of-sight of the viewer changes relative to a lattice model, the density of atoms viewed along certain directions is seen to be much greater than along others. The gaps or channels between the atomic centers provide a path for the beam to penetrate more deeply into the crystal before scattering. As a result, the backscattering coefficient is reduced when the beam is lined up with the crystal channels. For slightly different beam–crystal orientations, the channels are closed, the atom density is higher, and the beam electrons scatter more closely to the surface, which increases the backscattering coefficient. Although

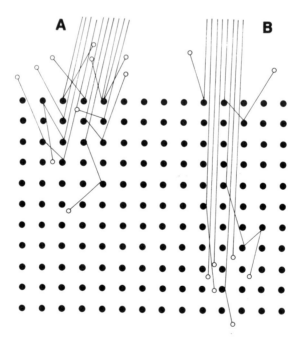

Figure 3.1. Schematic representation of a crystal lattice. Two different beam–crystal orientations are indicated, demonstrating (A) a nonchanneling and (B) a channeling situation.

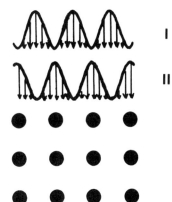

Figure 3.2. Bloch wave construction to describe the behavior of fast electrons in a crystal lattice.

the schematic diagram of Figure 3.1 appears to suggest that channeling is a strong effect, the actual difference between maximum and minimum channeling directions is only 3–5%. Channeling is thus a weak effect, and in order to make use of it as an imaging mechanism in the SEM, we must pay close attention to the strategy of preparing and imaging the specimen, following the guidelines described for imaging in *SEMXM,* Chapter 4.

3.3. Characteristics of Electron Channeling Contrast

The behavior of the beam electrons within the crystal can be described mathematically as a superposition of waves, known as Bloch waves, whose amplitude is related to the magnitude of the electron current, as illustrated in Figure 3.2 (Hirsch and Humphreys, 1970). The two types of Bloch waves of interest illustrated in Figure 3.2, are the type I wave, which has its current vectors aligned with the channels between the atoms and is thus weakly scattering, and the type II wave, which has its current maxima aligned with the atom positions and is strongly scattering. For any orientation of the incident beam relative to the crystal, the behavior of the electrons within the crystal can be described as a mixture of the type I and type II waves. For particular orientations, the relative mix changes sharply, i.e., from a strong channeling to a nonchanneling condition. These critical beam–crystal orientations are those which satisfy the Bragg condition for the various crystal planes:

$$n\lambda = 2d \sin \theta_B \qquad (3.1a)$$

where n is the integer order (± 1, 2, 3, . . .), λ is the wavelength of the incident electrons, d is the interplanar spacing, and θ_B is the Bragg angle.

For a particular crystal, the set of d values is fixed, and λ is fixed by the choice of the electron accelerating voltage, so that a unique set of Bragg angles exists which is characteristic of that crystal structure. For the cubic system, the Bragg angles can be calculated from the lattice spacing a_0, the electron wavelength, and the Miller indices (hkl) of the plane according to the equation

$$\theta_B = \sin^{-1}\left[\frac{\lambda}{2a_0}(h^2 + k^2 + l^2)^{1/2}\right] \tag{3.1b}$$

If we plot the intensity of backscattering as a function of angle relative to a particular set of crystal planes of spacing "d," the resulting inten-

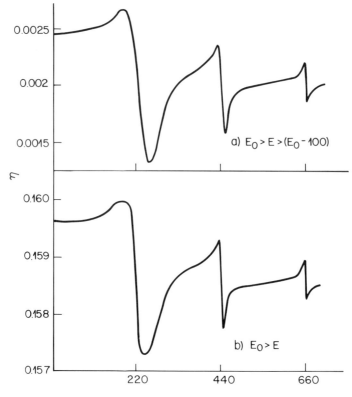

Figure 3.3. Plots of backscattered electron intensity as a function of beam angle relative to the crystal planes ("rocking curve"). The lower curve shows the magnitude of the signal when the full spectrum of backscattered electron energy is used, while the upper curve shows the decreased signal strength but greatly increased contrast when energy filtration is used to exclude all but those backscattered electrons which have lost less than 100 eV of energy.

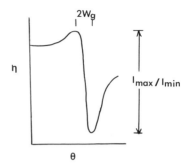

Figure 3.4. Characteristics of the rocking curve at a Bragg position which are useful measures of channeling contrast: signal ratio, I_{max}/I_{min}, and angular width, W_g.

sity distribution, known as a rocking curve, reveals sharp transitions in intensity at each order $n = \pm 1, 2, 3, \ldots$, as shown in Figure 3.3. Two parameters can be used to characterize these channeling transitions, as illustrated in Figure 3.4. The intensity ratio I_{max}/I_{min} measured at the maximum and minimum points of the transition gives a measure of the contrast. The apparent width of the transition is a measure of the apparent size of the channeling transition. Schulson (1971) derived the angular width of the transitions, $2W_g$, as

$$2W_g = 2/\xi_g|\bar{g}| \tag{3.2}$$

where ξ_g is the extinction distance for the reciprocal lattice vector g. The extinction distance is a parameter obtained from electron diffraction theory (Hirsch *et al.*, 1965) and is given by an expression of the form

$$\xi_g = \pi V_c \cos \theta / \lambda F_g \tag{3.3}$$

where V_c is the volume of the unit cell of the crystal and F_g is the structure factor for the particular crystal planes under consideration. Structure factors can be calculated appropriate to the particular crystal under study; formulas for calculating structure factors are given by Hirsch *et al.* (1965). The magnitude of the reciprocal lattice vector, g, is given by $g = 1/d_{hkl}$. The crystal spacing d for cubic crystals is given by

$$d = a_0/(h^2 + k^2 + l^2)^{1/2} \tag{3.4}$$

where a_0 is the lattice spacing and h, k, l are the Miller indices of the plane. The widths of the channeling transitions predicted by equation (3.3) become narrower as the indices increase. Moreover, as shown from the calculations of Spencer *et al.* (1972), the contrast of the transitions decreases as the indices h, k, l increase.

3.4. The Electron Channeling Pattern

3.4.1. Coarse Structure

If the stereographic projection of a crystal is constructed, the inter-section of a trace of a particular plane denoted by the Miller indices (h, k, l) on the stereographic plot is a line. To construct the geometry of the electron channeling pattern, we must consider the rocking curve for the particular family of planes. Ignoring the contributions from other planes, the same rocking curve should be obtained at any location along the trace of the plane. Moving a rocking curve such as that shown in Figure 3.3 parallel to the trace of a plane will generate a series of lines ("channeling lines") which correspond to the transitions at the Bragg angles. In a real crystal, many different planes can simultaneously contribute to the pattern for any given orientation. An example of the geometric construction of a channeling pattern for silicon is shown in Figure 3.5. The corresponding channeling pattern generated from a real crystal is shown in Figure 3.6. For a particular low-index plane, the pattern consists of a bright central band which corresponds to the central portion of the rocking curve and which has an angular width of $2\theta_B$, since the first transitions occur at $\pm\theta_B$. Parallel to this bright central band are the channeling lines which arise from the sharp transitions at $\pm n\theta_B$. The low-index channeling

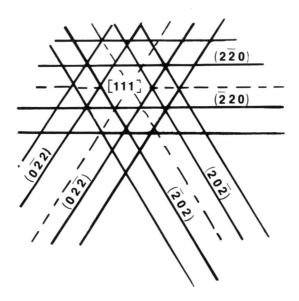

Figure 3.5. Geometric construction of a channeling pattern for a silicon crystal with the [111] direction parallel to the beam.

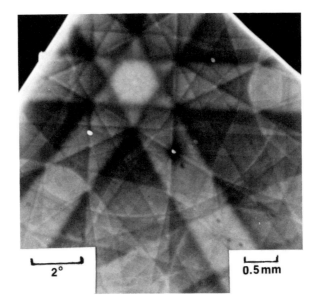

Figure 3.6. Electron channeling pattern which corresponds to Figure 3.5.

bands intersect in poles which correspond to low-index directions, denoted [m, n, o] in Miller indices, in the stereographic projection. If the crystal is tilted through all possible unique orientations relative to the beam, the individual channeling patterns can be assembled into a "channeling map" for the crystal. Examples of channeling maps for cubic and hexagonal crystals are given in Appendix 1.

The actual mechanism of producing the channeling pattern involves the scanning action of the SEM. For a particular orientation of the beam relative to the crystal planes, only one point on the rocking curve of Figure 3.3 is actually produced. In order to generate the complete pattern of Figure 3.6, it is necessary to vary the orientation of the beam relative to the crystal in a systematic fashion with the scan. Thus, the channeling pattern only exists as a result of scanning and cannot be recorded by placing a film in the chamber of the SEM, as is the case with x-ray Kossel patterns or electron backscatter patterns, both of which can be generated with a static beam. In the discussion of scanning action in Chapter 4 of *SEMXM*, the principal characteristic of the scan important in the generation of conventional images is the lateral motion of the beam off the optic axis. However, examination of the scanning action, shown schematically in Figure 3.7, reveals that at low magnification the beam undergoes a substantial change in angle as it moves laterally across the surface of the sample. The total angular excursion is given by the apex angle of

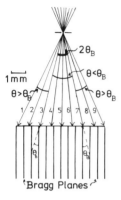

Figure 3.7. Scanning action in the SEM. At low magnification, the beam is deflected through both a spatial scan and an angular scan.

the scan cone in Figure 3.7 and depends on the magnification. For a 1-cm working distance, the scan angle at a magnification of $20\times$ is 28°, while at $50\times$ the scan angle is reduced to 12°. The scanning action covers the solid angle described by a pyramid while tracing out the matrix of points which form the base of the pyramid in the plane of the specimen. Note that the spatial scan which constructs the ordinary image and the angular scan which constructs the channeling pattern occur simultaneously in low-magnification operation. In order to construct the channeling pattern of a crystal by low-magnification scanning, it is necessary in the case of the scan shown in Figure 3.7 that the specimen be a large single crystal that will fill the entire field of the spatial scan. In this way, the atomic arrangement is the same no matter where the beam strikes the crystal, and the important consideration becomes the angle at which the beam meets the crystal. In Figure 3.6, the channeling pattern for a silicon crystal oriented with the [111] pole nearly parallel to the beam at the center of the scan is shown. Because this pattern has been generated by low-magnification scanning, it is appropriate to apply both an angular marker and a distance marker to the resulting micrograph, since both the spatial scan and the angular scan follow a regular pattern. If the magnification is progressively increased, the lateral extent of the spatial scan and the solid angle of the angular scan are both reduced. A smaller portion of the channeling pattern is imaged across the field, as shown in the series of images presented in Figure 3.8. Further increases in magnification serve to decrease the angular scan to the point that eventually only one gray level will be seen; the change in scan angle has become sufficiently small that no crossing of a critical Bragg angle occurs for any crystal plane.

3.4.2. Fine Structure

In addition to the coarse structure of the low-index bands which appear so prominently in the electron channeling pattern, e.g., bands associated with the {200} and {220} families of planes in the channeling map for face-centered cubic crystals shown in Figure 3.A1 in Appendix 1, fine structure can also be observed, particularly in the center of high-symmetry poles. This fine structure arises from high-index planes which lie in the first Laue zone of allowed diffraction conditions. Examples of the fine structure which lies near the [111] pole of silicon are shown in Figure 3.9.

A method for indexing fine-structure lines has been described by Madden and Hren (1985). Their analysis forms the basis for the following discussion. The fine structure around a low-index pole arises as shown in Figure 3.10. When a plane P' with an allowed reflection lies at an angle ϵ to the pole, channeling lines will appear at positions $\pm\theta_B$ on either side of the trace of plane P'. The planes which can contribute to the fine structure of the pattern around the low-index pole are those which meet two conditions: (1) The planes must satisfy the requirements of allowed reflections for the crystal system of interest. (2) The planes must be within an angle $\epsilon < \theta_{B(HKL)}$ of the pole to appear within the bright area surrounding the pole. The low-index bands which define the pole itself are those

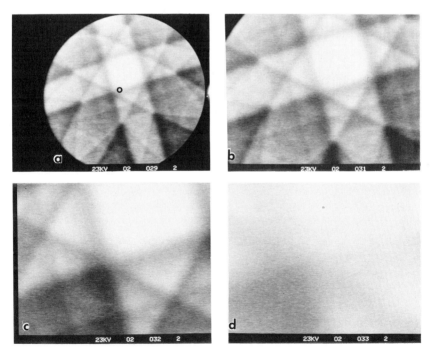

Figure 3.8. Effect of increasing magnification on the appearance of an electron channeling pattern. Silicon [001] pole; beam energy 23 keV. Note location of optic axis ("o") determined by noting point to which the scan collapses at high magnification.

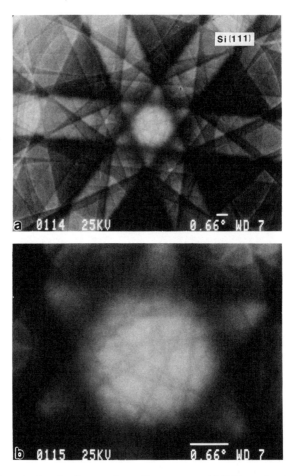

Figure 3.9. Fine structure in electron channeling patterns. (a) Wide-angle electron channeling pattern of [111] pole in silicon; beam energy 25 keV. (b) Reduced scan angle centered on the [111] pole; beam energy 25 keV. (b–d) Series of narrow-angle channeling patterns which illustrate the fine structure close to the [111] pole and how its form varies with small changes in the beam energy: (c) 24 keV; (d) 26 keV.

with $\epsilon = 0°$. The edges of the bands of these planes are located symmetrically at $\pm\theta_{B(HKL)}$ on either side of the pole. Thus, in order for fine-structure lines to appear within the pole, they must belong to planes which make an angle $\epsilon < \theta_{B(HKL)}$, where $\theta_{B(HKL)}$ is the Bragg angle for the low-index plane which defines the pole. For the cubic system, the angle ϵ between the plane (hkl) and the pole $[uvw]$ is given by the expression

$$\epsilon = \sin^{-1}\frac{hu + kv + lw}{(h^2 + k^2 + l^2)^{1/2}(u^2 + v^2 + w^2)^{1/2}} \tag{3.5}$$

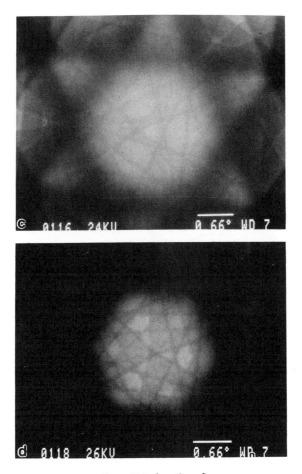

Figure 3.9 (continued)

The Bragg angles can be found for the cubic system by employing equation (3.1b). Indexing the fine structure for a particular low-index pole can be carried out by calculating the quantities ϵ and θ_B for allowed reflections such that $|\epsilon - \theta_B| < \theta_{B(HKL)}$.

The fine structure can be plotted for comparison to an experimentally determined channeling pattern by starting with the Laue zone map for the crystal system of interest as the basis for construction, as shown in Figure 3.11a. The values of the angles ϵ and θ_B for the possible high-index planes which can appear in the pole are first calculated, along with the Bragg angle for the planes which provide the coarse structure of the pole. Thus, for a [111] pole in silicon, the {220} bands form the coarse pole structure. The calculated parameters for silicon and a beam energy

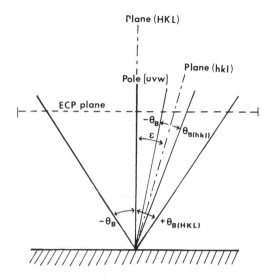

Figure 3.10. Origin of fine structure near a low-index pole.

of 25 keV are given in Table 3.1. Using the angular scale of the experimental pattern, e.g., 0.4°/cm, a circle of radius $|\epsilon - \theta_B|$ for a particular plane is drawn centered on the origin (000). The line which joins the point (*hkl*) with (000) is drawn so as to intersect the circle at two points. The trace of the band edge for (*hkl*) which corresponds to the condition $|\epsilon - \theta_B|$ is plotted as a tangent to the circle perpendicular to the line which joins (*hkl*) and (000). The choice of which of the two intersections with the circle depends on the sign of $|\epsilon - \theta_B|$. If this value is positive, the intersection nearest the point representing (*hkl*) is selected, while if the value is negative, the intersection opposite the point is selected. A completed construction for the 25-keV [111] silicon pole is given in Figure 3.11b.

The utility of the fine structure can be seen qualitatively by the radical change in the form of the fine structure with beam energy, as shown in Figure 3.9b–d. A change in beam energy of ±4% causes a remarkable change in the fine structure, while the width of the low-index {220] bands has not changed significantly. This is a direct result of the form of the relationship of θ_B upon the beam energy or wavelength and the crystal plane parameters given by equation (3.1b). The change in θ_B with a change in wavelength or lattice parameter can be found by differentiating equation (3.1b) appropriately. Differentiation with respect to wavelength yields the equation

$$\frac{d\theta_B}{d\lambda} = \frac{1}{[1 - (k\lambda)^2]^{1/2}} K \tag{3.6a}$$

where $K = (h^2 + k^2 + l^2)^{1/2}/2a_0$. Differentiation with respect to lattice parameter yields

$$\frac{d\theta_B}{da_0} = \frac{1}{[1 - (C/a_0)^2]^{1/2}} [-C/a_0^2] \qquad (3.6b)$$

where $C = (\lambda/2)(h^2 + k^2 + l^2)^{1/2}$. The presence of the multiplier $(h^2 + k^2 + l^2)^{1/2}$ in equations (3.6a) and (3.6b) causes the sensitivity of the Bragg angle to changes in $(\lambda/2a_0)$ to increase sharply with increasing Miller indices (hkl). Thus, the higher-index fine structure is more useful for measuring wavelength or lattice parameter.

3.5. Electron Optical Conditions to Observe Electron Channeling Contrast

Given a single-crystal specimen which has a strain-free, polished surface, it is necessary to follow a careful strategy in establishing electron optical and signal processing conditions in order to observe electron channeling effects. The following sequence of operations should be followed in initially establishing electron channeling contrast.

3.5.1. Beam Divergence

Electron channeling depends on the precise angle at which the beam meets the crystal. The effect of divergence in the beam is to reduce the contrast and to increase the apparent angular width of fine features in the channeling pattern. The visibility of these features is thus reduced. This effect of increasing divergence on the quality of a channeling pattern is shown in Figure 3.12. In order to detect fine-scale features in a channeling pattern, a divergence of 5 mrad or smaller is desirable. Thus, the first step

Table 3.1. Solution of Fine Structure Lines near [111] Pole[a,b]

Plane	$(h^2 + k^2 + l^2)$	θ_B	ϵ	$(\epsilon - \theta_B)$	Appearance in pole?	Number of planes
551	51	2.8882	4.6371	−1.7489	no	6
373	67	3.3109	4.0447	−0.7338	yes	3
751	75	3.5036	3.8226	0.3190	yes	6
375	83	3.6859	3.6334	−0.0525	yes	6
771	99	4.0261	3.3265	−0.6996	yes	6
359	115	4.3398	3.0862	−1.2536	no	6

[a] $E = 25$ keV; $\lambda = 0.00766$ nm. Silicon: $a = 0.54282$ nm; $\theta_B \{220\} = 1.14°$.
[b] Note that channeling lines which satisfy $h + k + l = 1$ appear near the [111] pole.

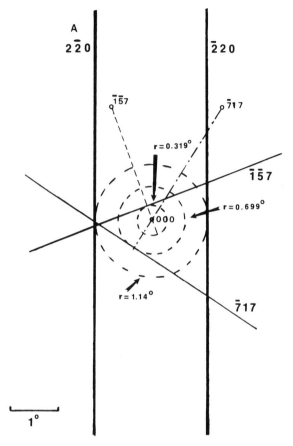

Figure 3.11. Construction of fine-structure map for silicon [111] pole at 25 keV. (A) Laue zone map and construction techniques following the method of Madden and Hren (1985). (B) Completed fine-structure map for {157} and {717} planes; note correspondence to experimentally determined fine structure shown in Figure 3.9b.

in obtaining channeling contrast is selection of a final aperture to reduce the beam divergence to 5 mrad or smaller.

3.5.2. Beam Current

Electron channeling produces a contrast level of the order of 0.05 (5%). This is a weak level of contrast, and from the concept of threshold current discussed in *SEMXM,* Chapter 4, it is necessary to establish a beam current of at least 5 nA to view a 5% contrast level in a rapid scan visual mode. Moreover, an efficient detector for backscattered electrons is also needed to keep the required threshold current as low as possible.

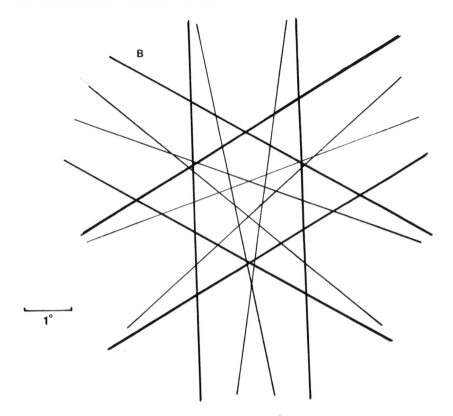

Figure 3.11 (*continued*)

3.5.3. Choice of Detectors

Electron channeling contrast is carried by backscattered electrons. Thus, a detector which is sensitive to backscattered electrons should be used. Since channeling contrast is a weak effect, it is especially important to utilize a detector with a high efficiency. If a conventional Everhart–Thornley scintillator/photomultiplier detector is used, it is important to bias the Faraday cage positively to collect secondary electrons, since secondaries produced by backscattered electrons which strike the chamber walls provide a reasonably efficient indirect collection of the backscattered electrons.

Greater geometric collection efficiency for backscattered electrons can usually be obtained by the use of a solid-state detector mounted above a specimen placed normal to the beam. However, because such a detector acts purely along the line-of-sight, it will be ineffective if the specimen is tilted so that much of the backscattered electron signal exits

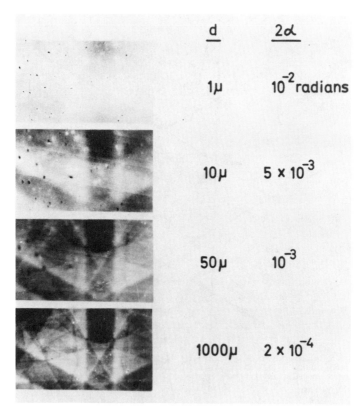

$\underline{d}$	$\underline{2\alpha}$
1μ	10^{-2} radians
10μ	5×10^{-3}
50μ	10^{-3}
1000μ	2×10^{-4}

Figure 3.12. Effect of increasing divergence on the appearance of an electron channeling pattern.

the specimen in a downward direction. A solid-state detector placed to receive the backscattered electrons offers another advantage for channeling contrast. As discussed below, channeling contrast resides primarily in the high-energy portion of the backscattered electron energy spectrum. Since a solid-state detector gives an energy-dependent response which emphasizes the high-energy electrons, channeling contrast is enhanced in the signal which leaves the solid-state detector relative to the contrast in the electron current received.

A third detection scheme which is very effective for use with channeling contrast is the specimen current. The specimen current signal has the advantage of being sensitive only to the number of backscattered and secondary electrons which leave the specimen and not to the direction which these electrons follow. Thus, specimen current can be used to form an image regardless of the tilt of the sample. Since the specimen current signal is sensitive to number effects only, there are no energy effects to enhance the contrast, which is a disadvantage.

Figures 3.A1 and 3.A2 provide a comparison of electron channeling maps of copper prepared with an Everhart–Thornley detector and with the specimen current signal, and demonstrate the reversal of the sense of the contrast between the two signals. That is, the low-order bands are bright against a dark background in the emissive mode signal and dark against a bright background in the specimen current signal.

3.5.4. Signal Processing

Another important consequence of the weak nature of channeling contrast is the need for signal processing in order to render the contrast visible to the eye when viewed on the final display. The most commonly applied signal processing techniques for viewing channeling contrast are differential amplification (also known as dark level or black level suppression, or contrast expansion) and time or spatial scan derivative operators. An example of differential amplification applied to a channeling pattern is shown in Figure 3.13. The unprocessed micrograph, Figure 3.13a, shows very little evidence of channeling contrast, whereas after differential amplification, Figure 3.13b, the channeling bands and fine-scale channeling lines of the pattern are clearly visible.

The application of time derivative processing is also illustrated in Figure 3.13. Since the channeling pattern contains many fine-scale linear features, which constitute the high-spatial-frequency portion of the image, the use of a spatial frequency filter such as a time derivative operator to emphasize the high spatial frequencies is especially effective. There are, however, two important consequences of applying conventional analog time derivatives to channeling patterns. The low spatial frequencies of the channeling pattern contain important information, particularly on the location of low-index channeling bands which are important in recognizing the orientation of a channeling pattern; these bands are lost in the time derivative image, as shown in Figure 3.13c and d. Second, in the case of an analog time derivative applied only parallel to the scan line, linear features in the image which run parallel to the scan line are lost since the value of the derivative along the scan line is about two orders of magnitude smaller than in a direction perpendicular to the scan line.

Both of these defects in analog time derivative images can be substantially eliminated through the use of the technique of signal mixing, in which the original signal, which contributes the low-frequency information that carries the bands and general shading of the pattern, and the time derivative signal, which provides enhancement of fine linear fea-

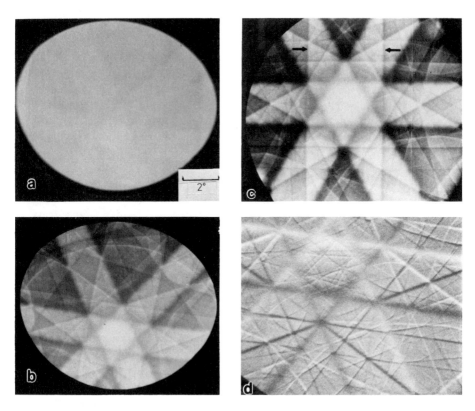

Figure 3.13. Signal processing techniques for enhancing the visibility of electron channeling contrast. Application of black level suppression (differential amplification) to enhance the visibility of an electron channeling pattern: (a) unprocessed signal; (b) black level suppression applied. Time derivative processing: (c) black level suppression; (d) first time derivative processing with vertical scanning lines; note loss of lines (denoted by arrows) which run parallel to the scan line.

tures of the pattern, are combined to give a final image (Heinrich *et al.,* 1970). In this combined signal image, the fine details of the channeling pattern are more pronounced than in the original image, and the important general shading is nearly fully retained.

3.5.5. Beam Energy

From the theory of Spencer *et al.* (1972), channeling contrast is found to vary as the reciprocal of the beam energy, $1/E$. The channeling contrast in the theory of Hirsch and Humphreys (1970) and Spencer *et al.* (1972) depends on two factors, the backscattering coefficients of the Bloch waves, which vary as $1/E^2$, and the mass absorption coefficients of the Bloch waves, which vary as $1/E$. The background upon which the channeling contrast resides is effectively independent of beam energy, as evidenced by the fact that the bulk backscatter coefficient is essentially independent of energy (Heinrich, 1966). The effect of all of these factors taken together is to give an overall $1/E$ dependence.

3.5.6. Backscattered Electron Energy

Electron channeling contrast is formed as a result of backscattering effects which occur in a thin layer at the specimen surface. As the beam penetrates further into the crystal, elastic scattering effects decollimate the beam and inelastic scattering reduces the energy of the beam electrons, leading eventually to the development of the interaction volume described in *SEMXM,* Chapter 3. As the initially highly collimated beam, which is sensitive to the orientation of the crystal, is decollimated, further scattering effects lead to the development of the bulk backscattering contribution, which is insensitive to crystal orientation, since the beam electron trajectories are effectively randomized. This backscattering due to multiple scattering from the bulk acts as a background which lowers the magnitude of electron channeling contrast. Since these backscattered electrons result from deeper penetration into the crystal, they are also more likely to have lost energy, and thus can be distinguished from the backscattered electrons which are carrying channeling contrast information on the basis of energy. The effect of energy filtration to exclude lower-energy backscattered electrons is shown on the rocking curve of Figure 3.3, where energy filtration to exclude electrons which have lost more than 100 eV of energy results in channeling contrast of 25% compared to 1.3% when the complete energy spectrum of backscattered electrons is utilized. Wells (1974) has demonstrated experimentally the use of energy filtration to form "low-loss" images of electron channeling with substantially increased contrast.

3.5.7. Specimen Tilt

The tilt of the specimen has a strong influence on the appearance of the shading of the low-order channeling bands and the higher-order channeling lines, as shown in Figure 3.14, which gives an electron channeling pattern for a silicon crystal which has been tilted by 20° to bring the [111] direction nearly parallel to the beam. If this channeling pattern is compared to the pattern obtained from a silicon crystal in which the orientation is such that the [111] direction is parallel to the beam at 0° tilt

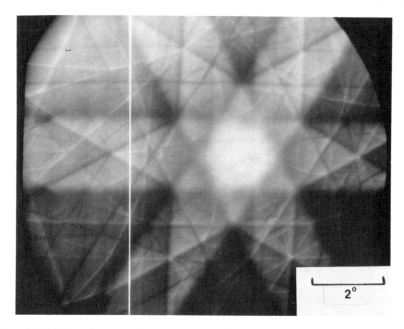

Figure 3.14. Effect of sample tilt on appearance of an electron channeling pattern. Electron channeling pattern of a silicon [111] pole obtained with a specimen tilt of 20°. Note loss of contrast in central bands and alteration of higher-order lines to pure black or white. Compare to Figure 3.13c, which shows the same orientation with a specimen tilt of 0°.

(Figure 3.13c), it can be seen that the low-order $\{222\}$ bands which intersect at the [111] pole have lower contrast relative to the general background of the pattern. Moreover, at normal incidence the higher-order channeling lines, e.g., $\{444\}$, $\{666\}$, and so on, appear to be black–white close pairs, while for the tilted specimen the higher-order lines change character to pure black or pure white lines against the general background.

3.5.8. Specimen Condition

As discussed below, electron channeling is extremely sensitive to the perfection of a crystal, particularly in the near-surface region. As a result of this property, it is necessary to ensure that a sample is carefully prepared to avoid introducing damage. At the same time, it is often important to reduce the surface roughness of a sample of eliminate topographic contrast which, being a stronger contrast mechanism, might tend to suppress the visibility of the channeling contrast of interest. Thus, mechanical polishing is often a necessary first step in the preparation of a suitable channeling specimen. A typical mechanical polishing procedure involves successive grinding through 100-, 200-, 400-, and 600-grit silicon carbide abrasives. The coarse and fine grinding is followed by polishing with diamond, alumina, or cerium oxide, depending on the nature of the material. Such a mechanical grinding–polishing procedure, while producing a mirror surface, results in the formation of a shallow region of extreme damage, the so-called Bilby layer. In order to detect channeling contrast from such a polished specimen, it is necessary to remove the Bilby layer by careful chemical or electrochemical polishing. Alternatively, certain proprietary final polishing agents incorporate a chemical polishing agent with the fine mechanical abrasive.

3.6. Channeling Micrographs

3.6.1. Polycrystalline Samples

With a satisfactory sample, the requirements for which will be discussed separately, the strategy of establishing the beam divergence, beam current, and signal processing should provide channeling contrast in the final image. If the specimen is a large single crystal, the image should be an electron channeling pattern (ECP) similar to that of Figure 3.5, but with the exact form appropriate to the crystal under study. If the sample is not a single crystal but is instead polycrystalline, the channeling contrast in the resulting image will reveal grain boundaries and similar crystallographic features. The following examples show the form of these channeling images as a function of crystal size.

Coarse polycrystal (grain size > 1 mm): Figure 3.15 is a low-magnification image of a coarse polycrystalline material with a grain size on the order of 5 mm. The scanning action is the same as that used to generate the single-crystal pattern shown in Figure 3.5. In the case of Figure 3.15, the individual grains are at different orientations relative to the beam, which results in a different channeling pattern visible on each grain. However, since the grains are substantially smaller in size than the scanned field, the change in scan angle across any of the grains is only a few degrees so that only a small portion of the channeling pattern of a particular grain is visible. Although specific information on the orientation of the individual grains has been lost, the shape of each grain can be recognized in the image, since the abrupt change in orientation at a grain boundary is revealed as a discontinuity in the channeling pattern.

Intermediate grain size (grains 0.1–1 mm): If the grain size is further reduced (Figure 3.16) so that the individual grains have a diameter in the range 0.1–1 mm, the magnification must be increased to make the indi-

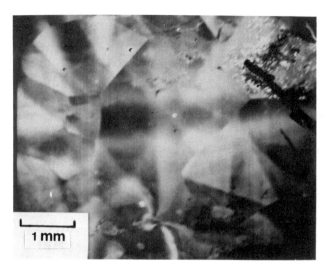

Figure 3.15. Electron channeling contrast image with conventional image scanning of a coarse polycrystalline sample of iron.

vidual grains occupy a significant fraction of the scanned field. As a result, the total scan angle is reduced, and the change in scan angle across any particular grain is small. Therefore, the portion of the channeling pattern visible on any grain is so small as to be unrecognizable. Many of the grains display a constant level of intensity across the entire grain, while a few show a mottled contrast. For these latter grains, a sufficient change in scan angle occurs to yield a change in channeling contrast which corresponds to a transition across a channeling band or fine line. Each grain displays a channeling pattern equivalent to the effect of increasing the magnification of a single-crystal pattern to some high value, as was illustrated in Figure 3.8.

Fine-grained polycrystals (< 0.1 mm): If the grain size is reduced below 0.1 mm, the magnification must be increased to the point that the change in scan angle across any grain is so small that the image of virtually all grains is a constant shade of gray, differing according to the particular orientation. The shading of each grain is controlled by its own channeling pattern in an analogous way to the magnification series of the channeling pattern shown in Figure 3.8 a–d. Since at high magnifications the change in scan angle is so small that the beam is effectively parallel at all points in the image, the shading of each grain is essentially that which would be seen at the exact center of the channeling pattern of each grain. The grain boundaries are easily discerned, and any crystallographic feature which produces a misorientation, such as a twin or a subgrain,

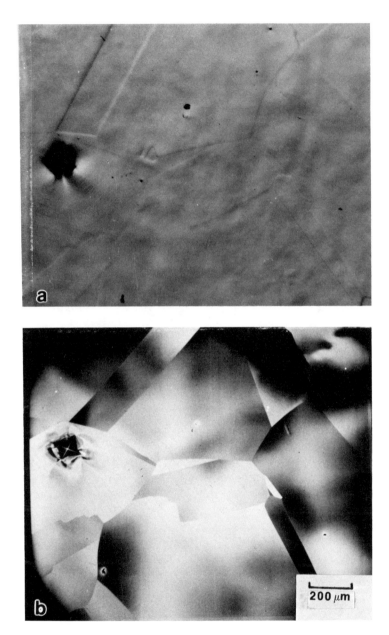

Figure 3.16. Electron channeling contrast image of a polycrystalline nickel sample with an intermediate grain size. (a) Optical micrograph and (b) scanning electron micrograph of the same area; note twin in both images and hardness indent for reference.

can be observed. Note that this allows the microscopist to discern the presence of crystallographic boundaries regardless of whether a topographic discontinuity exists at the boundary. This effect is shown in Figure 3.17, where many of the grain boundaries underwent etching during preparation by electropolishing. Unetched boundaries can be observed in channeling contrast even though there is no surface discontinuity to produce topographic contrast.

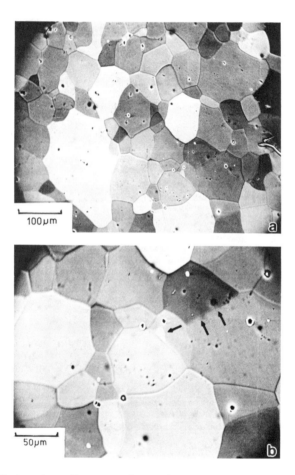

Figure 3.17. Electron channeling contrast image of polycrystalline tin with a fine grain size. Note uniform contrast of all grains and detection of boundaries which did not etch during electropolishing of the sample.

3.6.2. Limit of Spatial Resolution in Channeling Contrast Images

The requirements placed on the beam current and beam divergence in order to render channeling contrast visible in the final image exert a controlling influence on the spatial resolution as well. The relationship among beam current (i), divergence (α), and the beam size (d) is given by the brightness equation:

$$\beta = \frac{4i}{\pi^2 d^2 \alpha^2} \tag{3.7}$$

For a brightness (β) of 5×10^4 A/cm-sr, which is typical for a tungsten hairpin filament at 20-kV accelerating potential, the requirement for a beam current of 5 nA and a divergence of 0.005 rad results in a minimum beam diameter of 400 nm. Crystallographic spatial details of this order can be recognized at visual scanning rates (1 s/frame).

In order to improve the spatial resolution of a channeling contrast image, three strategies are possible:

1. Once a feature of interest has been located, the beam current can be reduced to approximately 1 nA and the recording time increased to 100 s or more to lower the threshold current sufficiently. A beam diameter less than 200 nm can be obtained in this way with a reasonable recording time.

2. From the series of channeling patterns taken at various beam divergences (Figure 3.12), it can be seen that the effect of increasing divergence on the pattern is to degrade the fine details while the coarse channeling features, such as bands, remain visible. In channeling micrographs, the effect of increasing divergence is to degrade sensitivity to misorientations. If the misorientation across a grain boundary is large, then it is possible by changing the orientation of the sample by means of tilting and/or rotation to bring the boundary into strong contrast even if the beam divergence is relatively large. The influence of divergence in the brightness equation is strong since it appears as a squared term. Thus, increasing the divergence to 0.01 rad in addition to reducing the beam current to 1 nA yields a minimum beam size of 90 nm. Spatial resolution of a channeling feature with dimensions on the order of 100 nm is demonstrated in Figure 3.18. In this case, the specimen is a polycrystalline nickel sample with fine-scale structures on an annealing twin boundary. The beam divergence, beam current, and recording time were optimized to obtain this image on an instrument equipped with a conventional tungsten filament.

3. The electron optical brightness sets the final limit to the minimum

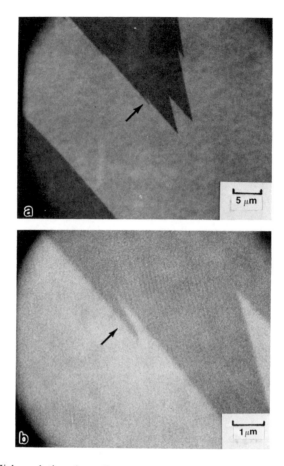

Figure 3.18. High-resolution channeling contrast image of crystallographic structures at a crystal boundary in nickel.

beam size which can be obtained. Operation with a higher-brightness source such as lanthanum hexaboride or field emission can yield substantial reductions in the probe size compared to a conventional source. With such illumination systems, it is possible to image crystallographic features down to a limit of 10–20 nm. Morin *et al.* (1979) have successfully imaged individual dislocations and stacking faults lying near the surface of crystals in a field emission-equipped SEM which was further refined to incorporate an energy-filtering backscattered electron detector to enhance channeling contrast.

3.6.3. Limit of Misorientation Detection

Because of the strong dependence of channeling on the orientation, it is also appropriate to consider the limit of angular resolution in terms of the misorientation of a pair of grains which can be detected in an image. Here the problem is not exclusively limited to the question of minimizing the beam divergence, but also to the position within the channeling pattern which each grain orientation represents. A small beam divergence is needed in order to maximize sensitivity to small misorientations between the crystallites. The minimum misorientation which can be imaged can be estimated by the angular width of the finest feature which can be seen in the channeling pattern which is obtained under the same beam conditions. However, in order to actually produce contrast between grains which are misoriented by an amount equal to this limiting angular resolution, it is necessary to tilt the sample to place the relative orientations of the grains on either side of a rapidly changing channeling feature, such as a band edge or a higher-index line. The orientations of the grains can be thought of as two closely spaced points in the channeling map. The spacing between the points in the channeling map represents the misorientation between the two grains. In order to bring the grains into contrast, the sample must be tilted so that these points in the channeling map fall across a band edge or a high-index line. In an arbitrarily oriented sample, this relative orientation will not be established by chance, and a particular boundary between two slightly misoriented grains may not be visible. Thus, the absence of a boundary in an image is not an immediate guarantee that the boundary does not exist. In order to check the possibility that a boundary exists but is not in contrast, a series of images taken at small tilt/rotation increments should be observed. An example of the changing visibility of low-angle boundaries with incremental changes in the tilt angle is shown in Figure 3.19.

3.7. Selected Area Electron Channeling Patterns

In conventional image scanning, the change in scan angle across a grain is too small to generate a sufficient portion of the electron channeling pattern to determine its orientation. In order to obtain channeling patterns from small grains, the scan must be modified to generate a selected area channeling pattern (SACP). Several techniques for the generation of SACPs have been utilized. We shall consider the "deflection-focusing" technique originally described by van Essen *et al.* (1970, 1971). If the conventional scan is examined (Figure 3.20a), the scan excursion

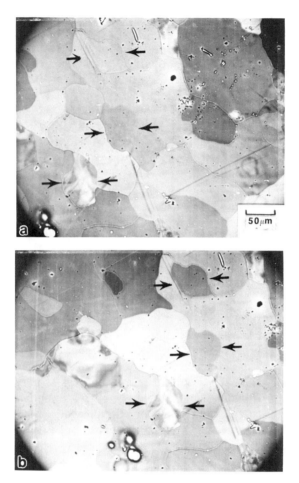

Figure 3.19. Appearance of subgrain boundaries in a polycrystalline iron sample with small increment of tilt (2°) applied. Note sharp contrast changes.

on the sample is obtained by double deflection scanning with the beam rocking about a point above the specimen. For the purpose of defining the beam divergence, this rocking point is placed on the optic axis at the level of the final aperture. In the deflection-focus SACP mode of operation (Figure 3.20b–d), the double deflection scanning action is modified to a single deflection whose purpose is to move the beam off-axis. The objective lens then acts by means of its focusing action to bring the off-axis beam back to a crossover, the position of which is adjustable according to the strength of the lens. Since the beam is far off-axis at the plane of the final aperture by a distance of as much as 2 mm, the final aperture must be removed completely to avoid cutting off the field of view. In order to define the divergence, a small aperture is placed at the position of the splash aperture above the scan coils. With three independent lenses operated with the deflection focusing mode, each lens has a separate function. The first lens operates to define the beam current. The second lens controls the divergence of the beam. The final lens acts to adjust the position of the crossover along the optic axis, and thus controls the size of the selected area, as well as focusing the beam.

In order to understand the operation of the deflection-focusing mode of SACP generation, consider the effect of altering the strength of the final lens, as illustrated schematically in Figure 3.20b–d. The images which result from such a "through-focus" series on a polycrystalline sample are illustrated in Figure 3.21. The conventional double deflection image, Figure 3.21a, which corresponds to the scanning action shown schematically in Figure 3.20a, shows a group of grains in a polycrystalline iron–3% silicon alloy. Note the central grain labeled "A," which is approximately 10 μm in diameter, and the small dark hole to the lower right in the grain labeled "B." Figure 3.21b shows a deflection-focus scanning action image which corresponds to the scanning schematic shown in Figure 3.20b. The crossover is above the specimen, which results in a normal matrix scan motion in the plane of the sample, creating a normal image, similar in appearance to the conventional scan. However, in deflection-focusing

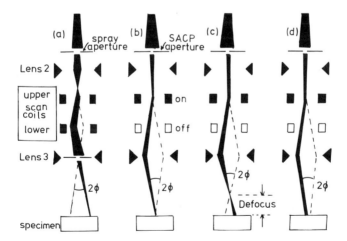

Figure 3.20. Schematic diagram of scanning action for (a) conventional image scanning and (b–d) selected area channeling pattern generation by deflection-focusing with the final crossover placed (b) above, (c) coincident with, and (d) below the specimen surface. The sequence (b), (c), and (d), which is controlled by adjusting the strength of the final lens, comprises a "through-focus" series.

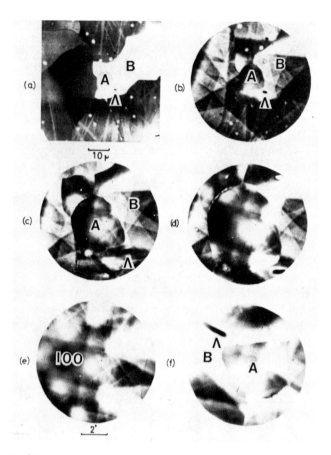

Figure 3.21. Conventional image scanning and selected area channeling pattern generation by "deflection-focusing". (a) Conventional image of grains in polycrystalline iron–3% silicon; (b–f) "through-focus" series with the strength of the final lens progressively weakened.

scanning the crossover is much closer to the specimen surface than normal, and the change in scan angle across the field is much larger than in the conventional scan. The image in Figure 3.21b is thus a composite image of normal scanning and rocking beam scanning, with the result that the image of the grains and hole appear similar in both Figure 3.21a and 3.21b, but in Figure 3.21b the larger angle of rock produces channeling patterns on each grain in the image. In Figures 3.21c and 3.21d the crossover has been brought progressively closer to the surface by weakening the objective lens so that the scan excursion on the sample is reduced and the magnification is consequently increased. The rocking angle remains the same, but since the lateral extent of the scan is confined to small areas, more of the channeling pattern of grain A is obtained. When the crossover coincides with the surface (Figures 3.20c and 3.21e), the magnification is a maximum, the image of grain A fills the field of view, and only the channeling pattern of grain A is seen. The scan angle is sufficiently large in the SACP mode to recognize the orientation of grain A. Further weakening of the objective lens moves the crossover below the surface so that lateral scan motion again takes place in the specimen surface plane. An image is again produced along with rocking action (Figures 3.20d and 3.21f), but the order of the scan positions is reversed relative to Figures 3.20a–c, so that the image, Figure 3.21f, is reversed, as evidenced by the relative positions of grain A and the hole in grain B.

The through-focus series can be performed rapidly, since the controlling parameter is the strength of the final lens. Such an image sequence, which can be observed on the visual display CRT, allows the microscopist to unambiguously identify the crystallographic region from which the SACP is obtained, an extremely useful feature when dealing with a complicated microstructure. Joy and Booker (1971) devised a sequential scan system in which images corresponding to the scanning action of Figure 3.20b and 3.20c could be displayed on alternate scans presented on the two visual CRTs, which provided both the image and the channeling pattern for simultaneous inspection.

3.8. Orientation Determination with ECPs

The ECP is a gnomonic projection of the crystal planes created by pairs of lines which run parallel to the traces of the planes and which are separated by multiples of the Bragg angles. Linear measurement L in the ECP image is related to the scan angle ϕ by the relation

$$L \cong \tan \phi \qquad (3.8)$$

If the cone angle of the scan is less than 15°, $\phi \cong \tan \phi$, and the ECP can be regarded as effectively equivalent to a portion of the stereogram of the crystal projected about the optic axis of the SEM. The ECP can be used in two different approaches to solving the orientation of the crystal, depending on the amount of information available to the microscopist. (1) If the crystal system is known in advance, e.g., face-centered cubic, then the ECP can be solved for the orientation with the aid of an appropriate electron channeling map and the stereographic projection. (2) If the crystal system is unknown, the bands in the ECP(s) can be measured to derive a set of lattice spacings and interplanar angles. From the overall geometry exhibited in a collection of ECPs from the unknown system,

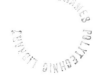

the symmetry elements, which include centers of rotation and mirror planes, can be recognized. From this information, the crystal system can be deduced, and the orientation determined.

3.8.1. Determining Orientation

We are generally interested in two types of orientation information: (1) What direction in terms of the crystal coordinates (Miller indices) is parallel to the beam when it is on the optic axis of the SEM? If the sample is set at a right angle to the beam, then the normal to the sample surface is parallel to the crystal direction of interest. (2) What crystallographic direction lies parallel to a selected feature of the sample as seen in the normal SEM imaging mode?

1. The crystallographic direction which lies parallel to the optic axis of the beam can be determined as follows. First, all scan deflections and rotations should be centered or returned to reference positions. Next, the position of the optic axis within the ECP image should be determined. It should not be assumed that the optic axis is invariably the center of the display CRT. Due to misalignments, both mechanical and electrical, the optic axis is likely to be located off-center. The exact position can be determined by progressively increasing the magnification control to collapse the scanned rays to the optic axis. Once the optic axis has been located by this procedure, it is useful to mark the location on the visual and the photographic CRTs. The optic axis point can then be transferred relative to recognized poles and bands in the ECP and plotted on a stereographic projection.

2. The crystallographic orientation of specific features which can be observed in the image can in principle be determined by overlaying the ECP on the conventional micrograph, which can be readily accomplished by using negatives on a light table. However, a rotation often exists between the conventional imaging mode and the SACP mode. Several authors have detailed the nature and magnitude of this rotation in different electron optical systems (e.g., van Essen and Verhoven, 1974; Joy and Maruszewski, 1975; Davidson, 1976). In a particular system, the rotation between the micrograph and SACP should be calibrated by using a sample with a feature which has a known crystallographic orientation such as a cleavage line or a facet. A series of images and SACPs should be obtained at different lens excitations to derive a calibration curve of relative rotation as a function of working conditions.

3.8.2. Channeling Maps

The main tool for solving the orientation of the ECP is the channeling map, which represents the collection of all unique channeling patterns for a crystal. The angular size of the channeling map depends on the symmetry of the crystal. For crystals of high symmetry, e.g., cubic, the existence of symmetry elements such as centers of rotation and mirror planes, actually reduces the number of unique orientations, since the structure is replicated by simple rotations or mirror reflections. Thus, for a cubic crystal, the symmetry leads to a "unit triangle" of unique orientations which encompass the regions bounded by the poles [100], [110], and [111] in Miller index notation. All other possible orientations of a cubic crystal can be produced from an orientation within this unit triangle by a sequence of rotations and/or mirror operations. Thus, an ECP from an arbitrarily oriented cubic crystal should be recognizable within this unit triangle.

Two techniques exist for constructing channeling maps. The experimental method involves tilting a crystal through all possible unique orientations and recording the individual ECPs in increments of approximately 15°. The crystal must be tilted through angles of 50° or more in order to cover all possible orientations for a cubic crystal, and even larger tilt angles are necessary for crystals of lower symmetry. At these high tilts, the effect of the 15° ECP rocking angle during the scan across a flat sample causes a substantial change in the gross backscattering coefficient across the image field, which results in uneven illumination of the ECP. At high tilts, fine-scale changes also occur in the sense of the contrast of the channeling band edges. The close white/black nature of the channeling lines changes to pure white or pure black lines at high tilts. In order to minimize these effects of high tilt, the single crystal used for generating the ECP map should have a spherical surface so that at any tilt the local surface is approximately normal to the electron beam.

Examples of channeling maps for copper (face-centered cubic) and other crystals are given in Appendix 1. Since the map is assembled from actual channeling patterns, the experimental map conveys important contrast information as well as the geometry of the map. However, distortions inevitably arise when assembling an experimental map because the relation $\phi \cong \tan \phi$ becomes inaccurate for angles larger than approximately 15°. Thus, the use of the channeling map for accurate measurement of larger angles and spacings is not recommended. The chief value of the experimental channeling map is the direct representation of the true ECP contrast, which is a great aid in recognizing the orientation of an unknown pattern and obtaining an approximate location of that orientation within the stereographic projection.

For accurate orientation determination, it is necessary to construct the stereographic projection of the channeling map. The major poles of the map are first plotted, and the traces of the planes through these poles can then be constructed. The channeling lines are plotted parallel to the traces of the lattice planes at angles of $\pm \theta_B$ and the appropriate multiples.

In Miller index notation, the planes $(U1, V1, W1)$ and $(U2, V2, W2)$ which intersect at a particular pole $[h, k, l]$ follow the relations

$$hU1 + kV1 + lW1 = 0 \qquad (3.9)$$
$$hU2 + kV2 + lW2 = 0$$

which yield

$$h = V1W2 - V2W1$$
$$k = W1U2 - W2U1 \qquad (3.10)$$
$$l = U1V2 - V1U2$$

In addition, not all channeling bands predicted by equation (3.1) are actually encountered. Due to certain scattering effects, only certain combinations of the Miller indices are actually allowed according to the particular crystal system. For cubic crystals, the allowed indices are given by the following relations:

Lattice type	Reflections
Simple cubic	All
BCC	$h + k + l = 2n$
FCC	h,k,l all odd or all even
Diamond cubic	h,k,l all odd or all even except $h + k + l = 2 + 4n$

The generation of stereographic projections of channeling maps by computation is made simpler by using the system of Cartesian coordinates derived from the Miller indices proposed by Christian (1956) for the cubic system. To produce a stereogram of radius R, the Cartesian coordinates (x,y) for the pole $[h,k,l]$ relative to the point $(0,0)$ placed at the $[0,0,1]$ pole are given by the expressions

$$x = RH/(1 + L) \qquad (3.11)$$
$$y = RK/(1 + L)$$

where H, K, L are the normalized Miller indices given by

$$H = h/(h^2 + k^2 + l^2)^{1/2}$$
$$K = k/(h^2 + k^2 + l^2)^{1/2} \qquad (3.12)$$
$$L = l/(h^2 + k^2 + l^2)^{1/2}$$

An example of a unit triangle for a cubic crystal plotted with Cartesian coordinates derived from normalized Miller indices is shown in Figure 3.22.

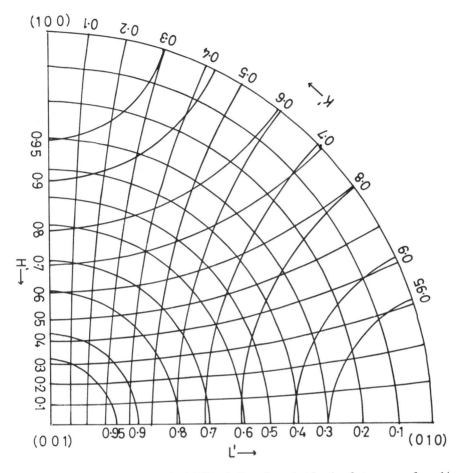

Figure 3.22. Plot of normalized Miller indices for unit triangle of stereogram for cubic crystals.

By making use of an experimentally determined channeling map to aid in the recognition of the orientation of an unknown crystal and an accurately constructed stereogram to actually plot the orientation, the experimental portion of the orientation determination task is complete. In order to make use of the information, it is useful to make further use of the concept of normalized Miller indices. Although many natural crystal faces will be found to lie on or near low-index poles such as [011], the orientation of the normal to a plane taken at an arbitrary orientation to the crystal will not necessarily have a low or even rational set of conventional Miller indices. Thus, an orientation plotted near a pole such as [321] may need to be expressed as [32 22 12] or [321 221 121]. It is often difficult to assign Miller indices to an arbitrary point in the stereogram.

The technique of expressing the orientation in Cartesian coordinates and normalized Miller indices becomes particularly valuable. After the (x,y) coordinates of the orientation have been located on the plot shown in Figure 3.22, the normalized Miller indices H, K, L are given by the expressions

$$H = 2Rx/(R^2 + x^2 + y^2)$$
$$K = 2Ry/(R^2 + x^2 + y^2) \qquad (3.13)$$
$$L = (R^2 - x^2 - y^2)/(R^2 + x^2 + y^2)$$

Once the normalized Miller indices have been obtained, the values can be directly incorporated into calculations. Thus, since the normalized Miller indices are direction cosines, the angle ψ between two poles [$H1$ $K1$ $L1$] and [$H2$ $K2$ $L2$] is given by

$$\cos \psi = H1H2 + K1K2 + L1L2 \qquad (3.14)$$

As shown in the plot in Figure 3.22, poles with the same value of normalized coordinates lie on small circles relative to the origin.

At first examination, it appears that a different channeling map is required for each crystal structure and lattice parameter. Fortunately, for crystals in the cubic system, which includes many metallic elements and alloys, the angles between planes depend only on the Miller indices and not on the lattice parameter. Thus, all cubic channeling maps have the same general form, with modifications as to which bands will be present according to the selection rules listed above. Within a given subclass, such as face-centered cubic, the channeling maps will have the same band structure. However, the Bragg angles and thus the bandwidths depend directly on the lattice parameter, which results in different band spacings according to the specific crystal. Nevertheless, if a single map is available for face-centered cubic crystals, generally it can be used to recognize the orientation of any face-centered cubic crystal regardless of the lattice parameter. In such cases, it is especially useful to have a calculated channeling map which accurately represents the particular crystal under study for accurate orientation measurements once the experimentally determined channeling map has been used to recognize the orientation.

For other crystal systems of lower symmetry, the angles between planes depend on the lattice parameters, so that the channeling map differs significantly depending on the composition. If a totally unknown crystal is to be solved, as many channeling patterns should be obtained as possible in order to increase the chance of recognizing major poles and bands at which symmetry elements can be deduced.

A worked example of an orientation determination utilizing the techniques described above is given in Appendix 2.

3.9. Deformation Effects on Channeling Contrast

3.9.1. Channeling Patterns

The phenomenon of electron channeling is extremely sensitive to the degree of perfection of a crystal. The presence of defects such as dislocations which distort the lattice has an effect which is analogous to an increase in the divergence of the beam. As demonstrated in Figure 3.12, an increase in divergence initially leads to a loss of fine-scale angular details in the channeling pattern, and for larger divergences, coarser features are lost as well. An example of the effect of plastic deformation (cold

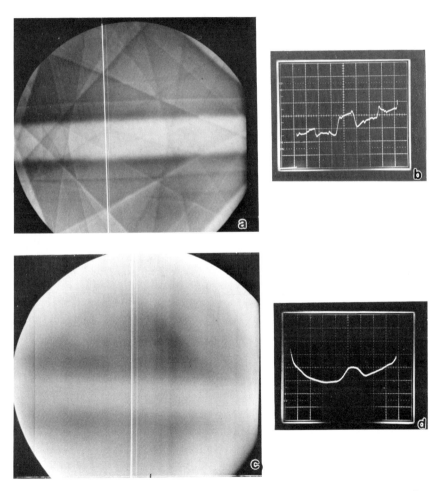

Figure 3.23. Effect of deformation by compression on the electron channeling pattern of an aluminum single crystal. (a) Annealed crystal; (b) corresponding line trace; (c) crystal compressed by 5%; (d) line trace.

working) on a crystal to introduce defects is shown in Figure 3.23. In this example, the application of a reduction in thickness of an aluminum crystal by 5% by cold rolling results in an almost total loss of fine detail in the channeling pattern, with only the central band structure remaining. In this case, the deformation process produced a wide variety of defects in the crystal so that the pattern degraded nearly uniformly. In experiments in which crystals were deformed so as to introduce parallel dislocations such that the crystal was preferentially distorted around one axis, the channeling lines parallel to the dislocations degraded while those perpendicular to the dislocations were not affected. Thus, close inspection of the quality of the channeling pattern can yield information on the nature of defects in a crystal.

Early experimental attempts to quantify the effects of crystal perfection upon the channeling pattern relied on visual examination of the pattern quality (Stickler *et al.,* 1971). To aid the direct visual interpretation of channeling pattern quality, a calibration sample can be produced by deforming a tapered tensile specimen of an annealed polycrystalline microstructure (D. L. Davidson, 1977). By using a tapered specimen, a range of strain could be applied to a single specimen with a common starting condition. Channeling patterns were then obtained from many of the grains in this sample and grouped according to the total strain at that point in the sample. Although the exact nature of the degradation of the pattern depended on the orientation and on local strain conditions, by averaging observations over many grains with randomly selected orientations for each strain increment, a useful strain calibration chart could be created. This chart could then be used to estimate the equivalent tensile strain in a deformed grain of the same material. An example of such a calibration chart is shown in Figure 3.24 and an application of the technique to assess the strain around a crack arrested in a sample is shown in Figure 3.25.

More detailed examination of the effects of crystal defects on channeling patterns has revealed that the channeling lines undergo two distinct changes. The angular width of the channeling lines increases and the contrast decreases as the crystal becomes less perfect. Quantification of these effects cannot be accurately assessed by visual observation of a photographically recorded channeling pattern. The apparent width of the channeling line depends on the perception of gray levels by the eye, which is subjective and irreproducible. Accurate measurement is now possible by the use of digital signal storage techniques. An easy way of obtaining such a system is to build it around a "personal" computer such as the APPLE since low-cost analog-to-digital convertors (ADC) for signal input to the computer and digital-to-analog convertors (DAC) for scan ramp generation are readily available. In one typical system, the signal from the backscatter detector which lies in the range 0–5 V is passed into the

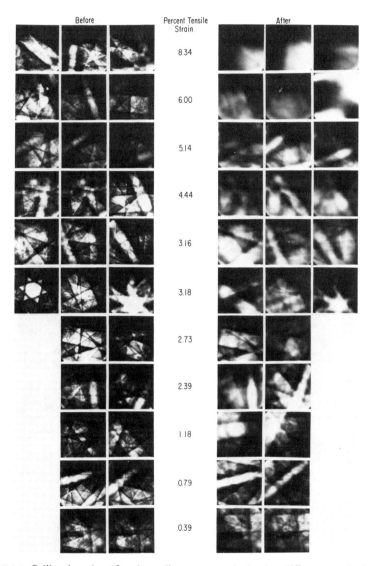

Figure 3.24. Calibration chart for channeling patterns obtained at different tensile deformations; material: stainless steel (courtesy of David Davidson).

ADC where it is converted to a digital signal with 12-bit resolution (1 part in 4096). The signal is sampled once at each picture point. The DAC generates a line scan containing 512 picture points, with a typical dwell time of a few milliseconds per picture point. In order to improve the signal-to-noise ratio, the scan can be repeated up to 256 times, with the mea-

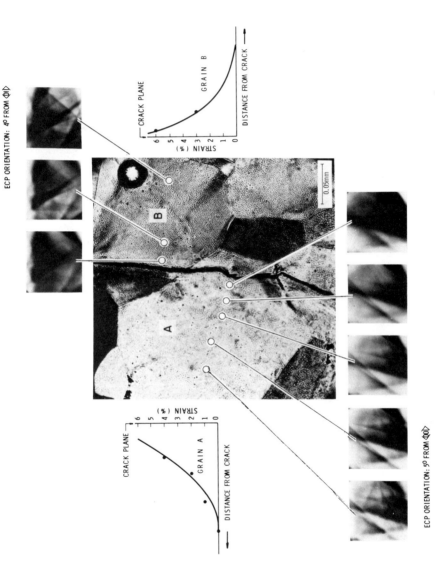

ECP ORIENTATION: 4° FROM ⟨011⟩

ECP ORIENTATION: 5° FROM ⟨001⟩

Figure 3.25. Electron channeling contrast image of a crack arrested in an iron–3% silicon transformer alloy and selected area electron channeling patterns obtained at indicated locations. By use of a calibration chart similar to that shown in Figure 3.24, the equivalent strain has been estimated as a function of distance ahead of the crack (courtesy of David Davidson).

sured signal at each scan point being added to the results of previous scans. The final result is then numerically averaged and displayed on the computer screen. The stored channeling profile data can now be quantified by using a software-generated cursor to identify points of interest in the profile, where angular width and contrast can be calculated. Angular measurements are made after an internal calibration against a known angular spacing such as that of a major band, and a precision of significantly better than 1 mrad is obtainable. Contrast is typically measurable to 1 part in 100. A complete experiment including data collection and analysis can be performed in less than 5 min.

Figure 3.26 illustrates an application of the technique to studies of damage caused by ion implantation into silicon. The sample contained 2.5×10^{15} As/cm^2 implanted to give a layer 50 nm deep. Figure 3.26a shows the computer measurement of linewidth for the implanted, and for perfect silicon as a function of electron beam energy. The difference between these two curves represents the broadening due to lattice damage. This term becomes less as the beam energy is increased because more of the channeling information is coming from the perfect crystal beneath the implant. Changing the electron beam energy is therefore equivalent to performing a depth profile. Figure 3.26b shows results of linewidth measurements in the implanted material after the area has been laser annealed at different power levels. At all three beam energies, the linewidth falls as the laser power is increased, indicating that the laser is annealing the damage caused by the implant. Again, less of an effect is seen at a beam energy of 25 keV that at 10 keV because the majority of the material sampled at the higher energy is perfect. However, at higher laser powers it can be seen that the linewidth starts to increase again. This is because the laser is now damaging the silicon. These results can be more easily interpreted by using the data of Figure 3.26a and subtracting from each curve the expected linewidth for perfect silicon; the difference then represents the damage sampled by the beam. Figure 3.26c shows how this appears; at all three beam energies the damage rapidly falls with laser dose and when a level of 60 mW/cm^2 is reached, all three measurements indicate perfect silicon. As the power is further increased, the 25-keV data start to rise showing that damage is occurring deep beneath the surface, because power is absorbed at a finite depth, followed by corresponding rises in the 18-keV and then the 10-keV data.

Dislocations and point defects introduced into a crystal at low relative temperatures ($T/_mT < 0.3$, where $_mT$ is the absolute melting point) by mechanical deformation or ion implantation cause a degradation of the channeling linewidth and contrast, but the patterns retain their original geometry and bands and lines remain straight. At higher relative temperatures, the defects introduced by deformation of a crystal are more

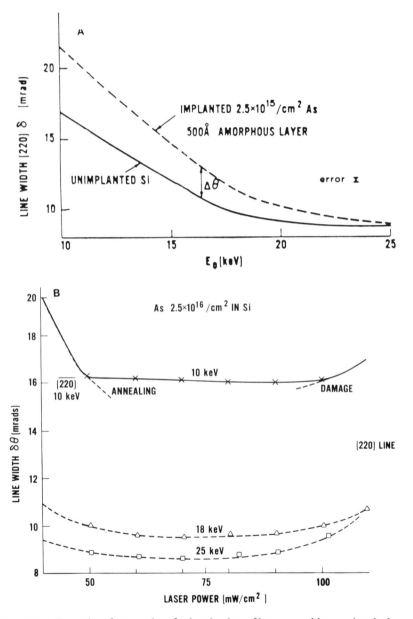

Figure 3.26. Examples of a crystal perfection depth profile measured by varying the beam energy and digitally recording and analyzing channeling patterns; sample: ion-implanted silicon.

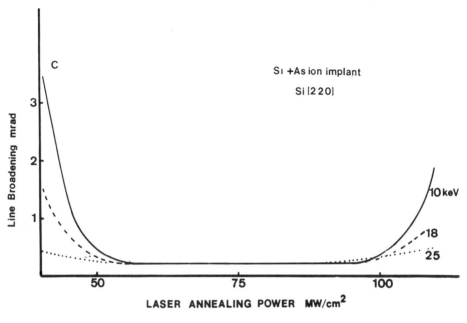

Figure 3.26 (*continued*)

mobile in the crystal and can organize into boundaries such that small units of the crystal are formed which are called subgrains. Adjacent subgrains, which range in size from tenths of a micrometer to a few micrometers, are misoriented by an angle of a few degrees or less. When an SACP is formed of such a group of subgrains, a distorted, wavy channeling pattern may be observed, with distinctly wavy bands, as shown in Figure 3.27. This form arises from the complicated way in which the channeling pattern is formed, combining angular scanning with a complicated spatial scan within the selected area. If the selected area of 10-μm diameter contains subgrains at the 1-μm size range, then as the selected area beam simultaneously rocks angularly and moves laterally, the orientation sampled by the beam will vary throughout the pattern.

3.9.2. Deformation Effects in Channeling Contrast Images

Channeling contrast images obtained with conventional image scanning can also contain direct evidence of deformation-induced effects in crystalline solids (Joy *et al.,* 1972). The origin of these effects can be understood with the aid of Figure 3.28. At high magnifications, the change in scan angle of the beam relative to the crystal is quite small, of

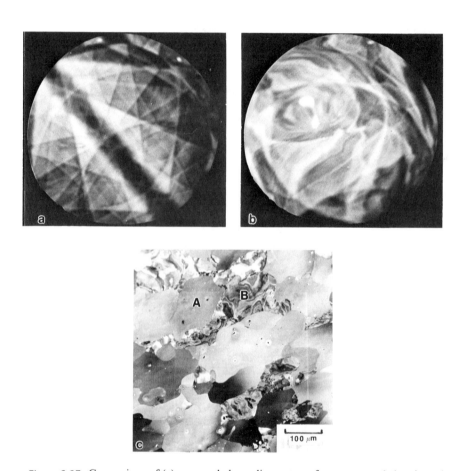

Figure 3.27. Comparison of (a) a normal channeling pattern from an annealed grain and (b) a distorted channeling pattern which arises as a result of plastic deformation. Both grains coexist in a partially recrystallized iron–3% silicon alloy shown in (c). Note direct observation of bend contours in the image of the grains.

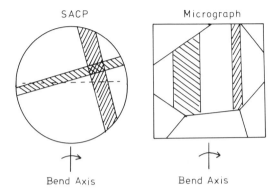

Figure 3.28. Illustration of the origin of bend contours observed in channeling micrographs.

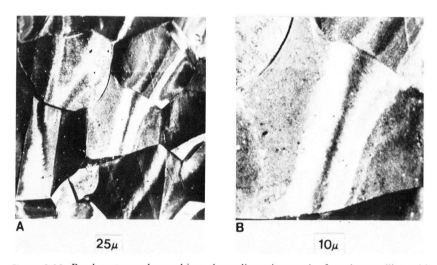

Figure 3.29. Bend contours observed in a channeling micrograph of a polycrystalline gold sheet which has undergone bending about a vertical axis.

the order of a few milliradians for a 20-μm-diameter grain imaged at a magnification of 500×. The beam is effectively parallel at all locations on the grain, and thus only a single beam orientation is sampled in the ECP. The average grain displays a constant signal intensity unless it is so oriented that the particular orientation which is sampled is exactly at a critical Bragg angle in which changing signal may be observed across the grain.

However, if the grain is itself bent about an axis parallel to the surface, the effective change in angle between the beam and the crystal lattice may be sufficient to produce a change in channeling and consequently in the signal intensity. A simple bend about a single axis is equivalent to a line traverse through the channeling pattern perpendicular to the bend axis, as shown in Figure 3.28. The resulting appearance of the grain can be referred to as bend contours, in analogy with the structures observed in transmission electron microscopy of thin crystals (Hirsch *et al.,* 1965). An example of the appearance of grains in a polycrystalline gold sample, which has been subjected to bending around a single axis, is shown in Figure 3.29. Contrast bands which run parallel to the bend axis are observed. The bend contours vary in exact appearance from grain to grain since the orientation changes sharply from grain to grain.

In polycrystals subjected to tensile or compressive deformation, the stresses applied to individual grains can be quite complicated. The distortions introduced into the grains can often be directly imaged. Complex bend contours can often be observed as a result of deformation, particularly at high relative temperatures where subgrains and long-range systematic misorientations can be produced. An example of such bend contours in grains in partially recrystallized polycrystalline iron–3% silicon steel is shown in Figure 3.27. Since the channeling contrast depends on the beam–crystal orientation, tilting the sample by a small angle can cause pronounced changes in the contrast, as shown in Figure 3.30. Such a tilt series is a good procedure to follow in order to confirm the suspected existence of bend contours in a sample. The development of bend contours during *in situ* deformation of a lead–tin alloy is illustrated in Figure 3.31. In the example of the crack arrested in a polycrystalline solid shown in Figure 3.25, the contrast adjacent to the crack arises through the formation of bend contours by the passage of the plastic zone which is associated with the crack. Finally, the hardness indent in the polycrystalline nickel sample shown in Figure 3.16 shows a complicated bend contour pattern which directly maps out the region of intense deformation around the indent as shown in Figure 3.32. The direct channeling image thus provides a powerful method to detect the effects of deformation on crystalline solids.

Bend Contours in Fe-3%Si (20 kv)
Effect of Tilt about Y-axis

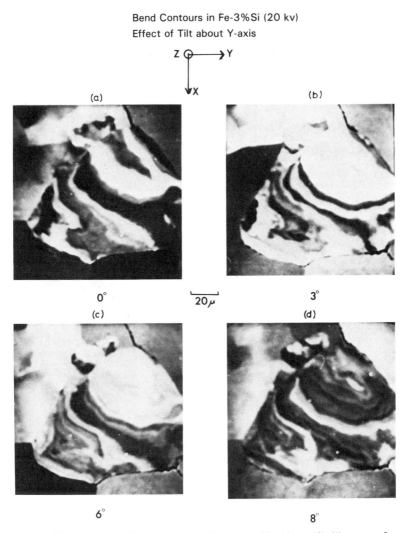

Figure 3.30. Bend contours observed on partially recrystallized iron–3% silicon transformer steel. Note the sharp changes in the relative contrast of the bend contours as a function of tilt about a horizontal axis.

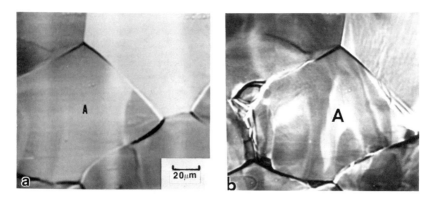

Figure 3.31. Development of bend contours during *in situ* deformation of polycrystalline lead–tin alloy.

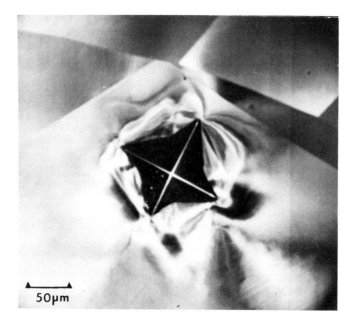

Figure 3.32. Bend contours revealing extent of zone of severe plastic deformation around a hardness indent in polycrystalline nickel; sample of Figure 3.16 viewed at higher magnification.

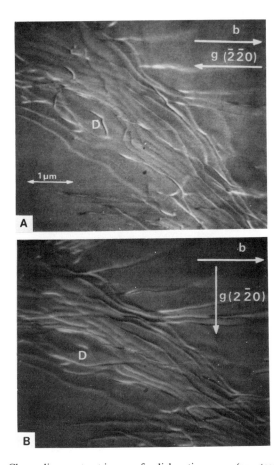

Figure 3.33. Channeling contrast image of a dislocation array (courtesy of P. Morin).

   The presence of a dislocation in a crystal acts to distort the crystal lattice planes in the immediate vicinity of the line defect. In principle, this distortion should be revealed in a channeling micrograph due to the direct effect on altering the channeling as a function of position in direct analogy to the bend contour illustrated above. In actual practice, the direct imaging of dislocations by channeling contrast in a conventional SEM has not proved possible because of threshold current/contrast limitations. Specifically, with a conventional electron gun, the beam size necessary to contain adequate current to exceed the threshold current for channeling contrast is substantially larger than the extent of the distortion zone around the dislocation. In order to image dislocations, Morin *et al.* (1979) had to resort to a high-brightness field emission source; in addition, to increase the magnitude of the channeling contrast in order to further reduce the threshold current and the beam size, energy filtering of the backscattered electron signal was employed. An example of the direct imaging of dislocations lying near a surface is shown in Figure 3.33.

Appendix 1: Electron Channeling Maps

The following channeling maps are included as an aid in solving crystal orientations by the ECP technique.

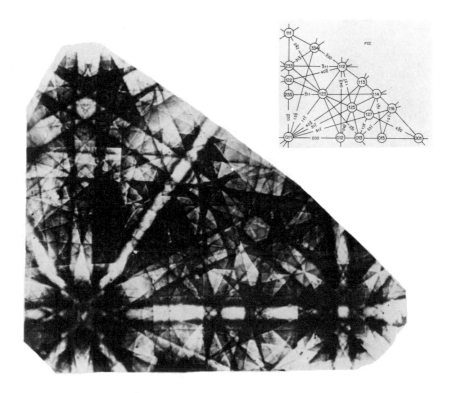

Figure 3.A1. Face-centered cubic: copper at 20 keV, backscattered electron signal; complete unit triangle map with indexing guide inset (courtesy of C. van Essen).

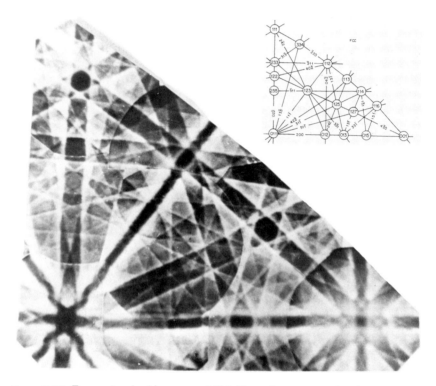

Figure 3.A2. Face-centered cubic: copper at 30 keV, specimen current signal; complete unit triangle map with indexing guide inset (courtesy of C. van Essen).

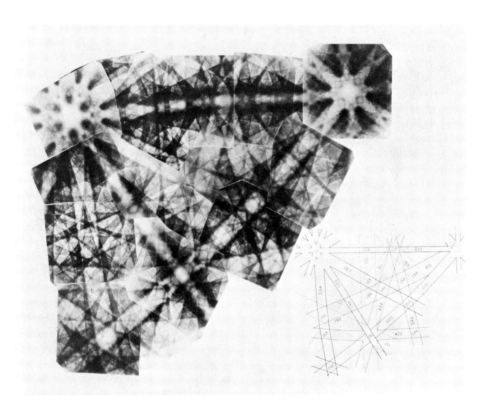

Figure 3.A3. Body-centered cubic: molybdenum at 30 keV, backscattered electron signal; complete unit triangle map and region reflected across (220) with indexing guide (courtesy of D. Davidson).

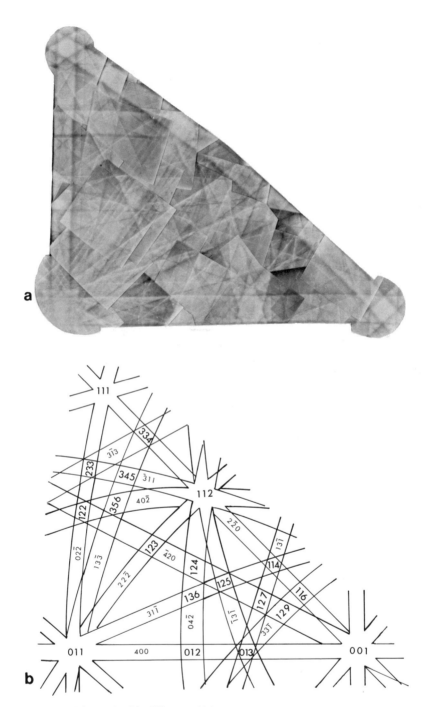

Figure 3.A4. Diamond cubic: Silicon at 30 keV, backscattered electron signal. (a) Complete unit triangle map; (b) indexing guide.

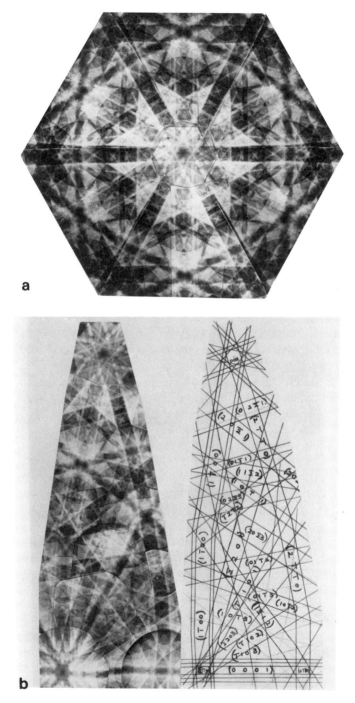

Figure 3.A5. Hexagonal close-packed (C/A = 1.63): Cobalt at 20 keV, backscattered electron signal (courtesy of D. Fathers). (a) Partial map centered on [0001]; (b) complete unit triangle map and indexing guide.

Appendix 2: Worked Example of Orientation Determination

In the ideal world, orientation determination would be easy because we would always have a perfect channeling map, whose scale corresponded to the scale of the experimental SACP that we wished to orient. In the real world, this is never the case because we invariably have imperfect maps, whose scale (for practical reasons) is usually quite different from that of the SACPs which we record. To obtain a good orientation determination, it is thus helpful to employ a systematic procedure.

1. Make sure that the correct map is used for the sample at hand, or at least a map for the same crystal type. If, for example, an FCC map must be used for BCC crystals, be aware of the differences in the allowed reflections for each crystal type. For cubic crystals, it is possible to make the SACP correspond to the scale of the map at hand by adjusting the accelerating voltage so that $\lambda/2d$ is the same. Note that $\lambda = 12.398/E_0$, where λ is in Å and E_0 is in kiloelectron volts.

2. Construct an accurate stereographic representation of the map to the same scale (Joy *et al.,* 1982).

3. Take the experimental SACP. It is obvious that the larger the angle covered by the pattern, the easier the analysis will be. On the other hand, a pattern covering only a few degrees will possibly allow a more accurate orientation determination since the angular distortions are then minimized. The pattern shown in Figure 3.A6 covers approximately $\pm 5°$ and is a reasonable compromise between the two extremes.

4. The first step in determining the orientation is to assess the major features of the SACP. Figure 3.A6 is the SACP of a silicon crystal, which is a diamond cubic structure. The SACP contains a significant band running across the pattern together with two poles and their associated bands. An initial temptation might be to identify the "hexagonal" pole as [111]. However, it is clear on detailed inspection that the fine detail on each band around the pole is not the same, and hence the pole cannot be [111], which has threefold rotational symmetry. We do note that the major band is a symmetry plane because the structures on either side of it are mirror images. This band must therefore be either {400} or {220} type since these are the only such mirror planes in the cubic system. Furthermore, we see that the bands are apparently converging at the right-hand side of the pattern, which suggests the presence of a major pole just out of the field of view. With appropriate tilting of the specimen, the nature of this low-index pole could be confirmed, if necessary, to increase confidence in the orientation which is assigned to the pattern of interest.

We now have sufficient information to localize the position of the

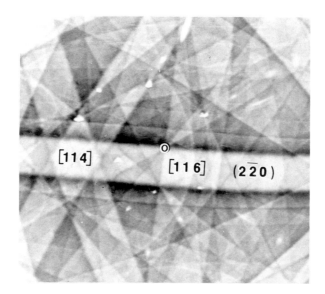

Figure 3.A6. Selected area channeling pattern of silicon. The poles and band noted were determined according to the procedure described in Appendix 2. The "o" marks the pattern center on the optic axis.

pattern. First, by calibrating the angular scale of the pattern in advance, we can determine that the band must be {220} type because the bandwidth spacing is substantially more narrow than the {400} bandwidth. Since the {220}-type bands meet at all three low-index poles, [111], [011], and [001], we must inspect the diamond cubic map, Figure 3.A4, along the (022) and (220) bands to look for a combination of two closely spaced poles, one starlike (pseudo-[111]) and the other rectangular. We find such a match near the [001] pole, with the pseudo-[111] pole identified as [114] and the rectangular pole identified as [116]. The rectangle drawn on the map in Figure 3.A7 shows the approximate limits of the experimental pattern.

5. Having found the general position, we must now locate the optic axis point since this represents the position where the beam is on-axis. We shall also assume that the surface normal of our sample is parallel to the optic axis, providing we have established this relationship by careful calibration of the stage. Given the positional uncertainties in most mechanical stages, it is a good idea to fix a reference crystal to the sample surface. An accurately oriented low-index pole of silicon in wafer form with the front and back surfaces accurately parallel is excellent for this task. The optic axis can be found as shown in Figure 3.8 by increasing

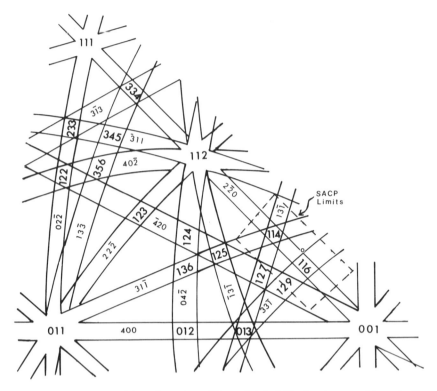

Figure 3.A7. Location of the orientation of Figure 3.A6 within the stereographic projection of the diamond cubic channeling map.

the magnification to collapse the scan to the optic axis. The optic axis is marked in Figure 3.A6.

6. In our case, the optic axis is on the edge of the band (220) so we can fix it exactly by measuring the width of the band, which equals $2\theta_B$ (220) and then comparing this distance to that from the center of the [114] pole. In a more general case, we need to measure the angle between the axis and two nearby features to measure it exactly.

7. The result shows that the surface normal lies close to [116]. For a more accurate representation of the result, the normalized coordinate trace can be used (Figure 3.22) to give (0.205, 0.123, 0.971).

8. Finally, we must remember that if a complete orientation is required, one direction on the surface of the sample must be specified. When doing this, attention must be paid to the rotation which exists between the SACP and the micrograph. This rotation can be readily cal-

ibrated for any microscope operating condition if the reference silicon wafer suggested above for establishing the parallel between the sample surface normal and the optic axis also contains a feature such as a scratch or a cleavage edge which runs parallel to a known crystallographic direction.

4

Magnetic Contrast in the SEM

4.1. Introduction

The magnetic microstructure of materials can be directly observed in the SEM by means of three different contrast mechanisms, which are designated by their chronological order of discovery. Type I magnetic contrast arises from the deflection of secondary electrons which have left the specimen by external magnetic fields and was first observed in recorded magnetic media by Dorsey (1969) and in natural magnetic crystals by Joy and Jakubovics (1968) and Banbury and Nixon (1967). Type II magnetic contrast originates from deflection of the beam electrons by internal magnetic fields; this contrast was first observed by Philibert and Tixier (1969) and the mechanism elucidated by Fathers *et al.* (1973a, 1974). Type III magnetic contrast arises from the polarization of the secondary electrons emitted from the surface of a magnetized material (Pierce and Celotta, 1981). The choice of the contrast mechanism to employ is determined by the type of magnetic microstructure which is to be imaged. In order to provide a basis for the discussion of the contrast mechanisms, the nature of magnetic microstructures will be discussed briefly. A more detailed description can be found in Craik and Tebble (1965) and Kittel (1966). This introduction will be followed by a description of the characteristics of the magnetic contrast mechanisms and the practical techniques required to obtain this contrast in images with the SEM.

4.2. Magnetic Microstructures

4.2.1. Magnetic Domains

A spinning electron generates a magnetic moment. In most atoms, the electrons are paired with opposite spins so that the net magnetic

147

moment of the atom is near zero. In certain atoms, the existence of unpaired spins in an incompletely filled inner electron shell can create a strong magnetic moment, and for three elements, iron, nickel, and cobalt, spontaneous alignment of the magnetic moments of large groups of atoms can occur, which results in the condition called ferromagnetism. Ferromagnetic materials which are not under the influence of an externally imposed magnetic field have a magnetic microstructure which consists of domains. Domains are regions in which the spins of the atomic electrons are aligned. The local magnetization is saturated within the domain, i.e., all magnetic moments of the atoms are aligned. Thus, the domain displays the properties of a magnet, with distinct north and south poles. In a macroscopic specimen, the orientation of the magnetization vector of different domains varies so that when the magnetization is integrated over a large volume of matter, the vectors tend to cancel, thus giving the specimen as a whole a net magnetization which is very much less than the saturation magnetization. The domains of different magnetic vector orientation are separated by a thin transition region, known as a Bloch wall, which has a thickness of tens to hundreds of nanometers, and across which the orientation of the magnetic moments of the atoms gradually change in alignment from one domain to another.

When an external magnetic field is applied to such a ferromagnetic

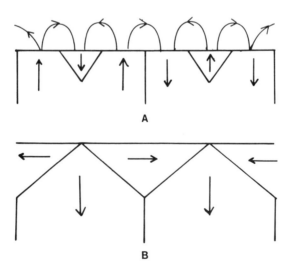

Figure 4.1. Schematic diagram of magnetic domain structures at the surface of: (A) a uniaxial magnetic material showing the leakage magnetic field above the surface and (B) a cubic magnetic material showing closure domains at the surface.

material, the volume of the domains with magnetization vectors favorably aligned to the applied field will increase at the expense of unfavorably aligned domains by the motion of the domain walls. With a sufficiently high external magnetic field, eventually only one orientation of domain will remain, and any further increase in the applied field will actually cause a rotation of the magnetic moments of the atoms to become parallel to the applied field. When the external field is removed, a domain pattern will again be formed as the sample minimizes its free energy by reducing the magnetic energy, $(\frac{1}{8}\pi) \int H^2 dV$ (Kittel, 1966), where H is the magnetic field and dV is the volume element, required to maintain long-range order among the magnetic moments, the so-called exchange interaction. The tendency to subdivide the microstructure further and further by forming domains is opposed by the increase in energy associated with forming the Bloch wall, which has an energy of about 1 erg/cm^2. Thus, an equilibrium domain structure is formed. The domain pattern which is formed will also be affected by the presence of residual stress in the solid.

With regard to the near-surface region of a magnetic sample which can be imaged in the SEM, two different kinds of domain structure are encountered, uniaxial and cubic, depending on the crystallographic nature of the sample and its magnetization.

4.2.2. Types of Magnetic Materials

4.2.2.1. Uniaxial

In a uniaxial magnetic material (e.g., cobalt), the magnetization lies along a single direction in the crystal. In the case of cobalt, which in its magnetic state has a hexagonal crystal structure, the magnetization vector lies along the c axis. Because of the limited choices for the alignment of the magnetization in the hexagonal crystal structure, the behavior of the magnetic flux at the surface will depend on how the crystal is sectioned. If the crystal is cut parallel to the c axis, the magnetization can lie in the surface plane so that no flux leaves the surface. If, however, the crystal is sectioned perpendicular to the c axis, then the flux cannot follow the c axis and remain inside the specimen. Instead, an external magnetic field is formed in which the magnetic flux exits the sample from one domain, a so-called "leakage field," and reenters the specimen at a nearby domain of the opposite magnetization, as shown in Figure 4.1a. The existence of a magnetic field outside of the sample actually increases the free energy of the sample, but the increase is not as great as would be the alternative of changing the crystallographic alignment of the magnetization at the surface. The leakage magnetic field above the specimen can perturb electrons passing through this region; this perturbation is the physical basis of type I magnetic contrast (Dorsey, 1969).

Besides uniaxial crystals, leakage magnetic fields are also character-istic of the important class of artificial magnetic structures represented by magnetic recording tape and magnetic storage media such as disks. In such a material, the effect of applying a magnetic field through the mag-netic writing head is to induce a permanent magnetic field in a region of magnetically "hard" particles, i.e., particles which retain the magnetiza-tion which is impressed upon them even when the applied field is removed. In order for the field to be detected by a reading head, the sense of the applied magnetization is perpendicular to the plane of the tape or disk. Such an arrangment creates a leakage field above the tape.

4.2.2.2. Cubic

The second type of surface magnetic microstructure of interest is that found in cubic magnetic materials such as iron and nickel. In cubic mate-rials, the magnetization is aligned along the cube edges, which provides a multiplicity of possible paths. Thus, when a domain which is charac-teristic of the interior of the specimen approaches a free surface, it is not necessary for the flux to leave the surface of the sample to maintain the continuity of the magnetic flux path. Instead, with the multiplicity of pos-sible cube edges for the magnetization to follow, a flux closure domain can be formed at the surface, as shown in Figure 4.1b, which is an ener-getically more favorable situation. Since the flux is contained entirely within the sample due to the formation of these closure domains, the magnetic microstructure cannot be observed by the type I contrast mech-anism, which depends on the existence of external leakage fields. Type II magnetic contrast arises from deflection of the beam electrons within the specimen by the internal magnetic field (Fathers *et al.*, 1973a, 1974).

4.3. Type I Magnetic Contrast: External Deflection of Secondary Electron Trajectories

4.3.1. Physical Origin

When a magnetic field, **B**, exists above the surface of a specimen, an electron with velocity **v** passing through this field experiences a force, **F**, given by the vector (cross) product:

$$\mathbf{F} = -e\,\mathbf{v} \times \mathbf{B} \tag{4.1}$$

where e is the electron charge. Because the leakage field from a natural magnetic material is highly localized to a few micrometers above the surface, the effect of this field on the incident high-energy electron beam is negligible. The beam thus reaches the specimen and interacts in the normal manner, causing the emission of secondary electrons, which are emitted with the usual cosine angular distribution. Under the influence of the positive bias applied to the Faraday cage of the Everhart–Thornley (E-T) detector, the secondary electrons are collected with high efficiency. However, while passing through the leakage magnetic field above the domain, the electrons are deflected by the magnetic field so that the effect, from the point of view of the detector, is to introduce an asymmetry to the apparent angular distribution of the secondary electrons, as shown in Figure 4.2. The deflection of the secondary electrons from domains of opposite magnetization will be in opposite directions so that if the specimen is rotated into the proper orientation relative to the detector, contrast will result between the domains. Domains of the one polarity will appear bright compared to domains of the opposite polarity. An example of type I magnetic contrast observed from the domain pattern in a cobalt crystal is shown in Figure 4.2b.

Note that although the same total number of secondary electrons may be produced at all locations in the domains, the number collected will differ because of perturbation of the trajectories between the specimen surface and the detector. Type I magnetic contrast is therefore an example of pure trajectory contrast, i.e., a contrast mechanism which depends entirely on the characteristics of the secondary electron trajectories and not on the number emitted from the sample. Since type I contrast is produced entirely by trajectory effects outside the specimen, the contrast cannot be detected in a specimen current image, which depends entirely on number effects. As noted above, the high-energy beam electrons and backscattered electrons are unaffected by their passage through the leakage field above the domains, so that no leakage field contrast effects are expected in a backscattered electron image. To demonstrate this point, Figure 4.3 contains images of magnetic recording tape taken with and without the secondary electron component of the signal. The magnetic domains produced by recording a square wave can be seen in the secondary electron image, but not in the backscattered electron image.

4.3.2. Characteristics of Type I Magnetic Contrast

4.3.2.1. Specimen–Detector Orientation

The formation of type I magnetic contrast depends on creating differences in the efficiency of collection of secondary electrons passing through the leakage magnetic field above the specimen. It is thus impor-

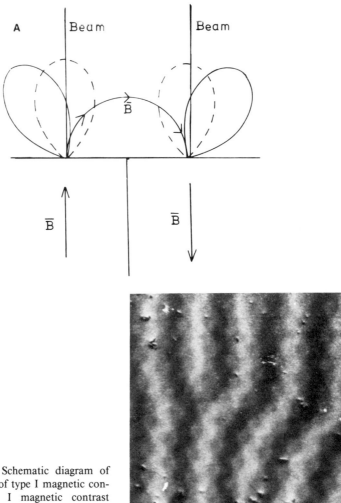

Figure 4.2. (A) Schematic diagram of the mechanism of type I magnetic contrast; (B) type I magnetic contrast observed from a cobalt crystal.

tant that the deflection be such that the difference in secondary electron collection is maximized between domains of opposite magnetization. The deflection should be such that domains of one polarization, e.g., north, deflect secondaries preferentially toward the detector, while domains of the opposite polarity deflect secondaries away from the detector. The strength of the contrast thus depends on the orientation of the specimen relative to the detector rather than the beam. If the specimen is rotated 90° from the maximum contrast position, the contrast will decrease to a minimum, possibly to zero, because in this case the deflec-

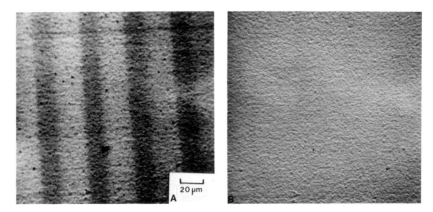

Figure 4.3. Type I magnetic contrast from a square wave recorded on magnetic tape. (A) Secondary electrons, E-T detector biased positively; (B) backscattered electrons, E-T detector biased negatively; note loss of contrast in (B), demonstrating that contrast is carried by the secondary electron component.

tion of secondaries from domains of opposite polarity is parallel to the face of the detector, which produces no net differences in collection efficiency. If the specimen is rotated another 90°, placing it 180° from the initial high-contrast position, the contrast will again be maximized, but with the opposite sense. Such a rotation experiment is illustrated in Figure 4.4, which contains images of type I magnetic contrast from magnetic recording tape. Contrast reversal between the 0° and 180° positions can be observed in these images.

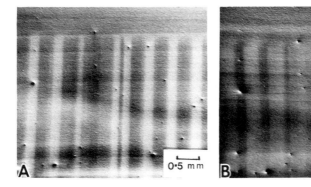

Figure 4.4. Type-I magnetic contrast from a wave pattern recorded on magnetic tape; the effect of sample rotation relative to the E-T detector is shown. (A) 0° rotation (stripe domain axis pointed toward the E-T detector); (B) 180° rotation from (A).

4.3.2.2. Tilt Dependence

Given that the contrast has been maximized by rotating the specimen relative to the E-T detector, the effect of specimen tilt will mainly be the modification of the total secondary electron yield according to the approximate expression $\delta(\theta) = \delta_0 \sec \theta$. Thus, specimen tilt will serve to increase the total number of secondary electrons, which will lower the threshold beam current for visibility.

The angular distribution of the emitted secondaries remains a cosine distribution relative to the local surface normal at all tilts, since this distribution results from the exit path length dependence relative to the surface normal. If the specimen plane is tilted toward the E-T detector, the effect may be to direct the major portion of the cosine distribution toward the detector from domains of both polarities, which will actually tend to reduce the contrast. Tilting the specimen plane away from the E-T detector, i.e., negative tilting angles, can actually serve to maximize the contrast, since with proper specimen rotation the deflection from one domain polarity will be distinctly away from the E-T detector.

4.3.2.3. Detector Dependence

Since the detection of type I magnetic contrast depends on creating differences in the number of secondary electrons which are collected by the E-T detector, the high efficiency of the conventional E-T detector is actually a hindrance, especially with the specimen plane tilted toward the detector. The contrast can actually be increased by reducing the collection angle of the E-T detector by using a foil aperture to reduce the acceptance area of the Faraday cage which surrounds the scintillator and thus decrease the collection efficiency. Contrast values as high as 20% can be realized, depending on the magnetic field strength of the material under study and details of the secondary electron detector.

A second factor to be considered in optimizing type I magnetic contrast concerns the role of backscattered electrons in the generation of secondary electrons at the polepiece and chamber walls, the so-called SE-III component of the secondary electron signal received by the E-T detector. The SE-III component is very efficiently collected by the conventional E-T detector, and for elements with a high backscattering coefficient the SE-III component can form 50% of the total signal. The SE-III component of the secondary signal actually carries backscattered electron information, and therefore does not contribute to type I magnetic contrast, which exists in the SE-I and SE-II signals. The SE-III signal actually represents a noise component of the signal which degrades the visibility of type I contrast. Type I contrast can therefore be improved by reducing the remotely produced SE-III component by shielding the polepiece and chamber walls with a material which has a low secondary electron coefficient, such as carbon.

4.3.2.4. Beam Energy Dependence

As noted in Section 4.3.1, type I magnetic contrast is carried exclusively by the secondary electron component of the signal. Moreover, due to the short range of the leakage fields, the high-energy beam electrons are not significantly perturbed during entry into the specimen. Over the typical operating range of the SEM, 1–30 keV, there is no direct effect of the beam energy on the character of type I magnetic contrast. However, since the secondary electron coefficient, δ, generally increases as the beam energy is lowered, the relative strength of the secondary electron signal which carries type I contrast will be increased by operating at low beam energy, e.g., below 10 keV, and thus the threshold current for visibility of a given level of magnetic contrast will be lowered. As an added benefit, lowering the beam energy will also reduce the lateral range of the backscattered electrons, which will increase secondary electron production near the beam impact area.

4.3.3. Quantitative Theory of Type I Magnetic Contrast

A quantitative theory of type I magnetic contrast has been given by Joy and Jakubovics (1969) and Wells (1983). These authors consider the deviation from the signal $S = 1$ obtained when the sample is in a nonmagnetic state caused by the presence of the specimen magnetization. The signal in the presence of the magnetic field, S_M, is given by

$$S_M = 1 - (2/\pi)[\sin^{-1} u + u(1 - u^2)^{1/2}] \tag{4.2}$$

The term u is given by

$$u = (e/mv) \int_0^\infty H_x \, dz \tag{4.3}$$

where e/m is the charge-to-mass ratio and v is the electron velocity. H_x is the horizontal leakage field component which is normal to the line which joins the beam impact point on the specimen to the detector. The integral is calculated along the electron trajectory, an element of which is given by dz. Since u is generally much less than unity, equation (4.2) can be approximated as $\sin^{-1}u \cong u$ and $(1 - u^2)^{1/2} = 1$. Equation (4.2) thus becomes

$$S_M = 1 - (2/\pi)(u + u) = 1 - (4u/\pi) \tag{4.4}$$

$$= 1 - (4e/mv\pi) \int_0^\infty H_x \, dz$$

Note that from equation (4.3), the magnetic contrast effect, u, on the signal given by equation (4.4) will increase as the electron velocity decreases and as the specimen magnetic field increases. Thus, secondary electrons with their low kinetic energy (< 50 eV, and predominantly < 5 eV) will be strongly affected by the specimen magnetic field, while the high-energy beam electrons ($E \sim 20$ keV) will experience a deflection which is several orders of magnitude less.

Equations (4.2) to (4.4) can be used to predict the magnitude of type I magnetic contrast from a particular material and domain microstructure if an expression is available for the magnetic scalar potential in the magnetic field integral, equation (4.3). Fathers *et al.* (1973b) described such a procedure for bubble domains, which are cylindrical structures of radius a. The radial field component of a bubble domain is described in terms of cylindrical coordinates (r, z) by

$$H_R = h \int_0^\infty a \exp(-uz) J_1(ua) J_1(ur) \, du \tag{4.5}$$

where $J_1(x)$ is the first-order Bessel function and h is Planck's constant. The component H_x needed in equation (4.3) is found by

$$H_x = H_R \cos \phi \tag{4.6}$$

where the angle ϕ is measured from the diameter of the domain which is perpendicular to the detector.

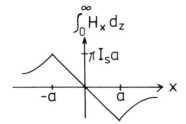

Figure 4.5. Calculation of type I magnetic contrast from a bubble domain (after Fathers *et al.*, 1973b).

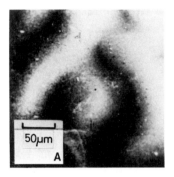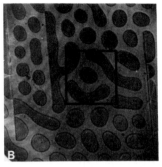

Figure 4.6. Magnetic domains observed from a crystal of yttrium orthoferrite. (A) Type I magnetic contrast image observed in the SEM; (B) same region observed by the Kerr magneto-optical effect, the boxed region corresponding to the region observed in the SEM.

A graphical plot of the contrast term for bubble domains is shown in Figure 4.5. A corresponding image of a bubble domain in yttrium orthoferrite is shown in Figure 4.6. Comparison of Figures 4.5 and 4.6 reveals good agreement between prediction and observation: the contrast reverses across the center of the bubble domain with the signal maximum and minimum at the edge of the bubble domain. In agreement with equation (4.6), there is no signal change along the tangent to the bubble domain which is perpendicular to the detector vector, since for that chord $\phi = 90°$ and thus $\cos \phi = 0$.

Figures 4.5 and 4.6 illustrate the limitations of the edge resolution available with type I magnetic contrast. Because the leakage field above the specimen surface does not change abruptly at the domain wall, the contrast function, as illustrated in Figure 4.5, only undergoes a change in slope at the domain wall without a sharp discontinuity. This effect is confirmed in the image shown in Figure 4.6, where the domain boundary is not distinct.

4.3.4. Strategy for Observing Type I Magnetic Contrast

Type I magnetic contrast can be observed in a relatively straightforward manner providing a suitable sample is available. While type I magnetic contrast can, in principle, be observed from any magnetic material which has leakage fields, the strength of the contrast, and hence its visibility, will depend on the magnitude and orientation of the magnetic field which is characteristic of the sample. Thus, for initial experiments to gain experience in observing type I contrast, it is recommended that a test specimen should be employed which produces strong contrast. Such a specimen can be obtained from ordinary magnetic recording tape upon which has been recorded a square wave with the maximum possible signal input amplitude. The spacing of the resulting domains can be calculated from the known frequency of the recorded square wave and the rate of tape transport:

$$\text{Spacing (cm/cycle)} = \text{Rate (cm/s)/frequency (cycles/s)} \qquad (4.7)$$

1. Beam parameters: A beam energy of 10 keV or less should be selected to maximize the emission of secondary electrons. For the initial search to locate suitable domains, the beam current should be set to at least 5 nA to ensure that the threshold current for visibility is exceeded.

2. Selection of detector: Since type I magnetic contrast can only be viewed with the secondary electron signal, the E-T detector should be employed in a positively biased mode. Since the contrast depends on preferentially losing some of the secondary signal from domains of one magnetization, it may be useful to reduce the value of the positive bias on the detector or to reduce its acceptance area and, therefore, efficiency, with an aperture made of a foil.

3. Signal processing: Although contrast as strong as 20% can occur, which should be directly visible without extensive signal processing, weaker contrast will necessitate the use of differential amplification (black level, dark level, contrast expansion) to improve the visibility in the final display.

4. The specimen should be mounted on a specimen stage which allows rotation of the specimen about its normal. If type I magnetic contrast is not visible after the above conditions have been established, it may be necessary to rotate the specimen to bring the domain pattern into contrast.

5. The specimen can be viewed at a tilt of 0°, or if it is necessary to increase the total secondary electron yield, the specimen can be tilted to increase the secondary electron coefficient. Since the contrast depends on excluding electrons preferentially from one set of domains relative to the other, it may be useful to tilt the specimen negatively, i.e., away from the detector.

4.4. Type II Magnetic Contrast: Internal Deflection of Primary Electron Trajectories

4.4.1. Physical Origin

Magnetic fields fully contained within the sample through the formation of closure domains can be detected through their effects on the beam electrons as they scatter within the target. The mechanism of type II magnetic contrast is illustrated in Figure 4.7a. The contrast arises through deflection of the beam electrons by the action of the magnetic force, $\mathbf{F} = -e\mathbf{v} \times \mathbf{B}$, on the electrons as they scatter elastically within the target (Fathers *et al.*, 1973a, 1974). Depending on the relative orien-

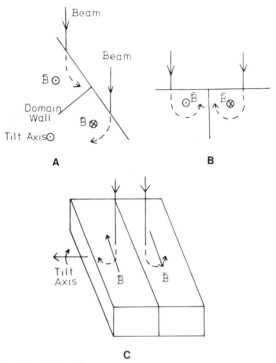

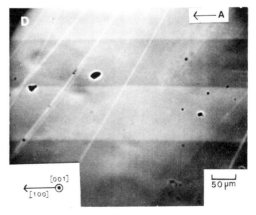

Figure 4.7. Mechanism of type II magnetic contrast. (A) Sample tilted to 55° and rotated to bring magnetization parallel to the tilt axis; (B) sample set to 0° tilt (normal incidence); (C) sample tilted to 55° and rotated to bring magnetization perpendicular to the tilt axis; (D) type II magnetic contrast image showing stripe domains in an iron–3.22% silicon alloy with the magnetization parallel to the long axis of the domains. The crystallographic directions indicated were confirmed with electron channeling patterns.

tation of the beam vector and the specimen magnetization vector, the cyclotron deflection due to the magnetic force can cause the beam electrons to travel closer to or farther from the sample surface than they would in the absence of the internal magnetic field, which modifies the backscattering coefficient. Thus, different numbers of beam electrons backscatter depending on the magnetization of the domain. An example of magnetic domains in iron transformer steel imaged by means of the type II contrast mechanism is shown in Figure 4.7d. Since type II magnetic contrast arises as a result of a number effect, the contrast is visible in both the backscattered electron signal, and the specimen (absorbed) current signal, as illustrated in Figure 4.8. This property of type II magnetic contrast provides a distinct test to distinguish it from type I contrast.

The magnitude of type II magnetic contrast is extraordinarily small. Experimental measurements of type II magnetic contrast in iron, the strongest natural ferromagnetic material, reveal that the maximum contrast at a typical SEM beam energy, 30 keV, is only 0.3%. This low value is a result of (1) the deflection due to the magnetic force is small and (2) due to the randomizing effect of elastic scattering on the trajectories of the beam electrons, only a small fraction of the trajectory of an individual electron is oriented to produce a net motion toward or away from the surface.

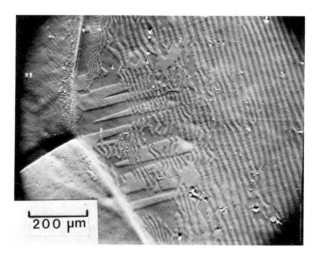

Figure 4.8. Type II magnetic contrast from iron–3.22% silicon alloy demonstrating that the contrast can be observed in the specimen current mode. The detection of the contrast in specimen current demonstrates that the contrast mechanism is a number effect. First time derivative signal processing.

4.4.2. Characteristics of Type II Magnetic Contrast

4.4.2.1. Effect of Sample Tilt

The magnetic force on the moving electron is produced according to equation (4.1); the magnitude of the force given by the vector product varies as the sine of the angle between **v** and **B** and is thus a maximum when the beam vector and magnetization vector are at right angles. However, even when this condition is satisfied, contrast between domains of opposite magnetization can only occur for certain orientations of the specimen relative to the beam. Consider the case in which this magnetization vector lies parallel to the tilt axis of the specimen. The beam will thus be perpendicular to the magnetization no matter what tilt angle is chosen, and the incident electrons will experience the maximum possible Lorentz force as they enter the specimen prior to elastic scattering. When the specimen is tilted to a high angle, e.g., 50°, the effect of the magnetic force will be to deflect the electrons either toward the surface, which will increase the backscatter coefficient, or away from the surface, which will decrease the backscatter coefficient, depending on the sense of the magnetization. When the specimen tilt is reduced to 0° so that the beam enters normal to the surface, as shown in Figure 4.7b, the magnetic force on the beam electrons remains at the same maximum value since the beam is still perpendicular to the tilt axis and the magnetization, but the effect of the magnetic force is merely to change the sense of the cyclotron action from clockwise to counterclockwise in domains of opposite magnetization so that there is no net difference in electron depth and therefore no contrast. These two conditions of tilt illustrate the strong dependence of type II magnetic contast on the specimen tilt. Experimental measurements of the effect of tilt are given in Figure 4.9, where it can be seen that the maximum value of the contrast occurs for a tilt of approximately 55°. Further increase in the tilt angle above this value causes the contrast to decrease because the beam electrons tend to backscatter out of the sample in a few events and thus do not spend sufficient time under the influence of the internal magnetic field to alter the backscatter coefficient as much.

4.4.2.2. Rotation

The effect of rotation of the sample magnetization vector relative to the beam can be understood with the aid of Figure 4.7a and 4.7c. For a tilted specimen, the maximum influence of the field occurs when the magnetic field vector is parallel to the tilt axis, thus producing the condition of perpendicularity which maximizes the vector product. As the specimen is rotated, the angle between the magnetization vector and the

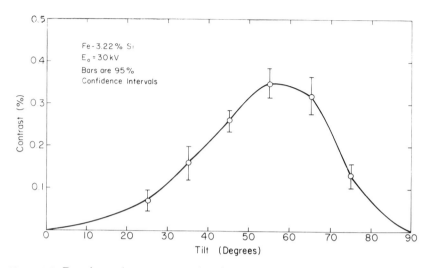

Figure 4.9. Experimental measurements (specimen current signal) of type II magnetic contrast as a function of specimen tilt for a sample of iron–3.22% silicon alloy with stripe domains oriented parallel to the tilt axis. Beam energy 30 keV.

beam vector decreases and becomes a minimum when the magnetization vector has been rotated to be perpendicular to the tilt axis. However, when the magnetic field vector is oriented perpendicularly to the tilt axis, Figure 4.7c, the symmetry of the situation becomes the same as that of Figure 4.7b; the effect of the magnetic field in the domains of opposite magnetization is only to change the sense of the cyclotron action so that no net change in depth occurs and therefore no contrast is produced. Thus, as the tilted specimen is rotated about an axis parallel to its surface normal, the contrast is maximized when the magnetization is parallel to the tilt axis and zero when it is perpendicular to the tilt axis. This behavior provides a test to determine the orientation of the magnetization in an unknown domain structure.

The effect of rotation on the appearance of a complicated domain structure, is illustrated in Figure 4.10 for a "fir-tree" domain structure in iron, which has the pattern of magnetization vectors illustrated in the schematic diagram. As the tilted specimen is rotated around its normal, as shown by the change in the position of the topographic surface feature, the portion of the domain pattern which produces contrast is that for which the magnetization vector is parallel to the tilt axis.

4.4.2.3. Beam Energy

Type II magnetic contrast shows a strong dependence on the beam energy. Monte Carlo calculations (Newbury *et al.*, 1973), which have been confirmed by experimental measurements (Yamamoto *et al.,* 1975; Newbury *et al.,* 1976), reveal that the contrast depends on the beam energy through a power law:

$$C \sim E^n \tag{4.8}$$

where the exponent n has a value of the order of 1.4. This relationship arises through the dependence of the electron velocity v on the beam energy, $(mv^2/2) = E$ for nonrelativistic energies. The magnetic force on the electron given by equation (4.1) thus increases with the beam energy,

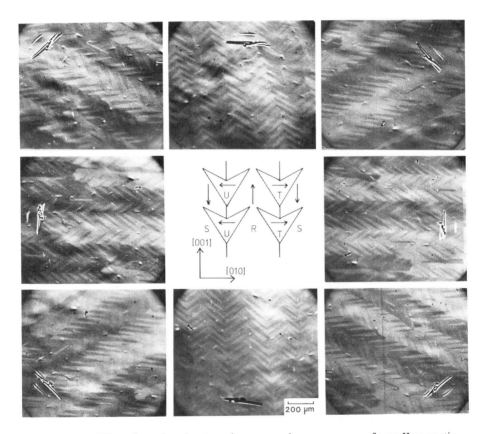

Figure 4.10. Effect of rotation about specimen normal on appearance of type II magnetic contrast. The "fir-tree" domain pattern from an iron single crystal is observed through a sequence of 45° increments of rotation as demonstrated by the successive positioning of the surface scratch. The portion of the fir-tree pattern for which the magnetization vector is parallel to the tilt axis is observed to be in contrast. Beam energy: 30 keV; tilt: 55°; tilt axis horizontal in all images. Schematic diagram of magnetization vectors in the fir-tree structure.

which leads to an increase in contrast. The high value of the exponent, n $\cong$ 1.4, is surprising since $v \sim E^{1/2}$, which would suggest n should be of the order of ½. A qualitative understanding of the high value of n requires consideration of the effect of elastic scattering. If there were no elastic scattering to cause the beam electrons to deviate from their initial trajectory along the beam vector and if there were no inelastic scattering to reduce the energy and eventually stop the electrons, then the effect of the magnetic deflection shown in Figure 4.7a would be to cause the beam electrons eventually to either intersect the surface or to penetrate more deeply into the specimen. However, both elastic and inelastic scattering are much stronger effects on the electron trajectories than the effect of magnetic deflection. The cross section for elastic scattering depends inversely on the energy, $Q \sim 1/E^2$, so that the mean free path for elastic scattering depends directly on the square of the beam energy, $\lambda \sim E^2$. Elastic scattering tends to randomize the electron trajectories so that electrons are scattered out of the initial trajectory which experiences the maximum magnetic force. Thus, when elastic scattering is reduced by operating at high beam energy, the electron mean free path becomes longer.

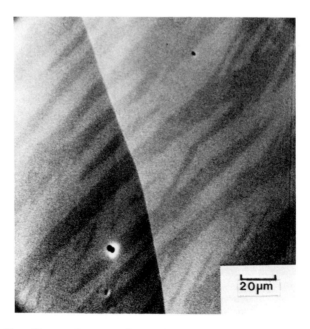

Figure 4.11. Type II magnetic contrast from polycrystalline nickel imaged at a beam energy of 50 keV. The domains are observed to cross a low-angle grain boundary; the grains are observed in contrast due to electron channeling contrast.

Near the surface of the sample, the electrons with trajectories aligned to maximize the magnetic force, $\mathbf{F} = -e\mathbf{v} \times \mathbf{B}$ have a greater opportunity to undergo significant magnetic deflection while traveling in the single or plural elastic scattering regime prior to the randomizing effects of multiple scattering.

The practical importance of the strong dependence of type II magnetic contrast on beam energy is that an increase in beam energy can increase the contrast, which may only be marginally visible at conventional SEM operating energies, e.g., 20 keV, and it may allow materials for which the saturation magnetization is lower than that of iron to be imaged. Thus, domains in nickel, which has a saturation magnetization which is only 29% that of iron (0.63 Wb/m^2 compared to 2.16 Wb/m^2 for iron), cannot be successfully imaged at 30 keV, where the contrast is below 0.1%, while by increasing the beam energy to 50 keV, domains in nickel could be successfully imaged, as shown in Figure 4.11 (Newbury *et al.*, 1974). Shimizu *et al.* (1974, 1976) and Yamamoto *et al.* (1975) have used very high beam energies in the range 150–200 keV to increase the contrast sufficiently in iron to enable them to view domains beneath an overlayer of glass used for stress control on iron–3% silicon transformer steel and to observe domains in Mn–Zn ferrite which has only one-fourth the magnetization of pure iron.

4.4.2.4. Backscattered Electron Energy

Monte Carlo electron trajectory simulation of type II magnetic contrast has been utilized to study the behavior of the contrast as a function of the fraction of the incident energy which is retained by the backscattered electrons, as shown in Figure 4.12. The maximum contrast is obtained with those electrons which have lost up to approximately 20% of their incident energy. Including backscattered electrons which have lost more energy lowers the contrast. This behavior can again be understood in terms of two opposing processes. The beam electrons must travel an adequate distance in the specimen for the magnetic field to deflect the electrons, and during this travel within the specimen inelastic scattering reduces the electron energy. Running counter to this increase in contrast with increasing path length in the sample is the effect of elastic scattering, which tends to randomize the direction of motion and reduce the effect of the magnetic field on the trajectories. Beyond approximately 20% energy loss, the randomization effects of elastic scattering dominate, and further contributions to the contrast are reduced. The practical value of this observation can be realized by increasing the weak contrast with an energy-filtering backscattered electron detector which could exclude a selected fraction of the backscattered electrons.

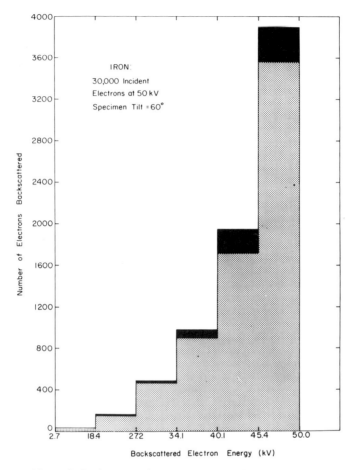

Figure 4.12. Monte Carlo electron trajectory calculation of the energy distribution of electrons backscattered from domains of opposite magnetization showing contrast development in the first 20% of the energy loss.

4.4.2.5. Resolution

The ability to resolve fine-scale features by type II magnetic contrast is limited by two effects. (1) Beam size: Because of the low value of the natural contrast, high beam currents and, hence, large beam diameters must be used for visual searching (100 nA) and for photo-recording (10 nA). With an ordinary tungsten hairpin filament, a probe size of 100 to 500 nm is required to carry these high currents. (2) Beam spreading: The spreading of the beam electrons through the specimen by elastic scattering also contributes to limit the resolution. Since the specimen must be highly tilted to maximize the contrast, the interaction volume has considerably different dimensions parallel and perpendicular to the tilt axis. This results in differences in the edge resolution of domain walls which run parallel and perpendicular to the tilt axis, as shown in Figure 4.13, since the walls are effectively crossed by beams with different dimensions. The resolution limit imposed by these effects is of the order of 500 nm. This limit could be improved by (1) using a higher-brightness electron source such as lanthanum hexaboride to reduce the probe size, and (2) using energy filtering to exclude backscattered electrons emitted from areas remote from the beam impact point as well as to increase the contrast.

4.4.2.6. Domain Wall Imaging

In all of the images of type II magnetic contrast considered so far, the contrast has been formed between the bodies of the domains, whereas the domain walls were only known as the discontinuity between the domain bodies. A special case exists in which the domain walls can be brought into contrast directly (Joy *et al.*, 1976; Fathers and Jakubovics,

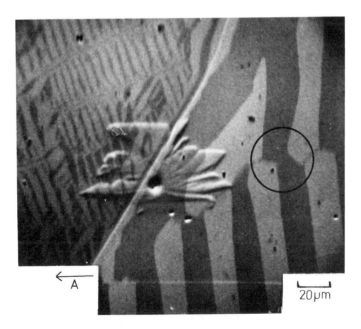

Figure 4.13. Effect of domain wall orientation on spatial resolution. Domain walls at right angles to the tilt axis display higher spatial resolution than domain walls which are parallel to the tilt axis, as shown in the circled region.

1976). The first requirement to realize this condition is to eliminate the contrast between the bodies of the domains, which can be conveniently achieved by setting the specimen tilt to 0°, which by the symmetry arguments given above, reduces the domain contrast to zero. However, in this condition a variant of type II contrast occurs when the beam exactly straddles a domain wall, as shown in the schematic of Figure 4.14. In this condition, the large convergence angle of the high-current beam leads to a situation in which rays which are not exactly parallel to the specimen normal are deflected through an angle which causes them either to penetrate more deeply into the specimen or to be scattered out of the specimen more efficiently. When the beam is not symmetrically placed on a boundary, the effect is suppressed. An example of domain walls imaged by this effect is shown in Figure 4.15. This wall contrast is an even weaker effect than that of bulk type II magnetic contrast.

4.4.3. Calculation of Type II Magnetic Contrast

Two different techniques for the quantitative calculation of type II magnetic contrast have been described. Newbury *et al.* (1973), Fathers *et al.* (1973a), and Ikuta and Shimizu (1974) have employed the Monte Carlo electron trajectory simulation method to model type II magnetic contrast. In this method, which is described in detail in Chapter 1, the

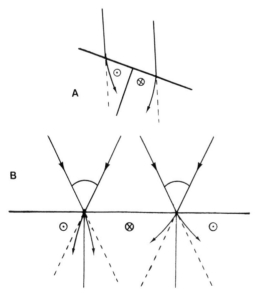

Figure 4.14. Schematic diagram of the technique for direct imaging of domain walls. (A) Conventional arrangement for type II magnetic contrast with a tilted specimen; (B) domain wall imaging at normal incidence with divergent beam placed symmetrically on the domain wall. The walls come into contrast only when the beam is placed symmetrically on the domain wall.

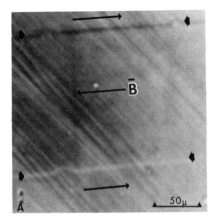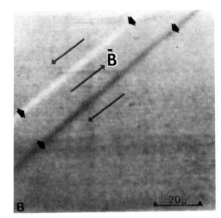

Figure 4.15. (A, B) Images of domain walls obtained at 0° tilt by the symmetric beam technique described in Figure 4.14. Magnetization vectors are indicated by long arrows. In (A), the walls are indicated by small arrows.

conventional Monte Carlo calculation is modified to include a magnetic perturbation to the trajectory. For each scattering event, the new location after elastic scattering is first calculated as usual. The perturbation of this location due to the influence of the magnetic force which acts on the moving electron is then calculated. The electron is considered to start its next scattering step at the new magnetically modified position. The strength of the Monte Carlo method is that it directly models the physics which underlies the formation of type II magnetic contrast and the multiple elastic scattering and inelastic scattering which accompanies the magnetic deflection. The Monte Carlo method can directly simulate the experimental parameters which can be varied: beam energy, sample tilt, rotation, backscattered electron energy distribution, and backscattered electron exit angle. The weakness of the Monte Carlo method is the necessity of calculating a statistically significant number of trajectories. Because of the weak level of the natural contrast, even with the expedient of making calculations with scaled-up magnetic fields within the linear response region, it is necessary to calculate 20,000 or more trajectories for each condition to be simulated in order to achieve statistically valid contrast calculations.

An alternative to the Monte Carlo method is modeling with analytic expressions which describe the phenomena of electron scattering and magnetic deflection (Fathers *et al.*, 1973a; Wells, 1976). The derivations of these models are quite complicated and the interested reader should consider the original sources. The chief difficulty of these methods is adequately modeling the effects of multiple elastic scattering which is clearly important as a controlling factor in determining the magnitude of the contrast.

4.4.4. Strategy for Observing Type II Magnetic Contrast

Type II magnetic contrast represents the weakest contrast mechanism which has been successfully imaged in the SEM. Because of the low value of type II contrast, approximately 0.3% for iron under optimum conditions with a 30-keV beam in a typical SEM, a carefully planned strategy must be followed to successfully image domains.

1. Specimen condition: Since a strong contrast mechanism tends to dominate a weak mechanism and greatly reduce its visibility in the final image, it is necessary to eliminate any surface roughness which might produce strong topographic contrast. Second, residual strains in the surface can cause extensive modification of the domain pattern. These two conditions generally lead to a requirement for chemical or electrochemical polishing as the final step in the preparation of a sample. A suitable test sample for initial experiments can be obtained by chemically polishing an iron–3.22% silicon transformer steel sheet to produce a highly polished flat surface.

2. Beam parameters: Type II magnetic contrast increases markedly with increasing beam energy. Since the contrast is so weak, even in the strongest magnetic materials, any effect which can increase the contrast is valuable. The maximum valuable beam energy should be selected; beam energies below 20 keV are inadequate for most materials. Since the natural contrast is low, of the order of 0.3%, calculation of the threshold current to observe the contrast indicates that for a visual search scan (e.g., 1 frame/s, 500 lines), a beam current of at least 100 nA is needed. The sample current should be measured to ensure this high beam current is actually reaching the specimen. Once a feature of interest has been located, the beam current and size can be reduced to 10 nA or less in the photograhic mode with a long scan time (100 s or more).

3. Specimen tilt and rotation: The specimen should be tilted to 55° to maximize the contrast. The specimen should be rotated about its normal to bring different domains into contrast.

4. Selection of detector: Since the contrast is carried by the backscattered electron component as a number effect, either a backscattered electron detector or specimen current can be selected. If an E-T detector is used, it should be positively biased in order to increase the efficiency for the collection of backscattered electrons through the production of remotely generated secondary electrons on the polepiece and chamber walls. The predominant portion of the backscattered electron signal may come through these remote secondaries. Since the specimen must be

tilted to a high angle, it is important that any backscattered electron detector be located in a position to collect the majority of the backscattered electrons. This position will not be in the conventional location near the incident beam but rather the detector should be located in a forward scattering direction, as shown in Figure 4.16.

5. Signal processing: In order to render the natural contrast level of 0.3% visible to the eye in the final display, it is necessary to apply extensive signal processing. A high level of differential amplification (black level suppression, dark level, or contrast expansion) is the usual choice to enhance the visibility of the contrast. On most instruments, the maximum available range of the black level suppression will be necessary. Note that this extraordinary level will make the image quality very susceptible to degradation by fluctuations in beam current and due to instability in the amplification caused by large contrast excursions which inev-

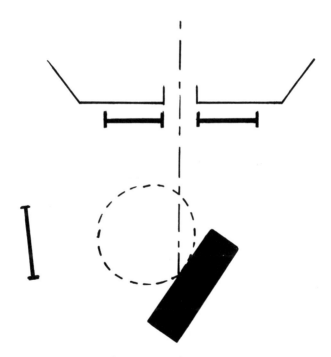

Figure 4.16. Detector placement for detection of backscattered electrons for observation of type II magnetic contrast. The annular solid-state detector or scintillator detector placed above the sample intercepts only a small portion of the backscattered electron angular distribution (shown by the dashed curve) while a backscattered electron detector (solid state or scintillator) placed in the forward scattering position has a much larger geometric collection efficiency due to the preferential scattering of electrons in the forward direction.

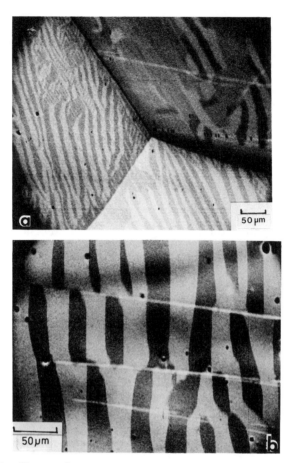

Figure 4.17. Type II magnetic contrast images of domain structures in iron–3% silicon transformer alloy. (a) Grain boundary triple point showing different domain patterns in each grain with the grain at the upper right showing islands of wide stripe domains in a sea of a domain structure which is not in contrast due to a sharp change in the orientation of the magnetization; (b) discontinuous domains observed as a result of interaction with residual stress field of surface scratches; (c) very fine-scale domain pattern; (d) a wide variety of domain patterns are observed in a grain which has a high and varying pattern of internal stress. All images obtained under optimum contrast conditions: beam energy, 30 keV; tilt, 55°; tilt axis horizontal in all images.

itably occur at small topographic features (e.g., inclusions, pits, scratches).

When the above conditions are satisfied, it is possible to obtain images with an extraordinary range of detail on magnetic domain structures. Examples of type II magnetic contrast from iron–3.22% silicon are shown in Figure 4.17. These images illustrate the detection of a variety

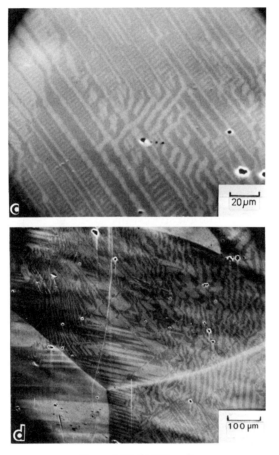

Figure 4.17 (*continued*)

of domain patterns, the fine scale of the features which can be observed, and the interaction of the domains with various features in the microstructure.

4.5. Type III Magnetic Contrast: Polarization of Secondary Electrons

4.5.1. Physical Origin

Recently, a new form of magnetic contrast in the scanning electron microscope has been reported (Celotta and Pierce, 1982; Unguris *et al.*, 1985). This new type of contrast mechanism, designated type III contrast, arises because of polarization of the secondary electrons generated at the sample. The low-energy secondary electrons passing near the surface ion cores are influenced by the exchange interaction. The exchange interaction occurs because the secondary electrons are subject to the exclusion principle and cannot occupy the same state, just as are the resident electrons of the ion core. This results in a large difference in the scattering cross section depending on whether the surface has a net spin-up or spin-down orientation. The local spin density varies from one domain to that of the opposite magnetization, with a continuous change occurring across the domain wall.

The interesting properties of type III contrast include its strong sensitivity to the surface of the material, since the secondary electrons can only escape with significant polarization information from the topmost atom layers, about 2–3 nm deep. Second, the sensitivity to changes in the spin density and orientation suggest that it should be particularly useful for direct visualization of the domain walls, which can only be seen otherwise in the SEM by means of the extremely weak variant of type II contrast described in Section 4.4.2.6. Third, the nature of the surface magnetization vector can be directly studied through detailed analysis of the polarization.

4.5.2. Experimental Techniques

In order to detect the polarization of the secondary electrons emitted from the surface of the magnetic material, an electron spin polarization detector of the type described by Pierce and Celotta (1981) can be employed. This detector involves the scattering of electrons with an energy of approximately 150 eV from the surface of a high-atomic-number crystal which leads to a strong difference in the scattering depending on the polarization of the incoming electrons. The secondaries emitted from the magnetic material are first accelerated to an energy of approximately 100–200 eV. An example of a type III magnetic contrast image obtained from an iron single crystal with a polarization detector of this type is shown in Figure 4.18.

This experimental detection of type III contrast is profoundly dependent on the properties of surfaces both at the emission of secondary electrons at the magnetic sample and at the scattering of these secondary electrons at the crystal surface of the polarization detector. To keep these surfaces atomically clean, it is therefore necessary to carry out the experiment in an ultrahigh vacuum environment. Moreover, if high-resolution images of domain walls are to be obtained, a field emission source is valuable to produce sufficient beam current in a small probe. Such a source is only compatible with an ultrahigh vacuum environment.

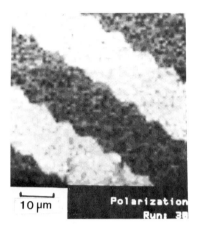

Figure 4.18. Type III magnetic contrast (detection of the polarization of secondary electrons) from iron–3% silicon grain in polycrystalline sheet. (From Unguris *et al.*, 1985.)

4.6. Dynamic Experiments

The classic techniques for the observation of magnetic domains in cubic materials involve the principle of observing domain features which have been decorated with magnetic colloid. A great advantage of observing magnetic domains in the SEM as compared with the colloid techniques has to do with the elimination of any inertia which the magnetic particles in the colloid have in responding to an impressed magnetic field or stress field. The beam electrons have no such inertia and can thus respond instantaneously to changes in the domain pattern, which makes dynamic experiments feasible, even at rapid scan rates. Examples of the dynamic experiments which can be carried out in the SEM are shown in Figures 4.19 and 4.20.

Figure 4.19 shows the change in the domain pattern which can be observed when a magnetic field is impressed on the specimen. In order to carry out this experiment, it was necessary to protect the beam from the magnetic field which was applied to the specimen. This was accomplished by making the specimen a closure element in the magnetic circuit of a small electromagnet which was placed below the specimen. Figure 4.19 shows the change in the domain pattern between conditions of no field applied (Figure 4.19a and a field of 25 Oe (Figure 4.19b). A substantial change in the domain pattern is observed; effects such as the inter-

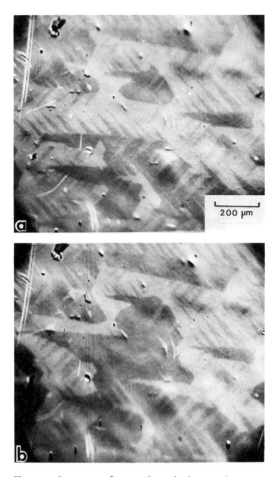

Figure 4.19. Type II magnetic contrast from an iron single crystal at two stages of an *in situ* applied magnetic field experiment; the specimen formed the closure element of a magnetic circuit surrounding an electromagnet assembly placed on the stage of the SEM. (a) No field applied; (b) magnetic field of 25 Oe applied; note expansion of dark domains.

action of domain walls with discontinuities such as inclusions and surface scratches could be studied in this way, as well as direct observation of hysteresis effects, in which the final domain pattern after removal of the applied field could be compared with the initial pattern.

Figure 4.20 records an *in situ* applied stress experiment in which a specimen of iron–3% silicon alloy was deformed in a straining stage which was equipped with a load cell to measure applied stresses. The image sequence shows the tremendous change in the domain pattern which is observed as the applied stress is first increased and long stripe domains are formed nearly parallel to the stress axis. Since the domain pattern is completely reorganized in the presence of the applied stress, a surface artifact was intentionally included to provide a point of reference in the field of view. As the applied elastic stress is removed, the domain pattern returns to its initial form, but close comparison of the initial and final images reveals a hysteresis effect.

Another aspect of imaging of magnetic domains in the SEM which increases the utility of the technique is the possibility of combining the domain images with other imaging and analysis techniques which are

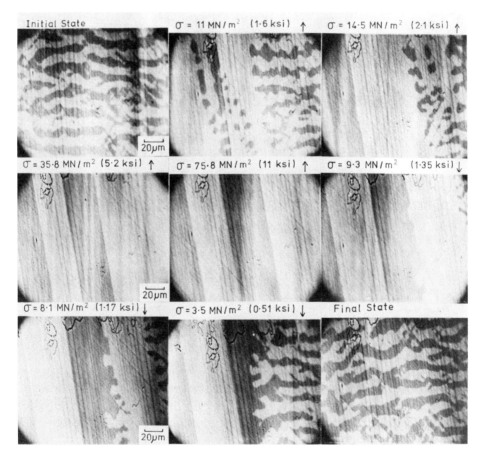

Figure 4.20. Type II magnetic contrast from iron–3% silicon alloy during *in situ* applied stress experiment performed on a special straining stage in the SEM. A surface artifact has been included in the field of view to provide a point of reference to compare changes in the magnetic domain pattern which totally reorganizes during the stress cycle. In all images, the axis of the applied stress is vertical.

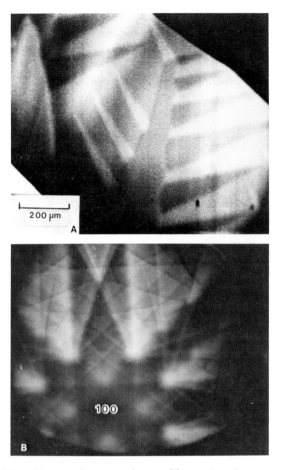

Figure 4.21. (a) Type II magnetic contrast image of fir-tree domain pattern observed on an iron single-crystal whisker; (b) electron channeling pattern from the iron whisker which reveals that the crystal orientation is approximately 4° off the [100] pole.

available in the SEM. For example, the immediate availability of x-ray microanalysis is a great aid in the study of inclusions and other compositional discontinuities which occur, particularly in alloys which are useful in industrial applications. In many cases, it is important to obtain crystallographic information to properly interpret the nature of magnetic microstructures. In this case, electron channeling patterns can be extremely useful in obtaining orientation information from areas as small as 10 μm in diameter. An example of such a study is shown in Figure 4.21, where a fir-tree structure on a single-crystal iron whisker is shown along with the electron channeling pattern which demonstrates that the crystal orientation is a few degrees off the [100] pole, which is consistent with the observation of the fir-tree structure.

Dynamic experiments involving magnetic contrast can also benefit by the use of "lock-in" phase-sensitive signal collection in which the image is composed by sampling the signal in phase with a periodic driving signal such as a a periodic applied field. Ikuta and Shimizu (1976), Wells and Savoy (1981), and Shimizu and Ikuta (1984) have described in detail techniques for phase-sensitive imaging of type II magnetic contrast.

Computer-Aided Imaging and Interpretation

5.1. Introduction

This chapter is concerned with the acquisition, display, and interpretation of the various images which can be obtained with the SEM—e.g., secondary electron, backscattered electron, x-ray—and how the modern digital computer can be applied in the process. We will be concerned with all aspects of SEM imaging from the generation of the signal when the electron beam interacts with the specimen surface to the perception and interpretation of this information in the mind of the observer. Indeed, we will view all steps involved as an information channel which has certain imperfections and nonlinearities which must be examined in the context of an SEM application.

We would like to believe that the part of the information channel comprised of the eye and mind of the observer is perfect and the part comprised of the various electron detectors, amplifiers, and display tubes is where all of the problems lie. In reality, most of the serious difficulties are in the eye and the mind. We are clearly taking some liberties when we use the word "mind." It is not our purpose to address the subjective and artistic aspects of SEM images. We as SEM operators have a large degree of freedom over the orientations of objects in our micrographs and the shading and "composition" of features. We should constantly question why we have arranged a micrograph in a certain way and whether our choice will affect the scientific fidelity. What we do wish to consider, however, are the known limitations of this visual information channel and the effect the various nonlinearities, distortions, illusions, and so on have on our ability to accurately "perceive" the sought-after physical (or other) properties of the specimen and what we might do to overcome these limitations.

5.2. Some Perceptual Limitations and Artifacts Due to Prejudice

Before proceeding, it would be useful to review some prejudices we bring to bear when we "interpret" a micrograph. From birth, we are inculcated with visual information about our environment. This information is transferred into our brain via a pair of eyes; a nontrivial portion of our mind's processing of this information involves stereo perception. That is to say, we perceive our environment in three dimensions. Furthermore, we see things with only one magnification, which we call unity for obvious reasons. The sources of illumination are usually overhead—the sun and room lights. We are familiar with direct lighting (the sunlight on a brilliant clear day producing harsh shadows) and indirect lighting (the lighting on a cloudy day, with soft or nonexistent shadows). Most of us see things in color and all of us have a logarithmic response to the intensity of light. Much of the process is a "bootstrap;" we learn that certain aspects of images mean certain things and when a new visual scene is presented to our eyes we draw on past experience to "interpret" it.

All of us have been brought up with the photographic "process" as a part of our daily lives—magazines, movies, and TV, among others. These media project a three-dimensional world onto a two-dimensional surface and we must call upon stored information in our brains to reconstruct the third dimension. It is a well-known fact in mathematics that a higher dimensional space can be projected uniquely onto a lower dimensional space—but there is no way to uniquely reconstruct in the opposite direction. Often, ambiguity results. We call upon our "data base" far more than we realize to make "reality" out of a two-dimensional photograph. When we view an SEM micrographic representation of nature at high magnification, using monoenergetic fast electrons as an illumination source and secondary or backscattered electrons or characteristic x-rays as a signal, we must be very cautious how we apply a word like "reality." We as human observers have no direct experience under such circumstances. Consequently, we come with prejudices and preconceived ideas in our interpretation of a micrograph. We must constantly suppress our "sense of reality" and recognize that the only "reality" which exists in a micrograph is the physics which governed its production. To give an example, we inquire as to which side of a secondary electron micrograph is "up"? The usual SEM specimen does not have a side which we would call "the top." However, an observer of an SEM micrograph will invariably prefer one orientation very much over the other three possibilities. And almost all observers of the same micrograph will have the same preference.

The answer is simple. Our "real world" experience is overhead illumination and we have a strong desire for the orientation of the bright and dark regions of an image to lie in one direction. Illumination from below, for example, is not "natural" even though it serves the same purpose in permitting us to "see."

In some cases, the "sense" of topography can be reversed by merely turning the micrograph upside down (Heinrich, 1981, p. 509). Objects which appear concave can be made to appear convex and vice versa. This phenomenon carries over into the world of pictures of macroscopic objects. If a picture of a well-known personality is turned upside down, very few people can identify the person without a very long look, and even then they might misidentify the subject.

5.3. Some Perceptual Limitations and Artifacts of the Eye and Mind

When one region of a specimen emits twice as many characteristic x-rays, or twice as many backscattered electrons for example, as some other region, we would, in general, like to look at a micrograph made from one of these signals and know this fact. Indeed, in general, if there are any differences in the signal from one region of the specimen to other regions, we would like to *quantitatively* elicit this from an examination of the micrograph. Unfortunately, for the purposes of looking at micrographs, our eyes have a logarithmic response to the intensity of light, and, furthermore, our ability to see different shades or brightness simultaneously is restricted to less than about 120 levels for black to white images under ideal conditions rarely attainable (Foley and Van Dam, 1982). We note that when one views a micrograph (on photographic film) in a lighted room, one will see fewer distinct shades of gray than viewing the same image directly from a cathode-ray tube in a dark room (or from a projected transparency in a dark room). In the first case, we will generally see a maximum of 16–20 levels (depending on the type and quality of the film), and in the second case, something over 120 under certain conditions with not many more than about 20 of any real use. The effect is demonstrated in Figure 5.1, which was made by photographing a graphics display terminal connected to a digital computer. The computer can control the horizontal and vertical coordinates of the focused electron beam of the display terminal and it can discretely control the intensity of the electron beam (and hence the brightness of the display). In this particular display, there are 512 discrete horizontal points and 512 vertical points (a "point" is where the display beam briefly dwells before it is "instantaneously" displaced to the next "point"). The brightness of the display at each point is adjusted by the computer over 256 levels from full black (no light) to full white (display emitting maximum usable light). The 256 levels are due to the use of one computer "byte" (i.e., 8 bits) for

Figure 5.1. Intensity wedges. See text for details.

each point. The 256 levels in this particular display device are distributed linearly with respect to light output from the cathode-ray tube, i.e., level 200 at a given point emits twice as many light photons as another point at level 100. In the top third of the photograph, there are 64 equal-size rectangles with the brightness of each rectangle increased by 4 over the rectangle to its left. In the middle third, there are 32 equal-size rectangles with the brightness of each rectangle increased by 8 over the rectangle to its left. In the lower third, there are 16 equal-size rectangles with the brightness of each rectangle increased by 16 over the rectangle to its left. Within each rectangle, all points are emitting the *same* brightness. There are three important points to be made concerning Figure 5.1: (1) We cannot see all of the rectangles. (2) It is easier to tell one rectangle from another at the left side than the right side of the picture. (3) The rectangles in the lower third have a pronounced "venetian blind" appearance and do not seem to have uniform brightness. Each of these three points must be discussed since each can have a profound effect on our interpretation of electron and x-ray micrographs.

1. There is a limit to how many distinct levels of brightness we can perceive. When we observe photographic prints in a lighted room, the number of levels is determined more by the properties of the film than any limitation of the eye. When we directly observe the display tube in a dark room, the limit is determined more by the eye but is still finite.

Experience would lead us to believe that we could distinguish very many more levels than the values stated above. For example, on a brilliant day with the sun overhead, a typical illuminance would be 100,000 lumens/m^2. On a clear moonless night, the stars alone provide an illuminance of 0.0003 lumen/m^2. This is a dynamic range of some ten powers of ten. Clearly, then, we should be able to distinguish more than 20 or so levels of brightness! A moment's reflection reminds us that we do not *simultaneously* have this dynamic range. It requires many minutes to go from one extreme to another to permit the eye to "adjust." Under typical ambient conditions of illuminance, the hard fact remains—we can only usefully distinguish 20 or so levels. We stress this point because it determines the number of levels of information we can simultaneously "distinguish" coming from the specimen. If we wish, for example, to display an image derived from some elemental signal such as characteristic x-rays from a bulk specimen over the full range of possible concentrations (0–100%), each detectable level would correspond at best to about 5 wt%.

2. Our perception of light is logarithmic. Even over the limited range of light output of a display oscilloscope, the effect is very pronounced. Figure 5.2 is a plot which graphically shows this effect.

The horizontal axis is proportional to the number of light photons entering the eye and the vertical axis is proportional to the "perception" of this light. Since the slope of the curve increases as the amount of light entering the eye decreases, it stands to reason that the darker rectangles in Figure 5.1 will appear to be further apart in brightness than the brighter rectangles.

3. The last artifact, the perception of nonuniform brightness of uniformly bright objects, is due to the sharp transition from one rectangle to the next. The eye is more sensitive to those regions of an image where abrupt changes in brightness occur than to those regions where brightness changes more slowly. The exact cause of the effect is not completely understood. For a detailed discussion, see Ratliff (1972). Even though the cause of this perceptual artifact may not be understood, the results are dramatic and clearly have implications for interpreting micrographs, especially those which convey elemental concentration such as backscattered electron or x-ray micrographs. There are large classes and varieties of specimens which will produce sharp boundaries with uniform signal

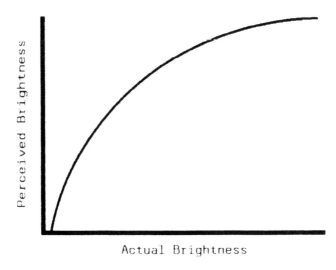

Figure 5.2. Plot of perceived brightness as a function of actual brightness.

on either side of the boundary. If it is important to the investigator to know even *qualitatively* that homogeneity exists on either side of a sharp interface, he cannot trust his eyes to provide the information.

For all of the above three reasons, quantitative information cannot be obtained unaided from the brightness information of a micrograph or display screen. Later we will show that quantitative information can be obtained from an image in other ways: line scans and histograms are two methods which will be demonstrated.

5.4. The Image Acquisition and Display System

In the conventional display system used on scanning electron column instruments, we move the electron beam over the face of the recording oscilloscope in synchronism with the beam over the specimen surface. When a detector in the vicinity of the specimen receives an increase in its signal (e.g., secondary or backscattered electrons or x-rays), the beam on the recording oscilloscope is increased in brightness. Consequently, an "image" is "painted" onto the face of the display tube. The synchronous beams are displaced by imparting horizontal and vertical velocity components V_x and V_y. V_x is typically between 500 and 2000 times V_y. The direction in which the velocity component is greater is historically called the line direction and the other direction is called the frame direction.

When the beam reaches the end of a line on the oscilloscope, it is inhibited from producing light (blanked), moved to the beginning of the next line, and the scan repeated. The "conventional" display system has been used since the earliest days of scanning electron column devices since only simple analog electronic devices are required.

An alternative method to continuous beam rastering is discrete rastering accomplished with what is usually called a "digital scan generator." In this technique, the x and y velocity components of the synchronous electron beams are not constant but remain zero for a finite period of time and then the beam is rapidly stepped to the next point. The displacements along the line direction are equal. When the end of the line is reached, the beam is moved back to the beginning of the line and displaced one step along the frame axis with the step equal to the line step. Each point in the image at which the beam dwells is called a "pixel." Digital scan generators as used in the SEM typically use between 500 and 4000 pixels along the frame and line directions. The digital method of scan generation is very convenient for applications with the digital computer. Images contain an enormous amount of information and so mathematical manipulations involving images require the use of a computer. It can be expected that the digital technique will replace the "conventional" method in most future microscopes. We are presently in a transition period.

The application of an on-line and interactive computer results in a substantial improvement in several key capabilities of the SEM. These capabilities derive mainly from the ability of the computer to record most of the information generated and detected when the primary electron beam interacts with a location on the specimen. Consequently, beam-induced radiation damage is minimized (an important consideration in biological or polymer applications). The recorded information may be modified, and most importantly, combined, in a great variety of ways before presentation to the operator-analyst; permitting structural and/or analytical information to be seen in a micrograph where none could be seen before.

Until quite recently, the majority of computer applications in electron or scanning electron microscopy involved the digitization of a micrograph recorded on a photographic emulsion. Such digitization (Saxton, 1978) is carried out by a device such as a rotating drum or flat bed microdensitometer or a flying spot scanner. Subsequent processing of the digitized image is carried out in a large central computer. It was obvious from the beginning that the output from a scanning mode microscope could be directly digitized. There have recently been several reports of such work now that computers with sufficient memory, mass storage, and speeds have become available at an acceptable cost (see, e.g., Strahm and Butler, 1979, 1981; Zubin and Wiggens, 1980; Llimas *et al., 1979*; Jones and Smith, 1978; Fiori *et al.,* 1981; Gorlen *et al.,* 1982, 1984; Leapman *et al.,* 1983). The floodgates are opening as cost decreases and computer power increases.

5.5. General Considerations for a Computer and Its Microscope Interface

We will describe the advantages of an "on-line" and "interactive" computer. By "on-line" we mean that the computer does more than just record and process signals produced by the microscope; it also actively controls how the signals are acquired. Once the analytical requirements have been specified by the operator, the computer controls, for example, the position of the electron beam, the acquisition parameters for the x-ray spectrometers (EDS or WDS), and gain and integration times of the secondary or backscattered electron detectors. By "interactive" we mean that the computer returns an answer quickly enough to be useful in the analytical strategy of the operator. For example, if the operator requires an x-ray analysis, the computer can process the acquired spectra to obtain elemental concentrations. Also, images may be processed by modifying or combining information content in such a way as to permit the operator to see features in the image that the unprocessed image did not reveal. The operator can utilize the results of such rapid calculations on data to decide whether a particular feature of a specimen should be further examined.

We need to clarify a possible confusion in terminology. An "image" ("micrograph," "picture," "area scan," among others) of an "area" is obtained by scanning the primary electron beam over a usually rectangular area of the specimen and changing the intensity of the electron beam of the display oscilloscope (which is scanning in synchronism with the primary beam) by a signal derived from some component of the beam–specimen interaction process. Confusion can result when more than one type of signal (e.g., secondary or backscattered electron, characteristic or continuous x-ray) is recorded simultaneously. We can now, obviously, have different "images" of the same area all derived from one and the same raster scan. Consequently, it becomes necessary to specify which signal (or combination of signals) was used and the area scanned for each "image." Indeed, in some situations it is desirable to record more than one regular scan of the same area to provide a measure of, for example, differential mass loss. It is then necessary to identify the raster scan in addition to area and signal.

5.5.1. Considerations for the Microscope

There are several features which are desirable to have on a computerized SEM; also, there are limitations of the microscope itself which need to be recognized in the design of the interface.

When the computer has completed a task, control of the microscope electron beam should be returned automatically to the conventional sweep circuits so that an image can be viewed on the microscope display. While the computer is processing data, the beam can be turned off to avoid unnecessary specimen irradiation. Devices which accomplish this are referred to as beam blankers and typically consist of an electromagnetic or electrostatic deflector located above the first condenser lens. These devices should be designed so that the electron beam can be moved on or off the specimen in a few microseconds or less. When the beam is moved back on the specimen, there should be no spatial hysteresis. Such beam blankers permit the use of a "pulsed tube" mode of operation in conjunction with the energy-dispersive detector (Jaklevic *et al.*, 1972). Pulsed tube mode EDS can increase x-ray count rates by as much as a factor of four. At the present time (1986), no implementations of this potentially powerful mode of imaging are known, and for no good reason.

Long data acquisition times (many hours) are sometimes required because of the nature of the samples being analyzed and the physical processes involved. If standards are being used in a quantitative scheme, significant periods of time might elapse between standard measurements. During these times, it is possible that the current in the electron probe will change and some measure of this change is required. A device which will accomplish this task is a small insertable Faraday cup located preferably just above the specimen or between the condenser and objective lenses after any beam-limiting apertures. This device can also serve as a slow beam blanker. Both the insertable Faraday cup and fast beam blanker are examples of what might be called "premium" accessories. That is, they are not yet on the standard accessory list of all microscope manufacturers but can be had at the time of initial purchase by "special" request (i.e., before final submission of a purchase order).

Computer control of the electron beam in the microscope is accomplished by the use of digital-to-analog convertors (DACs). Due to noise and magnetic and electrical nonlinearities in the microscope scan coil circuits, it is not meaningful to use DACs which convert more than 12 bits (Jones and Unitt, 1980). This conversion corresponds to a spatial resolution of one part in about 4000.

To avoid electrical ground loops, it is desirable to exclude the metal of the microscope column from any signal circuit. Consequently, it may be required to convert coaxial-type vacuum feed-throughs to triaxial or other multiple-pin types. Examples of signal lines for which this modification may be required include the solid-state detectors for backscattered electrons and the induced specimen current signal feed-through.

5.5.2. Considerations for the Computer

As is well known to this generation of workers adapting computers to the laboratory, the development of computer and related technology is proceeding at a staggering pace. As soon as a "state-of-the-art" device is announced, it is superseded. However, when one has work to be done and a need for some device to do this work, one has to select the best equipment affordable and proceed. A lot of good work gets done with "outmoded" equipment and one can console oneself that producing results is more important than finding design errors for the manufacturer of the "latest" state-of-the-art gadget. The following paragraphs describe equipment that is available at reasonable cost at this time (1986). It is a certainty that better devices will soon be available to do many of the things discussed below and so we have attempted to be as general as possible.

Image processing requires large amounts of main memory and disk storage. Even a simple operation such as subtracting one $512 \times 512 \times$ 8-bit image from another would require 512 kilobytes of main memory to hold the data. Many 16-bit minicomputers (the most ubiquitous variety at the time of writing) cannot be equipped with this much memory, and most of those which can must resort to address mapping tricks to access all of it. This situation exists because the instructions of 16-bit processors usually produce 16-bit addresses, which allows only 65K words or bytes of data to be accessed. Given this constraint, it is necessary for programs to operate on images in small pieces which must be moved between disk and main memory or in and out of a program's addressable memory. Even with these restrictions, a number of commercial products of great power exist at reasonable cost and performance. However, 32-bit computers with more than sufficient memory capability have recently become available at quite reasonable cost and speed; these are definitely more suitable for image processing.

Scanning a specimen in an SEM can produce a large quantity of data. For example, a 512 by 512 picture element scan of a specimen while collecting data from EDS, backscattered and secondary electron detectors would require multiple megabytes of disk storage for raw data. Depending on the nature of the various signals, different amounts and types of storage are required for the data. An absolute minimum amount of storage, at each pixel, in SEM applications would be 12 bits which corresponds to a resolution of one part in 4096. Other signals might require two full 16-bit "words" to store the data at each pixel in the image. Usually, these data will be stored on large-capacity disk units with either removable or fixed media packs. The latter units are often called "Winchester" disks and are presently available, for example, with 400 to 800 megabyte capacity for a total hardware cost of $15,000. Versions of 5–30 megabytes are available for several thousand dollars. These disks have an average access time of about 40 ms and can transfer or accept data at a rate of about a megabyte per second (i.e., about an image a second). These units are also used to store the "operating system" of the computer, user programs, and small data files. After the acquisition of only a few images, however, it becomes apparent that some form of main archival storage is required. Reel-to-reel nine-track tape drives (capable of storing on the order of 100 images) are excellent for this purpose ($15,000). Recently, "streaming" tape units and tape cartridges have become available at greatly reduced cost which are equally as effective, and more convenient, for archiving purposes. However, most computer centers have nine-track units and very few today (1986) have "streamers" or cartridge units. Standardization between the various computer manufacturers and, especially, peripheral manufacturers, is not very common.

An EDS or WDS x-ray spectrum can be mathematically described by a vector (one-dimensional array). Similarly, an image may be described by a matrix (an M by N dimensional array). There is a computer accessory, generally called an array processor, which can speed up operations on vectors and matrices by several powers of ten. For example, a typical array processor can perform a complex fast Fourier transform of a 1024-point x-ray spectrum in several milliseconds. The present cost of an array processor is approximately $5000–15,000. However, an array processor can be tricky to program.

Displaying digital images involves much more than exhibiting processed data on a screen. One should be able to alter contrast or brightness, perform pseudocoloring, annotate with arrows, text, and other graphical notation, superimpose graphs (line scans), outline areas of interest, zoom, pan, or combine several images. To have the central processor (CPU) of the main computer do these functions is slow and burdensome and difficult to program. The computer is unavailable for anything else while any of the above is being performed.

There are commercial products available which are usually called image display systems. These systems have enough memory to store multiple 512×512 or 1024×1024 by 8-bit images and a number of similarly sized several-bit overlays for alphanumeric and graphical information. Remember that 8 bits (i.e., 256 "levels") is totally sufficient for display purposes even though the data displayed, for example, were acquired with 16 bits of resolution (65,000 "levels"). It is a trivial matter to "map" the "acquired" resolution into the "displayed" resolution to display all, or only certain parts, of the data. Output can be produced on a standard red–green–blue (RGB) color monitor, refreshed at 30 frames/s directly from the display system memory. The main computer is free to perform other tasks, such as data acquisition, while all of the above-mentioned display functions are being performed on previously acquired images by the display system. The display system is also considerably faster at performing the above since there is usually special hardware included to make the display truly interactive with the operator. One such piece of hardware is an extremely fast integer array processor which operates directly on the 8-bit image planes. This processor can, for example, add one image plane to another in less than one frame time (i.e., 1/30 s). The cost of this "built-in" array processor is several thousand dollars. In the next section we will demonstrate a powerful application for such a processor.

At present, the cost of an image display system is between $20,000 and $50,000. Since a principal component of the cost of these devices is memory, the next few years should bring a reduction in price.

5.6. Color Display Systems

The motivation for the use of color in the display systems of scanning and analytical scanning electron microscopes is simple. Whereas a human observer can simultaneously distinguish no more than about 15–20 useful levels of monochrome light intensity, the same observer (who is not color blind) can distinguish 350,000 distinct colors. The latter figure is based on experiments where many pairs of colors are compared side by side by many viewers who are asked if the colors are different. When we intend to transfer information into the mind of the observer concerning the chemistry of the specimen under observation, we find that 15–20 levels is insufficient and 350,000 levels is excessive (the mind cannot make any sense out of that amount of information). The wide use of computer graphics has made it essential to understand color and gray scale. The theory of color is extremely complicated and is still a subject of intense research. There is still no one theory of human color perception that is universally accepted. The following paragraphs will highlight only these aspects which are germane to our subject. The development is derived from an excellent and considerably more detailed treatment of the theory of color by Foley and Van Dam (1982, Chapter 17).

Given a first exposure to the theory of color perception it is not unreasonable to think that we could specify any color by its wavelength and, perhaps, by its intensity. If we do this, we discover that many familiar colors such as brown, pink, and sky blue are not attainable. We find that it is necessary to add certain amounts of "white" to single-wavelength colors to achieve the "pastel" colors.

The average human eye is sensitive to electromagnetic radiation from about 700 nm (red) down to about 400 nm (violet). The "pure" (single frequency) colors that we can see range between these extremes from red through orange, yellow, green, blue, indigo, to violet. Since there exists a continuum of wavelengths between 700 and 400 nm, there are infinitely many colors, of which we have mentioned several of the well-known ones. But the vast majority of colors, the pastel colors, are not present. We now consider "colors" which are composed of more than one wavelength.

A typical spectral energy distribution from a light source might look like that shown in Figure 5.3.

The light source in Figure 5.3 is emitting a continuum of wavelengths in the visible part of the spectrum. Our perception of the light coming from this source is that it is one, specific color. An important point to remember is that another spectral distribution from another source (which could look completely different than Figure 5.3) could seem to us to be the identical color! That is to say, many different spectral energy distributions produce the same perceived color. It has been found that one way we can quantify the *visual effect* of any given spectral distribution is with three quantitites called hue, saturation, and brightness.

Hue corresponds to the *perceived* wavelength of the light source. We can think of the horizontal axis of Figure 5.3 as being hue. *Saturation* corresponds to the proportion of pure light of the perceived wavelength (hue) and white light needed to define the color. A completely pure color, which is 100% saturated, contains no white light. A half-and-half mixture would be 50% saturated. White light and hence all gray levels are 0% saturated. *Brightness,* as might be suspected, corresponds to the intensity of the light.

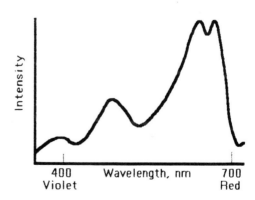

Figure 5.3. Typical spectral energy distribution. We perceive this source as having one, well-defined, "color."

Figure 5.4 is an idealized diagrammatic representation of a spectral distribution, which, like that in Figure 5.3, will be perceived by the observer to have a unique wavelength, the "perceived wavelength," and a "pastel" appearance due to the presence of "white" light. The "white" component is represented by the unform distribution at level L1 of all wavelengths in the visible part of the spectrum (erroneously assuming a uniform sensitivity of the eye between 400 and 700 nm).

It is agreed that the human eye has three sets of cones in the retina, each set of which has a relatively broad spectral response centered about the three wavelengths (hues) coresponding, approximately, to red, green, and blue (Figure 5.5A). It is interesting to note, however, that there is no histological confirmation of the existence of more than one type of retinal cone.

This observation forms the basis of the tri-stimulus theory of color and is the primary reason that color cathode-ray tubes (CRTs) have three electron guns each of which excites a phosphor emitting a narrow distribution of light having a wavelength centered at either "red," "green," or "blue." We note from Figure 5.5A that the eye is relatively insensitive to wavelengths in the region around blue. The sum of the three response curves, one for each type rod in the eye, gives the eye's response to a constant-intensity light while we change the wavelength of the light. This response is given in Figure 5.5B.

It turns out that by adding together different amounts of the three hues red, green, and blue, we can generate most of the colors to which the eye is sensitive (including white). Not all colors are attainable but there are certainly enough to convince people to buy color TV sets. The fact that we cannot achieve with a standard RGB display all the colors which the eye is capable of seeing has no relevance for applications in scanning and analytical scanning electron microscopy. Later in the chapter we will comment further on the use of color in our field.

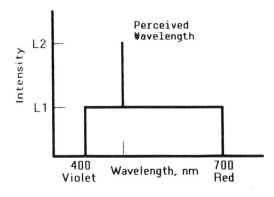

Figure 5.4. Idealized diagrammatic representation of a spectral distribution showing the "perceived wavelength" and a "white" component, responsible for the "pastel" colors.

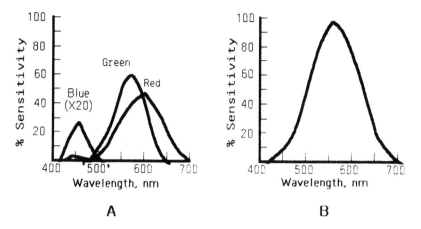

Figure 5.5. (A) Relative sensitivitiy of the three types of cones of the eye. (B) Response of the eye to equal intensities of light of different wavelengths.

5.7. The Photography of Color Displays

Until recently, the usual procedure for getting computer graphics onto photographic film was to use a hood which fits over the display terminal, blocks out ambient light, and positions the camera the proper distance from the display tube. There are several drawbacks to this procedure none of which prevent its use. The usual CRT used in display terminals has a curved surface. This curvature does not create problems when the tube is observed directly but does create a pronounced distortion when the image is directly focused onto flat photographic film. It is also difficult to avoid "darkening" at the corners of the photograph.

There are incompatibilities between the wavelength of the emitted light from the display tube and the spectral sensitivity of color film. The "purity" of the red, green, and blue guns of the display tube is usually poor. If just one of these guns is turned on, it would be expected that only that color would be emitted from the tube. In reality, a nontrivial amount of the other two colors leaks through. The effect of the leakage is unexpected colors produced on the film from what one "saw" on the display screen. For example, red can become orange. Or any pure color that strongly exposes the film will produce "white," which would be impossible if the primary colors were pure. The best color pictures are produced when the film is triple exposed one exposure for each primary color, individually displayed, with an appropriate color filter between the CRT and the camera. Lastly, the hood procedure is inconvenient.

Recently, these problems have been corrected in a relatively inexpensive ($2000–$6000) accessory called a CRT film recorder. These film recorders accept analog RGB signals in parallel with the display monitor. The RGB signals are displayed sequentially on a flat-face, high-resolution black and white CRT sealed within the unit. A fixed camera faces the monochrome tube, and a rotating color wheel with red, green, and blue filters matched to the characteristics of color photographic film is placed between the camera and the tube.

The camera photographs three exposures for each color image. The monochrome CRT displays the R information, the red portion of the filter rotates into place, and the camera records the red data. The display then brings up the G signal, the green section of the wheel moves into position, and the green signal is recorded on the same exposure. Finally, the procedure is repeated for the blue signal. There is generally a small, integral, dedicated computer or digital programmer which will correctly expose the film for each color and will do this for a number of different film types and formats.

5.8. Satellite Processors

Positioning the microscope electron beam, controlling the various detectors, and reading data from the analog-to-digital convertors during data acquisition are time-consuming tasks that are uneconomical to perform with a minicomputer. There are at least two efficient ways to handle these tasks: build special-purpose hardware or program a satellite microprocessor (a microcomputer) to do these jobs. Special-purpose hardware permits faster acquisition of the various signals, but a programmable microprocessor is substantially more flexible. The satellite processor will have a reasonable amount of its own memory (e.g., > 64 kilobytes) and a high-speed parallel link into the host computer. A typical transfer rate would be 150 kilobytes/s. The link is used to load the microprocessor with any one of a large number of possible data acquisition programs, depending on the mode of operation desired. The microprocessor acquires data which are sent in large blocks over the link to the host computer where they are processed and/or stored.

A computer system such as described will undoubtedly be asked to perform many functions in the laboratory: support applications program development, monitor instrument operating conditions, acquire and process data, display results, and play "Zork" and "Pacman." It is frequently desired to perform several of these concurrently; to simplify this job, it is desirable to use a multitasking/multiuser operating system. This would allow data to be processed (a CPU-intensive task) while acquiring new data (an I/O-intensive task) from the microscope. We will describe in the next few sections several powerful procedures which utilize an on-line and interactive computer.

5.9. Ways to Obtain Quantitative Intensity Information from Digital Images

Several times in the preceding sections we have commented that it is impossible to obtain quantitative intensity information from direct observation of a micrograph or display screen. We noted such problems as the logarithmic property of the human eye and "edge enhancement" effects. What is required is a way to transfer information into the brain in such a manner that bypasses the part of the "information channel" responsible for nonlinear effects. The most obvious way to unambiguously transfer intensity information is to print out a column of "three-tuples," i.e., the x and y coordinates of each pixel in the image and the corresponding numerical value of the "intensity" of each pixel. Considering that some images could easily have on the order of a million such "three-tuples," it is obvious that this form of data presentation, while absolutely unambiguous and quite thorough, it also essentially useless. We will discuss several "data presentation" procedures in the following paragraphs which have proven to be simply implemented and practical in SEM applications. The field of display technology is relatively new and we can expect profound changes in the coming years. Even now, for example, there are commercially available three-dimensional color displays using vibrating mirrors. However, these are temporarily out of the price range of the usual SEM application.

5.9.1. Line Scans

Let us take an SEM image and draw a straight horizontal line through any part of it. The resulting line will consist of a row of pixels all having the same "y" value. We could now plot on a piece of graph paper, if we were so inclined, the intensity in each pixel along the line as a function of the x coordinate of that pixel. For historical reasons, we will call such a plot a "line scan." We have transformed, for one line of the image, information which otherwise would have entered our mind as "brightness" information into "vertical displacement" information. There are several significant advantages which accrue from this transformation. To begin, the information reaches our mind via a linear path. The eye does not take the logarithm of the information and there are no "edge enhancement" artifacts at sharp transitions. The information is quantitative, especially if we label the axes of the plot with meaningful numbers. We may see more than the 20 or so levels we would see if the information had been transferred as "brightness." Indeed, if the plot is spread out sufficiently in the vertical direction, it is possible to see hundreds of levels. It is usual practice to superpose the plot onto the micrograph itself. This procedure permits the mind, using the information it knows absolutely from one line in the image, to extend this knowledge to neighboring lines and even other regions of the image.

It is, of course, unnecessary to restrict the direction of the line scan to the horizontal. The "line" can have any angle through the micrograph. The set of pixels which define the "line" we will call the "locus" of the line scan. The width of the plot is the horizontal width of the locus. The actual superposition of the locus on the micrograph tells us where the data for the plot have come from. The plot itself can be located anywhere on the micrograph. If the angle of the locus with respect to the horizontal is greater than 45°, the plot can be rotated 90°. Consequently, the length of the plot will not be reduced by more than 30% at most. An example of this type of line scan will be presented later (Figure 5.16).

The "line scan" we have just discussed assumes that we have a digital image already in computer memory and that the data for the line scan come from this image. Sometimes a particular signal, such as an x-ray signal, is so noisy that it is not possible to obtain a meaningful image. If another signal, such as secondary or backscattered electrons, is available from which it is possible to make an image, we can use the "line scan" in another way. The data for the line scan are obtained by causing the electron beam to move along the locus in a separate "acquisition" of the "noisy" signal from that required to obtain the image signal. The time spent acquiring data along the locus is relatively long and might exceed substantially the time required to obtain the image itself. The resulting "line scan," with greatly improved statistics, is superposed onto the "image" just as above. The amazing processing capabilities of the mind then "merge" the information content of both signals in such a manner that is more meaningful than viewing either signal separately.

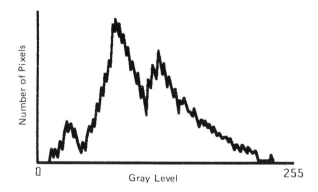

Figure 5.6. Intensity histogram of an image exhibiting three regions of distinct brightness level and good usage of the available display range.

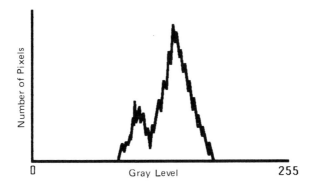

Figure 5.7. Example of image histogram indicating inadequate usage of the available display range.

5.9.2. Image Intensity Histograms

An intensity histogram of an image, or some part of that image, displays on the horizontal axis the intensity value, and on the vertical axis the number of pixels which have a particular intensity value. Image histograms are a particularly effective way to transform and condense an important aspect of the information content of an image and present it in an easily digestible form for the human mind. The abscissa of the image histogram is usually presented in units of the "display" scale (e.g., 0 to 255 which represents full black to full white of a standard display monitor). Figure 5.6 is a diagrammatic representation of such a histogram.

An image histogram of an excessively dark image will indicate this fact, as an example, by having a large peak in the lower gray level range. If the image data have been incorrectly acquired or inappropriately mapped into the display range, these facts will manifest themselves as excessive numbers of gray levels being unused. In Figure 5.6, there are relatively few (i.e., acceptably few) grays at the very darkest and brightest levels which are unused. Figure 5.7 is an example of an image histogram indicating inadequate usage of the display range.

Before proceeding with the various operations—generally referred to as histogram modification—it will be useful to clarify some potentially confusing terminology.

In much of the current literature on the subject, one finds statements such as "histogram modification," "histogram equalization or normalization," "histogram stretching," "histogram hyperbolization," and so on. These statements do not reflect what actually occurs and are, frankly, misleading. A histogram is merely one way to plot a data set. In our case, the data set resides in a computer memory. However, what we are concerned with is the histogram of what actually is *displayed,* i.e., the *image histogram.* It is possible with most display systems to read a particular memory location in the computer and by means of a look-up table assign this value to a particular intensity to be displayed. This operation is performed time-serially at each pixel in the image and does not alter what is stored in computer memory. The look-up table method can perform very rapidly such operations as contrast reversal (what is dark becomes bright and vice versa), "gamma" corrections such as exponentiation or logarithmic transformations, and so on. Consequently, the "image histogram" we "see" and work with in a display system usually does not have a data set in computer memory.

We now consider the various things that can be done to an image by working with its histogram. We will use the terminology that is already firmly established.

5.9.3. Histogram Stretching

Histogram stretching consists of assigning the darkest pixels in an image to pure black and the brightest pixels to full white (or full pure color if a color display is being used). Intermediate intensities are linearly varied between these extremes. The result of this particular operation is to fully utilize the available intensity range of the display system.

5.9.4. Histogram Normalization

When an image has a preponderance of pixels having nearly the same intensity, as manifested by a histogram with a particularly large and narrow peak, it is sometimes beneficial to "normalize" the histogram. To accomplish this operation, we define a transfer function, $H(k)$, as

$$H(k) = \frac{1}{T} \sum_{i=0}^{k} n_i \qquad (\text{for } k = 0, \cdots, 255) \qquad (5.1)$$

where T is the number of pixels, k is the original pixel value, and n_i is the number of pixels with intensity i.

The result of this transfer function is a new image (and histogram) such that pixel intensities are as evenly distributed as possible. It should be noted that $H(k)$ is the normalized cumulative histogram of the original image. Indeed, if the original histogram was a continuous mathematical curve, then $H(k)$ would be its integral.

5.9.5. Density Slicing

Density slicing is a display option where only those pixel intensities between certain values are displayed. Intensity values that fall outside of the specified range are set to full black. This operation is used to highlight structures in an image that have certain intensities and eliminate other details which might interfere with interpretation. A variant of this option sets the pixels within the chosen intensity range to full intensity.

5.9.6. Primary Coloring and Pseudocoloring

Primary coloring consists of assigning a primary color (red, green, or blue) to a particular signal, such as three different characteristic x-ray signals. Pseudo-, or "false," coloring consists of taking a single signal and assigning different intensity ranges of this one signal to a particular color selected from a continuum of colors. In its most commonly used form with inexpensive color display systems, only hue is varied and the "colors" are fully saturated with full intensity.

The basic idea of using an additive combination of several x-ray area scans in a multicolored image came from Duncumb (1957). A number of others have used color to display x-ray micrographs using various techniques (Fiori *et al.,* 1981; Gorlen *et al.,* 1982, 1984; Leapman *et al.,* 1983; Jones *et al.,* 1966; Statham and Jones, 1980; Pawley and Fisher, 1977; Ficca, 1968; Ingersol and Derouin, 1969; Yakowitz and Heinrich, 1969; Heinrich and Fiori, 1984).

The power of primary coloring lies in the fact that three (or only two if so desired) "images" are superposed over each other. Two important advantages accrue from this superposition. First, it is easy to see spatial correlations between the signals. Second, if the signals remain in fixed proportion to one another over regions of the "image," this is evidenced by a unique color in these regions. Since the eye is extremely sensitive to small changes in color, the technique is well suited to reveal, for example, mineral phases in geological specimens, or intermetallic phases in metallurgical specimens. Primary coloring produces the full continuum of colors since hue, saturation, and intensity are varied.

The power of pseudocoloring lies in the fact that the eye can discriminate more colors than it can intensities. For those display systems which can only vary hue, it is possible to display the signal with approximately 128 fully saturated and intense colors. If the image is, for example, a secondary electron micrograph of a three-dimensional object with pronounced "topography," the resulting pseudocolored image will fail to provide the impression of "depth" and may be difficult or impossible to interpret. Pseudocoloring with control over intensity and saturation will reduce or eliminate the deficiency (Heinrich and Fiori, 1984). The latest display systems in our field are beginning to include this capability. Later in this chapter we will present examples of primary and pseudocoloring.

5.10. Transformations for Electron and X-Ray Micrograph Processing: The Contrast Problem

As we have mentioned several times, a recurring problem in the making of a scanning electron micrograph is the fitting of the image signal into a range of intensities which will correctly expose the film in the display camera. In the conventional technique, the brightness of the oscilloscope beam is modulated over a range of gray tones, from black to white, in such a fashion that the gray level of the image is a monotonic function of the corresponding signal level. If the span of signal intensities within an image is contained within this range of gray tones, then small variations of the signal intensity may not be observable in the image. Alternatively, one can adjust the image signal intensity in such a way that the range of gray levels covers less than the full range of signal intensity. In this case, small intensity variations of the signal are enhanced, but picture areas in which the signal intensity exceeds the available grayness range will appear either white or black. The operator can thus choose between low contrast over the entire range of signal intensity, or high contrast within a restricted range of signal intensity. The problem just posed is, of course, not unique to electron micrographs and plagues many applications of photography. A number of procedures and algorithms have been devised over the years and a large body of literature exists on the subject. In our own field, most commercial electron column instruments have analog controls which implement a "gamma" correction (Fiori *et al.*, 1974a), the "derivative" correction (Heinrich *et al.*, 1970) whereby the original signal and its first time derivative are mixed together, and the homomorphic filter correction (Baggett and Glassman, 1974) which is commercially available from one manufacturer of accessories.

What we discuss here is motivated by the successful application and wide acceptance of the derivative methods in our field and by certain constraints imposed by the typical computer used to acquire and process x-ray and electron micrographs. There are certainly more flexible methods, e.g., Fourier transforms, but speed is a primary consideration. With the size of the digital images we consider, i.e., up to 512×512 pixels, computation times for a Fourier transform procedure can exceed several minutes—when all is said and done—for a single image even with the fastest laboratory computer available today. An integral component of many commercial image systems is an array processor which operates directly on the image planes. This class of array processor will not do Fourier transforms but will perform any of the mathematics discussed below in several seconds per 512×512 image. We discuss here certain image transformations which are sufficiently powerful to accommodate the contrast problem stated above and are fast enough to be considered "interactive" with the current generation of laboratory computer, and are based solidly on known properties of the human visual perception system.

5.10.1. Some Preliminaries

The following definitions will be required in the development.

Homogeneity: If a transformation is independent of translation of the coordinate system, i.e.,

$$F(x, y) = Tf(x, y) \Rightarrow F(x + x', y + y') = Tf(x + x', y + y') \quad (5.2)$$

for every (x, y) and $(x + x', y + y')$ in the domain of definition, then the transformation is said to be homogeneous.

Isotropy: If a transformation is homogeneous and satisfies

$$F(x, y) = Tf(x, y) \Rightarrow F(x', y') = Tf(x', y') \quad (5.3)$$

where

$$x' = x \cos\theta \mp y \sin\theta + k_1$$
$$y' = x \sin\theta \pm y \cos\theta + k_2$$

for every (x, y) and (x', y') in the domain of definition, then the transformation is said to be isotropic.

Linearity: A transformation is linear if it satisfies

$$T(k_1 f_1 + k_2 f_2) = k_1 Tf_1 + k_2 Tf_2 \quad (5.4)$$

where k_1, k_2 are arbitrary constants and f_1, f_2 are arbitrary functions.

Homogeneity is implied from isotropy but not vice versa. Isotropy does not imply linearity or vice versa.

Isotropy is an especially desirable (but certainly not required) property for an image transformation to possess. Clearly, for most applications in SEM, any transformation which is invariant to image shift or rotation is easier to interpret than one which is not. Indeed, isotropy corresponds to the property of human vision whereby an image which has been shifted and rotated remains the same except for the shift and rotation.

While isotropy is a desirable property, anisotropy is not necessarily undesirable. Indeed, shadowing in the emissive signal in the SEM enhances the spontaneous "three-dimensional" effect in a two-dimensional image. Anisotropy which results from specimen geometry and/or signal collection effects is an inherent feature of the SEM imaging process.

An SEM photomicrograph may be mathematically described in the following way. Let the surface of the micrograph be a cartesian plane (x, y) bounded by the edges of the micrograph. The subject of the micrograph can then be considered a scalar function, $f(x, y)$, having a domain consisting of the set of all valid (x, y), and a range consisting of the set of all gray levels between full black and full white. We will assume in the following discussion that $f(x, y)$ is well behaved and contains no singularities, i.e., we will not consider the digital nature of the image. We will include in a later section several discrete approximations to continuous derivatives which, in the context of our application and requirements, are more than sufficient.

5.10.2. Derivative Transformations

We have observed that in fitting the image signal into the range of usable gray levels for a correct film exposure the operator can choose between low contrast over the entire range of signal intensity or high contrast within a restricted range of signal intensity. This dilemma can be avoided if one modulates the brightness of the display not by the original signal but by a derivative of the signal. Modulation of brightness by the derivative signal produces an image in which all areas of constant signal have the same gray levels regardless of constant signal intensity. Pure derivatives of SEM images, however, do not give the usual impression of depth, since the static levels of the signal which provide general shading are no longer distinguishable from each other. For this and other reasons to be discussed, it is better to mix, in variable proportions, depending on the subject and purpose of the image, the original signal with the derivative signal. The major reason for mixing the derivative with the original signal is to reduce large gray level differences in the image and to provide increased contrast in regions of rapidly changing signal level. Figure 5.8 demonstrates this effect. Figure 5.8A is the original image with regions conceded to saturation in full white and black in order to see detail in the middle intensity regions. Figure 5.8B is the first space derivative with respect to the x axis of A. Note the "flattening" effect of the transformation, but detail over the entire image is seen. Figure 5.8C is a mixture of A and B. Note the restored perception of depth and the greatly improved

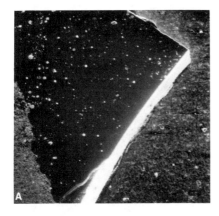
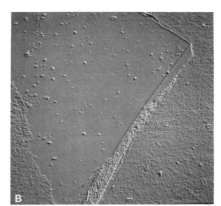
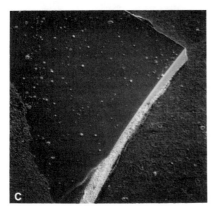

Figure 5.8. (A) Example demonstrating difficulty in fitting the image signal into the range of usable gray levels for a correct film exposure. The operator can choose between low contrast over the entire range of signal intensity or high contrast within a restricted range of signal intensity. (B) The first space derivative with respect to the x axis of A. Note the "flattening" effect of the transformation, but detail over the entire image is seen. (C) A mixture of A and B. Note the restored perception of depth and the greatly improved visibility of detail over the entire image.

visibility of detail over the entire image. We will consider first the "pure" derivative operators of the image function.

5.10.3. The First Derivative

Consider the first derivative of the image with respect to the x (line) axis,

$$F(x, y) = \partial f(x, y)/\partial x \qquad (5.5)$$

where $F(x, y)$ is the differentiated image. This transformation is anisotropic in that a rotation of coordinates of $f(x, y)$, i.e., rotating the specimen with respect to the scan frame or electronically rotating the scan frame relative to the specimen surface, will change the value of $F(x, y)$ at any (x, y). Indeed, all detail parallel to the scan line is lost in such a purely derivative image and all detail at an angle θ relative to the scan line produces a derivative signal multiplied in intensity by a factor of sin θ from that value when the detail is perpendicular to the scan line. Consequently, the nature of the derivative image is a function of the orientation of the specimen relative to the scan line. The derivative image will appear to be obliquely illuminated by a single point light shining along the x axis. If the original subject of the micrograph were three dimensional, i.e., a secondary electron micrograph of an irregularly shaped object, the derivative image will appear "flattened." This is the derivative operator used for years in many commercial electron column instruments (Fiori *et al.,* 1974a,b; Heinrich *et al.,* 1970).

5.10.4. The Space Gradient

If we add the effects of the first derivatives with respect to x and y, we obtain the gradient of the image function

$$F(x, y) = \partial f(x, y)/\partial x + \partial f(x, y)/\partial y = \nabla f \qquad (5.6)$$

The image transformation ∇f is also anisotropic. The subject will appear to be flattened—the effect very similar to that of the first derivative with respect to the x axis.

5.10.5. The Space Laplacian

The Laplacian operator ∇^2, sometimes called the curl operator, is defined as

$$F(x, y) = \nabla^2 f = \partial^2 f(x, y)/\partial x^2 + \partial^2 f(x, y)/\partial y^2 \qquad (5.7)$$

The spatial Laplacian, unlike the spatial gradient, is an isotropic image operator. The transformed image will appear to be vertically illuminated from a point source.

5.10.6. Isotropic, Nonlinear, Differential Operators

It is also possible to define an isotropic, but nonlinear, differential operator. Indeed, only even-order derivatives appear in isotropic linear differential operators. Odd-order derivatives can occur only in the form of their even functions. A good example is the square of the gradient

$$F(x, y) = (\nabla f)^2 \qquad (5.8)$$

This operator is nonlinear but isotropic and is useful, for example, in outlining the features of an image, and suppressing superfluous information, prior to determining the periphery, area, aspect ratio, and other parameters of these features. A reasonable approximation is to take the absolute value rather than the square. The resulting operator is only weakly anisotropic and strongly resembles equation (5.8) in effect. The absolute value operator is easier to implement than a squaring operator and is less prone to dynamic range limitations and saturation problems.

5.11. Application of the Derivative Transforms to the Contrast Problem

Now that we have demonstrated the effects of the pure derivative transforms, we return to the primary purpose of generating the various derivative signals, i.e., to mix them with the original signal. We will call this procedure derivative processing. The problem may be stated as

$$F(x, y) = K_1 f(x, y) + K_2 Df(x, y) \qquad (5.9)$$

where D represents a differential operator, K_1 and K_2 are scaling coefficients chosen by the investigator, f is the specimen function, and F is the derivative processed image. A basic characteristic of derivative processing is to apparently sharpen edge details in the image; some derivative operators are referred to as "crispening" operators in television technology (Goldmark and Holywood, 1951). Observers have an overwhelming preference for crisper images and thus some derivative processing may be esthetically pleasing (Goldmark and Holywood, 1951). However, crispening must be carefully evaluated with certain types of images so that false interpretation of specimen features does not occur. In general, crispening can be viewed as a beneficial or at worse, neutral, by-product of derivative processing. In television technology, a relatively small amount of first time derivative with respect to the horizontal direction is mixed back with the original signal to achieve the "crispening" effect. With derivative processing in our application the amount of derivative signal mixed back can considerably exceed the contribution of the original.

Image crispening parallels a process that is performed by our own visual system. When we view a scene, we perceive the intensity of light in a logarithmic manner compared to its actual intensity distribution at our eye. However, our visual system is more sensitive to the higher spatial frequencies of the image than to the low ones. Consequently, when we view an image we "see" the logarithm of the image with the higher spatial frequencies enhanced (Ratliff, 1972). Derivative image processing in many respects does the same thing and so it assists the human visual system. This effect plays a major role in the "venetian blind" appearance of Figure 5.1.

This is an appropriate point to consider the frequency distribution of micrographs from an SEM and microprobe. We proceed by noting that in terms of the spatial frequency distribution of the majority of images, the investigator is generally interested in the mid to high-mid components. The magnification of most micrographs is chosen to communicate information to the observer when the micrograph is held 1 or 2 feet away. Very fine detail in the image is not seen, and, indeed, if the investigator had been interested in the fine detail, he would have used a higher magnification in the first place. Consequently, high frequencies, whether from fine specimen detail or from quantum noise, can be filtered or "smoothed" from the image without serious loss of information. If low frequencies are significantly present they modulate the information we wish to see and in many cases obliterate the mid to the high frequencies at the bright and dark excursions of the low-frequency components. The low frequencies are often important components of the image since they communicate, for example, the perception of depth in a secondary electron micrograph. However, this same perception can be communicated just as well by suppressing to some degree the low frequencies and enhancing the mid to mid-high components. This is percisely what equation (5.9) can accomplish. Such a procedure is perfectly legitimate in the vast majority of cases where the investigator is concerned with the shapes and sizes of objects in the image and only secondarily with the quantitative distribution of brightness levels. As we saw earlier, quantitative information about the signal responsible for brightness is impossible to obtain directly from the photographic film or display tube. When the investigator requires numerical information from a digital image, he must use regional histograms or quantitative line scans. We must not make the mistake of thinking that by derivative processing an electron micrograph we are destroying some sacred "reality" of the micrograph. We are merely rearranging the information content in such a way as to more efficiently utilize the information bottleneck of the photographic film and the human eye.

5.12. Discrete Approximations to Several of the Derivative Operators

The derivative operators discussed above were developed in terms of continuous mathematical functions. However, when we scan the specimen surface with a digital acquisition system such as described earlier, we do not continuously sample the specimen surface. Rather we sample the specimen with a fixed number of discrete points arranged in a uniform array. All our mathematical operations must involve these points since values between them have no meaning (in terms of the original image). A great number of useful mathematical functions, including the above derivatives, may be approximated by the application of "kernel" operators (Pratt, 1978).

A kernel is defined (for our purposes) to be a square array of adjacent elements. We require (again for our purposes) that the array have an odd number of elements which means that there will be a "middle" element. The importance of this middle element will become apparent. We will call the value of each element the "weight" of that element.

We apply a kernel to an image in the following way. We "lay" the kernel on the image in one of its corners, say the top left, such that the top left element of the kernel is laying on the top left pixel of the image. We multiply the value of each pixel under the kernel by the "weight" of the corresponding kernel element. We then sum all the products, perform a suitable scaling, and place the resulting number in a new image at the pixel corresponding to the location of the center of the kernel. We then move the kernel one pixel to the right and repeat the process until we have progressed through the image and the kernel is located at the bottom right of the image. Obviously, the new image will be slightly smaller than the original. The original image is unaltered by this procedure. The "scaling" operation is usually done after the entire image has been transformed since it is impossible, in general, to predict the range of values which can result from a particular transformation. The sole purpose of the scaling operation is to fit the transformed image into the available display range. Those transformations which produce negative values, such as the derivative transforms, will also require a "shift" such that the middle range point of the display (e.g., "middle gray") will become "zero."

We catalog here the unscaled weights of several useful kernels:

$$\frac{\delta F(x, y)}{\delta x} = \begin{array}{rrr} -1 & 0 & 1 \\ -1 & 0 & 1 \\ -1 & 0 & 1 \end{array} \qquad \frac{\delta F(x, y)}{\delta y} = \begin{array}{rrr} 1 & 1 & 1 \\ 0 & 0 & 0 \\ -1 & -1 & -1 \end{array}$$

$$\nabla = \begin{array}{rrr} 0 & 1 & 2 \\ -1 & 0 & 1 \\ -2 & -1 & 0 \end{array} \qquad \text{i.e., the sum of the above}$$

$$\nabla^2 = \begin{array}{rrrr} 2 & 2 & 1 \\ 2 & 0 & -4 \\ 1 & -4 & -12 \\ 2 & 0 & -4 \\ 2 & 2 & 1 \end{array} \quad \begin{array}{rrr} 2 & 2 \\ 0 & 2 \\ -4 & 1 \\ 0 & 2 \\ 2 & 2 \end{array} \quad \text{or} \quad \begin{array}{rrr} 0 & 1 & 0 \\ 1 & -4 & 1 \\ 0 & 1 & 0 \end{array}$$

The 5×5 kernel is the convolution of ∇ with itself. Since ∇^2 is sensitive to any noise in the image, this version is more appropriate, than the 3×3 equivalent, under those conditions, e.g., x-ray images. To derivative process with this operator, the scaling coefficient K_2 is negative in equation (5.9).

It is possible to perform the effect of equation (5.9), with a Laplacian operator, directly with "chosen" values of the scaling coefficients which suffice for the "average" image. The kernel is

$$
\begin{matrix}
0 & -1 & 0 \\
-1 & 5 & -1 \\
0 & -1 & 0
\end{matrix}
\quad \text{or, similarly,} \quad
\begin{matrix}
-1 & -1 & -1 \\
-1 & 9 & -1 \\
-1 & -1 & -1
\end{matrix}
$$

These are also called "high pass" filters.

$$
\text{Sobel} =
\begin{bmatrix}
-1 & 0 & 1 \\
-2 & 0 & 2 \\
-1 & 0 & 1
\end{bmatrix}^2
+
\begin{bmatrix}
1 & 2 & 1 \\
0 & 0 & 0 \\
-1 & -2 & -1
\end{bmatrix}^2
$$

The Sobel kernel is similar to the absolute value of the del in that it is a "contouring," or "edge detecting," operator. A suitable approximation to the square of each component is to take the absolute value. This approximation works in many applications and is often easier to implement.

5.13. "Smoothing" Kernels

When a scanning electron micrograph is obtained under high-resolution conditions, the image is often modulated by noise. Similarly, x-ray micrographs are universally noisy due to the low quantum efficiency of the process. These SEM images often can benefit from the application of a "smoothing" kernel. The simplest of these is the so-called "block" kernel in which the center pixel under the kernel is replaced with an unweighted average of all the pixels under the kernel, e.g., for a 3×3 kernel

$$
\begin{matrix}
1 & 1 & 1 \\
1 & 1 & 1 \\
1 & 1 & 1
\end{matrix}
$$

The size of a block kernel can be any odd value greater than 3×3. A more useful set of smoothing kernels are the weighted variety such that the center value has the greatest effect. These are usually called "tent" kernels for an obvious reason. A 3 × 3 example is

$$
\begin{array}{ccc}
1 & 1 & 1 \\
1 & 2 & 1 \\
1 & 1 & 1
\end{array}
$$

The useful size of tent kernels in SEM applications can exceed 27 × 27. When the image-plane integer array processor described earlier is employed, such a large smoothing operation (which involves a staggering amount of arithmetic) will take only a few seconds. If such an array processor is not available, alternative procedures such as Fourier transform methods can be considered.

In general, the smoothing of images is the two-dimensional equivalent of smoothing an x-ray spectrum. And just as that tool has been considerably abused, we can only expect the same with image smoothing. Smoothing produces artifacts. Under the right circumstances (easily achievable in the SEM), smoothing can convert an image with "correct" but difficult-to-see information into an image with easy-to-see nonsense. However, under appropriate circumstances, smoothing can produce spectacular improvements in an image but the artifacts are always present. The difficulty often is in the display of the final image. We strive to get an acceptable balance between an improvement in the original image against the induced artifacts. Smoothing artifacts usually manifest themselves as a "wormy" pattern in the image with the width of the worms about the size of the smoothing kernel. Figure 5.9 is a series showing the effects of various size tent smooth operations. Figure 5.9a shows the original unsmoothed data. The original image is a 512 × 512-pixel computer simulation using an accurate Poisson random noise generator (Pun and Ellis, 1985). In this image, each pixel in the "background" has a mean of 50 counts and the "object" is a 50 × 50-pixel square with a mean of 52 counts per pixel. The contrast in Figure 5.9b–d is slightly enhanced to put an emphasis on the smoothing artifacts rather than the desired enhancement and visibility of the object. Figure 5.9b is a 3 × 3 smooth, c is a 9 × 9 smooth, and d is a 21 × 21 smooth. Figure 5.9e is identical to d except the contrast is adjusted to emphasize the "object" and suppress the "background." The "power" of smoothing is readily apparent. This final exercise of suppressing the "background" and enhancing the "signal" is very easy to do when one knows what it is one is looking for and very difficult to do when one does not. The acid test is, as always, to take several identical micrographs of the same area under identical conditions. If the smoothing operation produces the same result, then, obviously, one can believe the structure in the smoothed image. This is good

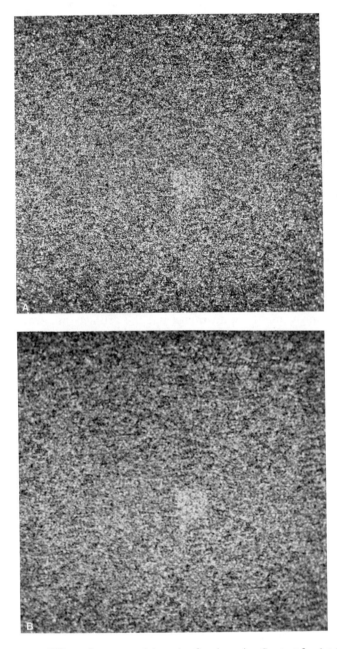

Figure 5.9. Effects of tent smooth kernels of various size. See text for details.

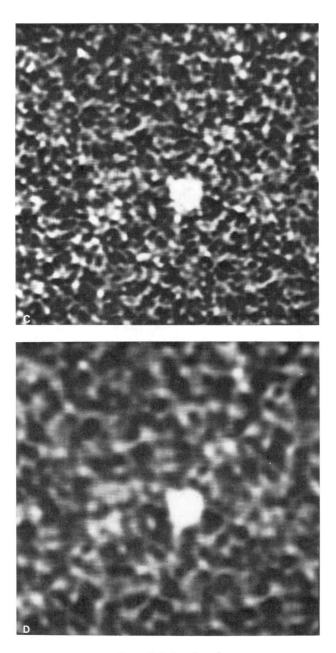

Figure 5.9 (*continued*)

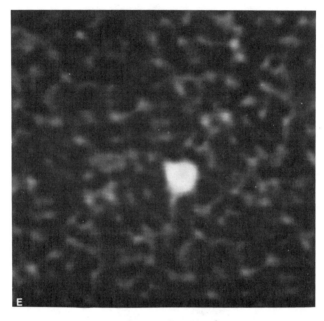

Figure 5.9 (*continued*)

advice to anyone using smoothing techniques for the first time (or the one-thousandth time). In general, the size of the smoothing kernel should be the same size, or somewhat smaller, than that of the image structure one is attempting to visualize.

Further useful references on the subject of this section are Moik (1980), Gonzalez and Wintz (1977) and Castleman (1979).

5.14. The Acquisition and Display of X-Ray Images in Scanning Electron Column Instruments

An x-ray image in the "conventional" SEM or electron beam x-ray microanalyzer is usually formed in a manner analogous to the secondary or backscattered electron images. A focused electron beam is scanned over an area of a specimen surface in synchronism with the electron beam of a CRT. The area which is scanned by the CRT beam is fixed (usually 10×10 cm) while the area scanned by the beam on the specimen surface is variable, resulting in useful magnification of typically 10 to 10,000 times when the specimen is "bulk." In an x-ray map from bulk specimens, the magnification is limited primarily by the size of the excitation volume.

The intensity of the beam in the CRT is modulated by the short rectangular voltage pulse caused by the detection of an x-ray photon. The effect of a pulse is to cause a single "dot" of light to appear on the CRT screen, hence the term "x-ray dot map." When an x-ray image is produced using an EDS in an analytical electron-column instrument, a potentially serious artifact occurs due to the poor peak-to-background ratio. The purpose of this section is to discuss this artifact and describe a procedure to reduce its effect to a negligible level (Fiori *et al.*, 1984). We will also discuss continuum correction when the detector is a WDS (Fiori *et al.*, 1984).

5.14.1. Statement of the Problem

X-rays result from two types of inelastic or energy-loss interactions between fast beam electrons and target atoms. In one case, a beam electron interacts strongly with a core electron and imparts sufficient energy to remove it from the atom. A characteristic x-ray is occasionally emitted when the ionized atom relaxes to a lower energy state by the transition of an outer shell electron to the vacancy in the core shell. The x-ray is called characteristic because its energy equals the energy difference between the two levels involved in the transition and this difference is characteristic of the element. By counting characteristic x-rays, we obtain a measure of the number of analyte atoms present in the interaction volume defined by the deceleration of the beam electrons in the specimen.

The second type of inelastic interaction occurs between a fast beam electron and the nucleus of a target atom. A beam electron can decelerate in the coulomb field of an atom, which consists of the net field due to the nucleus and core electrons. Depending on the deceleration, a photon is emitted which can have any energy ranging from near zero up to the total energy of the beam electron. X-rays which emanate due to this interaction process are commonly referred to as continuum or bremsstrahlung x-rays.

In the usual procedure of forming an x-ray image with the EDS system, two channels of the multichannel analyzer are defined as limits such that the channels between include slightly more than one-half the height of an x-ray peak of the analyte. Whenever an x-ray is detected and its resulting voltage pulse falls between the limits specified by these channels, a single pulse is sent to the display CRT to form a single "dot" of light. Any x-ray photon within the energy of interest, whether a characteristic or continuum x-ray from the specimen, or continuum from the environment, is processed since there is no way to tell one from the other.

When the height of a characteristic peak in an x-ray spectrum is in the same order as the height of the continuum at the same energy, it should be obvious that the contrast of the resulting x-ray image is as much a function of the physical processes responsible for continuum generation as it is of the desired characteristic generation. Consequently, a serious artifact can result which, in the worst case, manifests itself as a high-contrast x-ray image of an element which is not even present in the specimen. Indeed, any "bulk" specimen which has phases differing in average atomic number by more than several percent (depending on the number of x-ray counts in the image) can produce convincingly apparent images for any element the operator wishes. In the case of "thin" specimens, the problem is compounded since the number of generated continuum photons at any given energy is also proportional to the mass-thickness of the specimen.

5.14.2. Discussion

In the "conventional" x-ray dot map technique which has been used for years, we move the electron beam over the face of the recording oscilloscope in synchronism with the beam over the specimen surface. The synchronous beams are displaced by imparting horizontal and vertical velocity components, V_x and V_y. V_x is typically between 500 and 2000 times V_y. The direction in which the velocity component is greater is commonly called the line direction and the other direction is called the frame direction. When the beam reaches the end of a line on the oscilloscope, it is inhibited from producing light, moved to the beginning of the next line, and the scan is repeated. When an x-ray photon selected for mapping is detected from a location on the specimen, a bright dot appears at the corresponding location on the CRT. The dots comprising the image can be stored photographically, each dot saturating the film. Since the usual photographic film is capable of approximately 15 shades of gray from black to white, the dot map technique considerably underuses the capability of the film. Variations in the x-ray production and hence the analyte concentration can only be deduced from variation in the spatial distribution of the dots. This problem has long been recognized and very early on Heinrich (1962) developed an ingenious device called a "concentration mapper." This device essentially mapped two to ten predefined and known concentration ranges (in terms of x-ray count rate) into distinct gray levels by means of analog discriminator circuits.

As discussed above, there is an alternative to continuous beam rastering. Discrete rastering is accomplished with what is usually called a "digital scan generator." In this technique, the x and y velocity components of the synchronous electron beams are not constant but remain zero for a finite period of time and then the beam is rapidly stepped to the next point. The displacements along the line direction are equal.

When the end of the line is reached, the beam is moved back to the beginning of the line and displaced one step along the frame axis with the step size equal to the line step. Each point in the image at which the beam dwells is called a "pixel." For x-ray imaging purposes, it is common to use between 128 and 512 points along the "line" and the same number of lines in the "frame." It is desirable to have at least 8 counts, on the average, per pixel in the image (Eden, 1985). If this cannot be achieved, then fewer pixels (with a corresponding increase in acquisition time per pixel) should be used.

Discrete rastering is convenient for application with the digital computer. Since the area on the specimen surface is scanned point by point, in computer memory we can define this matrix of points as a two-dimensional array. If the beam remains at any given pixel long enough for a given beam current, beam voltage, and specimen type, it is probable that many pulses will be generated during the dwell time. These pulses can be counted and the value of the count stored along with the pixel coordinates. With appropriate circuitry, the counts in this array can be displayed at the appropriate coordinates on the CRT with the brightness at each point proportional to the number of counts. We will call such a display an x-ray intensity map (to distinguish it from the x-ray dot map). An intensity map can fully utilize the gray scale of photographic film. Figure 5.10 compares the acquisition of an x-ray image using both the "dot" method and the "intensity" method. The number of detected photons is the same in both cases. Note the considerably improved visibility with

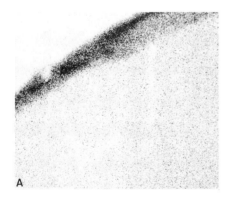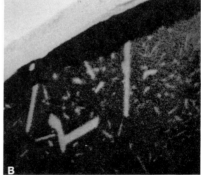

Figure 5.10. (A, B) The element being imaged is scandium using the K_α line at 4.088 keV. Scandium is not present in the specimen so the image is pure artifact with the contrast mechanism being average atomic number. (A) Dot map and (B) an intensity map; both images contain the same number of counts. Note the considerably greater visibility in the intensity map. The nature of the specimen will be explained in Figure 5.12.

the "intensity" map. The specimen is an iron and iron–aluminum alloy with intermetallic phases and the element being imaged is scandium using the K_α line at 4.088 keV. Since scandium is not present in the specimen, we know that the images are pure artifact; the contrast mechanism is average atomic number.

With discrete rastering and the digital computer to store and process the data, it is possible to produce an x-ray intensity map with the contribution of the background removed at each pixel. The following section will describe a procedure to accomplish this.

5.15. Methods to Separate the Characteristic and Continuum Radiation: EDS

Procedures that accomplish removal of the continuum contribution to x-ray EDS spectra can be classified into one of two catagories: modeling or filtering. Background modeling (see, e.g., Fiori *et al.,* 1976) consists of measuring a continuum energy distribution or calculating it from first principles and combining this with a mathematical description of the detector response function. The resulting function is then used to calculate an average background spectrum that can be subtracted from the observed spectral distribution. Background filtering ignores the physics of x-ray production, emission, and detection; the background is viewed as an undesirable signal to be removed by modification of the frequency distribution of the spectrum by digital filtering or Fourier transform methods.

Either continuum modeling or filtering will suffice for our purposes. However, a method that does not require an explicit model is more flexible and is clearly advantageous in applications such as imaging of irregular specimens and applications in the analytical electron microscope operating in the energy region above 50 keV. In the latter case, one can in principle calculate specimen continuum from a model. However, in practice the calculated continuum rarely accounts for the background since a significant proportion of the background does not originate from the impact point of the primary electron beam but rather from such sources as the specimen support or holder (Fiori and Newbury, 1981). Fiori *et al.* (1984) have described an imaging method using the top-hat digital filter.

The top-hat filter was first applied to energy-dispersive x-ray spectra by Schamber (1977). The algorithm is both simple and elegant; calculations can be performed very quickly by a computer. The latter point is extremely important since we require the calculations to be made on the fly at every pixel and within the pixel dwell time. Briefly stated, counts in a group of adjacent channels of a spectrum are "averaged" and the "average" assigned to the center channel of the group; the procedure is repeated at each channel as the filter is stepped through that part of the spectrum from which we wish to remove the continuum. One may describe the averaging by the following equation, using the notation of Statham (1976b):

$$y_i' = \frac{1}{2M + 1} \sum_{j=i-M}^{i+M} y_j - \frac{1}{2N} \left[\sum_{j=i-M-N}^{i-M-1} y_j + \sum_{j=i+M+1}^{i+M+N} y_j \right] \quad (5.10)$$

where y_i' is the contents of the ith channel of the filtered spectrum and y_j is the contents of the jth channel of the original spectrum.

The filter is divided into three sections: a positive, central section consisting of $2M + 1$ channels centered in turn at each channel in the region of interest, and two side sections each containing N channels. The average of the counts in the side sections is subtracted from the average in the central section.

The effect of this particular averaging procedure is as follows: If the original spectrum is curved concave upward across the width of the filter centered on a particular channel, the average will be negative; if the curvature is convex, the result is positive. The greater the curvature, the larger is the value.

In order for the filter to respond with the greatest measure to the curvature found in spectral peaks, and with the least measure to the curvature found in the spectral background, the width of the filter must be carefully chosen. For a detailed treatment of the subject, see Schamber (1977) and Statham (1976b). In general, we choose the width of the filter to be twice the full width at half the peak maximum amplitude (FWHM) of the x-ray peak being used for imaging, with the number of channels in the central section equal to the combined number of channels in the side section (see Appendix). Using the above filter dimensions with a standard-resolution EDS detector, it is possible to image the adjacent elements Mg, Al, and Si with negligible interference even when the adjacent element is the pure element and the imaged element is present at zero concentration.

The final step in the application of the digital filter is to extract a quantity which will be assigned to the coordinates of each pixel to represent the characteristic intensity. We choose the sum of the averages of counts in the central section computed at each channel in the filtered region since this quantity provides the highest peak-to-background ratio.

5.16. Deadtime Correction for Digitally Acquired EDS Images

The Si(Li) detector amplifier system produces an output pulse which can be many tens of microseconds long for each processed x-ray photon. Consequently, deadtime losses are high and we can easily attain a condition whereby the amplifier cannot process the detected x-ray photons fast enough and the output count rate for the analyte *decreases* for an *increase* in total input count rate. If we spend the same time at each pixel during the acquisition of an image under high count rate conditions, several bizarre artifacts can occur. A particularly insidious artifact is that regions of a specimen which contain higher concentrations of analyte can appear darker in the image than regions which contain less. This, and other contrast reversal problems, can be avoided by a simple logic gate whereby pixel dwell time is determined not by "real" time but rather by amplifier "live" time.

5.17. Methods to Separate the Characteristic and Continuum Radiation: WDS

Since the WDS is a single-channel device, it is not possible to obtain a measure of both continuum and characteristic signals simultaneously on the same spectrometer. However, there are several other ways to obtain a measure of the continuum. If time and radiation damage are not considerations, it is possible to sequentially record two images under identical conditions from the same spectrometer: one characteristic and one continuum. These images are then subtracted, leaving a net characteristic image. Before subtraction, it is best to "nearest neighbor" smooth the continuum image with, for example, a tent smooth.

Rather than record the two images separately, it is possible to interleave the acquisition such that the spectrometer is moved between characteristic and continuum wavelengths at the end of each "line" of the image—which is then repeated for the other signal. If the electron column has two spectrometers, it is, of course, possible to obtain a measure of the continuum for one spectrometer from the other. It is a trivial matter to scale the efficiencies of the two before the subtraction. The single-spectrometer approach has the significant advantage of viewing the specimen from a single direction. Specimen self-absorption effects will then be minimized. Whenever possible, the energy of the chosen continuum band should match as closely as possible the energy of the characteristic x-ray line.

If the second spectrometer is an EDS, the differences in deadtime correction must be reconciled. One of several ways to accomplish this is by dedicating a separate high-speed amplifier (< 0.5-μs shaping time) to the EDS channel. Since high count rate capability is the only requirement in the above application, loss of spectral resolution is not a problem. It is sometimes useful to place a beryllium or carbon absorber between the EDS and specimen to remove superfluous photons lower in energy than the measured continuum band.

Figure 5.11 is an example of a WDS characteristic image, continuum corrected from a simultaneously acquired EDS image. The specimen is from a human brain (the hippocampus) and the elements being imaged are aluminum [which is present *in the most intense* regions at approximately the 200–500 ppm level (dry weight after probe analysis)] and calcium (present in the most intense regions at approximately the 7000 ppm level) (Garruto *et al.,* 1984). The images were simultaneously acquired with 256×256 pixels over a 4-h period. The current was 2×10^{-7} A and the accelerating potential 15 kV. The specimen was nominally 20 μm thick mounted on a carbon substrate. In these images, it was extremely important to remove the possibility that the contrast was due to average atomic number or mass thickness effects and so a background correction was imperative. These remarkable images could not have been obtained with the "dot" map technique and, indeed, exploit both computerized acquisition and display, and the excellent current stability of the present-day electron column.

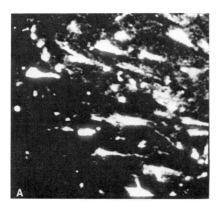
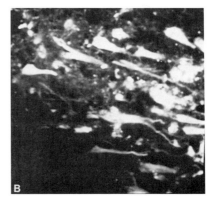

Figure 5.11. (A) Background-correcteed WDS Al image (200–500 ppm Al) from human brain, ¼ mm full field; smoothing was used here. See text for other details. (B) Same as A but Ca (present at about 7000 ppm). Both smoothing and Laplacian enhancement were used in this image.

5.17.1. Regional Variance in Background-Corrected Images

Background-corrected images remove the artifact due to average atomic number and mass thickness effects but, naturally, another artifact is created which is fortunately very much less serious. The background-corrected count at each pixel in the image is proportional to the elemental concentration at the corresponding point in the specimen. Since the average effect of the continuum is removed, its only contribution to the image is increased noise. If, however, the contribution of the continuum varies greatly from one part of the image to another, it would be expected that the variance, due to the continuum, in the corrected image will be greatest from those regions with the greatest continuum contribution. The effect is shown in Figure 5.12, which gives *digitally filtered intensity maps* of the same specimen and area as in Figure 5.10. Part "A" of the image is background-corrected aluminum, part "B" is background-corrected iron, part "C" is background-corrected scandium, and part "D" is background-corrected copper. Since scandium is not present in the alloy, we note that in the background-corrected image there is no "contrast" but there is increased variance correlated with those regions of the specimen with higher average atomic number. The increased "noise" in these regions attracts our attention to them but we are not inclined to attribute the presence of scandium, as we would in an image not background corrected such as Figure 5.10B. This "speckling" of an image is an unavoidable artifact and should not be a cause for concern. Indeed, once one understands the origin of the increased variance, the feature can be used as a tool.

5.17.2. Choice of Scale for Background-Corrected Images

When we remove the average effects of the background from a region of an image which does not contain the analyte, the mean count of the region is zero. A mean of zero implies that half the pixels have negative values. We would like to be able to assign the "zero" regions of an image to the darkest gray of the gray scale, i.e., "black." The observer can immediately interpret a region of dominant black as having no analyte. However, by this assignment we essentially "clip" the negative values since there is no shade of gray to assign to them. The net result of neglecting the negative values is to "bias" the regions which do not contain analyte to a mean which has a positive value. The greater the original variance, the greater will be this biased mean. An alternative procedure is to set the minimum pixel intensity in the entire image to be black. The latter method of setting the brightness scale of background-corrected images

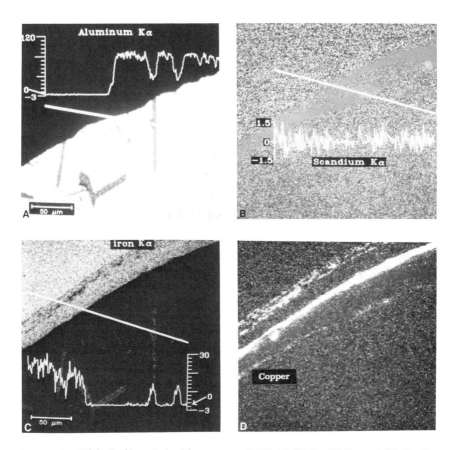

Figure 5.12. Digitally filtered, deadtime corrected, (A) Al, (B) Sc, (C) Fe, and (D) Cu. See text for details. Same specimen and area as Figure 5.10. The specimen is from a failed household electrical junction box. The iron-rich area is a part of the steel plate which held the Al wire, the Al-rich area is part of the wire (note the iron–aluminum intermetallic phase), and the copper region is from the coating on the plate. The line scan through the images shows the signal variance along the line. The numbers on the vertical axis represent counts per pixel. By the nature of the digital filter algorithm, the numbers are real rather than integer and have much less variance associated with them than their absolute value would suggest. Note that the mean is zero throughout the Sc image.

requires the author of the micrograph to identify those regions which are "zero" with some symbol on the micrograph or comment in the figure caption. The observer must then be able to interpret certain gray levels as representing zero and negative values but numerical information is not compromised.

5.17.3. Conversion of Background- and Deadtime-Corrected Intensity Maps to Quantitative Maps

The required first step in a traditional quantitative microprobe analysis of a single point on a specimen surface is to form a deadtime- and background-corrected intensity ratio of the counts from the specimen to the counts from a reference standard. After this ratio is formed (the ratio is traditionally called the k-factor or k-ratio), certain mathematical corrections are applied to it which account for specimen and standard matrix effects. It should be obvious that a similar procedure may be applied to the images we have been discussing. In general, however, the complete mathematical correction (e.g., a ZAF, Cliff–Lorimer, Hall, or other correction) would not be applied at each pixel in the image. A better procedure is to interpolate along a hyperbolic calibration curve. For a description of the hyperbolic correction for single points, see Heinrich (1981, pp. 208–216, 389, 405) which has been precalculated for various regions of the image.

We must consider the situation which will occur in images in which phases exist with mutually exclusive elements. In such situations, all elements occurring in the entire image should not be included in an analytical treatment at each phase in the image. This follows from a simple propagation of errors argument: one should not include elements known not to be present in, for example, a ZAF procedure.

5.18. An Example of Computer-Aided Imaging and Interpretation

We present in this section an x-ray imaging and interpretation example which utilizes many of the topics discussed in this chapter. The specimen is a polished meteorite section (carbonaceous chondrite) with many different silicate and metallic phases in the 1×1-mm area which was imaged. The accelerating voltage was 15 kV and the probe current (total current in probe) 1 nA. The acquisition time was 100 ms, detector livetime, per pixel (consequently the images are deadtime corrected). The images are 512×512 pixels. The detector was a 140-eV (at Mn K_α) Si(Li) energy-dispersive detector located 3 cm from the specimen at a takeoff angle of 40°. The elemental signals were continuum corrected at each pixel by the digital filter method described earlier. A total of 11 elements were imaged (Mg, Al, Si, P, S, K, Ca, Mn, Cr, Fe, Ni). It is clearly not possible to include here all the combinations of image processing which have been discussed. Those signals, however, which significantly benefit from a particular operation, or combination of operations, are demonstrated along with the untreated image.

The series of x-ray micrographs in Figure 5.13 are as follows: A is the Mg signal, contrast stretched to reveal as much structure as possible. B is the Mg signal but a 3×3 tent smooth and Laplacian enhancement applied. Note the visibility of structure at all levels of intensity. C is the Si signal, contrast stretched to reveal as much structure as possible. D is the Si signal, but with a 3×3 tent smooth and Laplacian enhancement applied. As with the Mg case, note the considerably greater visibility of detail at all levels of intensity. E is the Fe image, unprocessed, and F is the Fe image, smoothed and Laplacian enhanced. Note that Fe in the mineral phases becomes apparent in the enhanced image. G is the S image, smoothed. H is the K image, smoothed. I is the Ca image, unprocessed. Normally, the K_β line of K interferes with the K_α line of Ca. It is possible, however, to determine the degree of overlap in the digital filter procedure and subtract a fixed percentage of the K image from the Ca image. It is sometimes best to smooth the K image before the subtraction. This procedure is equally as effective in biological specimens where the K–Ca interference is a serious problem. J is the Cr image, smoothed. K is the Mn image, smoothed. Some smoothing artifacts are apparent. L is the Al image. No processing was required for Al due to its restricted dynamic range over the field and good signal-to-noise ratio. M is the P image, smoothed. No further processing is required since there is only one phase with P. Lastly, N is the Ni image, smoothed.

In interpreting these images, it must be remembered what the rational was in "processing" them. Since quantitative information cannot be obtained by direct observation of the intensity levels, we "process" to aid the visual system in seeing the structure, detail, and qualitative intensity information in the images. Contrast stretching, smoothing, and derivative enhancement are particularly effective for these purposes. To obtain quantitative intensity information from the images, we resort to line scans and regional histograms. Figure 5.14 is the same as Figure 5.13F, the Fe image, but with a line scan through some regions of interest. The data for the line scan came from Figure 5.13E, the "unprocessed" Fe image, but the line scan is superposed onto the derivative-enhanced image for purposes of clarity. The vertical axis is in terms of x-ray counts per pixel (as obtained by the digital filter operation described above) but can directly be turned into quantitative chemical numbers by reading the appropriate standards and performing the appropriate "correction" (e.g., ZAF or Bence–Albee) to the numbers on the vertical scale.

Figure 5.15 is, again, the same as Figure 5.14, but the quantitative information is obtained from a regional histogram. Unlike the line scan, the regional histogram provides numerical information about a region. The region can be any arbitrary shape or size, usually defined on the graphics monitor displaying the image by a "light pen" or "mouse" or a

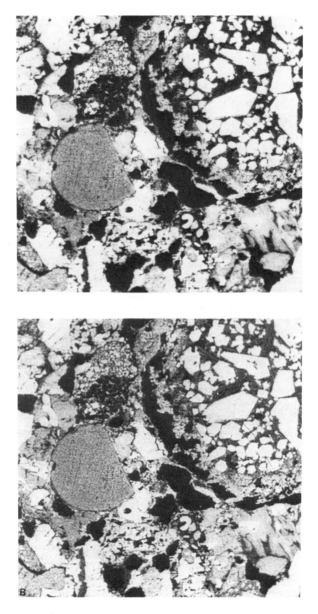

Figure 5.13. Series of elemental x-ray images of a carbonaceous chondrite meteorite. (Specimen courtesy of Kurt Fredriksson, Smithsonian Institution.) See text for full details. (A) magnesium, original; (B) magnesium, Laplacian enhanced; (C) silicon, contrast stretched; (D) silicon, Laplacian enhanced; (E) iron, original; (F) iron, Laplacian enhanced; (G) sulfur, original; (H) potassium, smoothed; (I) calcium, original; (J) chromium, smoothed; (K) manganese, smoothed; (L) aluminum, original; (M) phosphorus, smoothed; (N) nickel, smoothed.

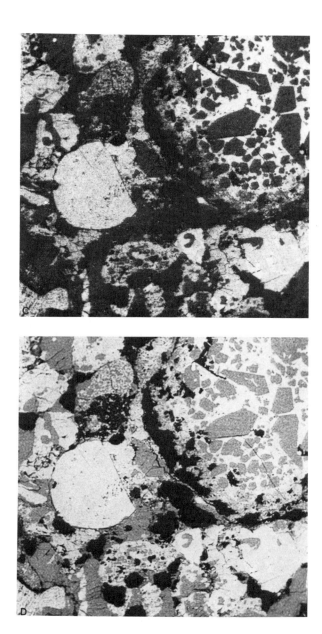

Figure 5.13 (*continued*)

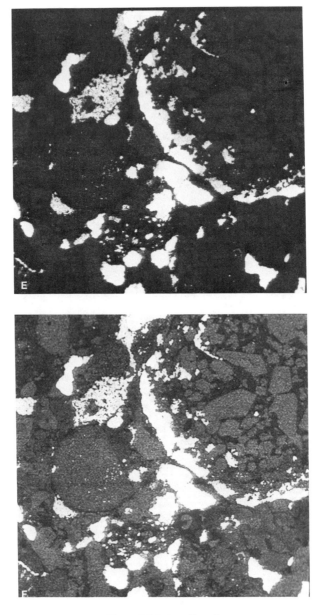

Figure 5.13 (*continued*)

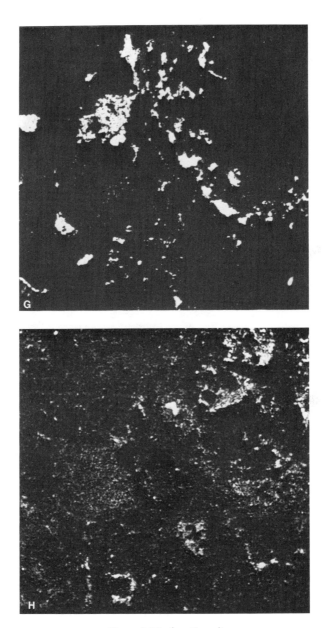

Figure 5.13 (continued)

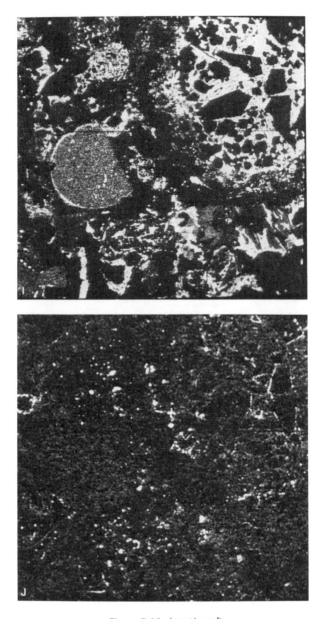

Figure 5.13 (*continued*)

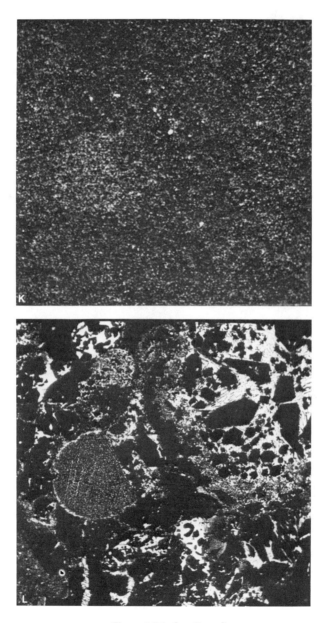

Figure 5.13 *(continued)*

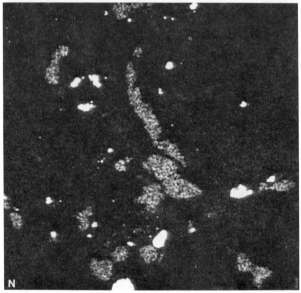

Figure 5.13 (*continued*)

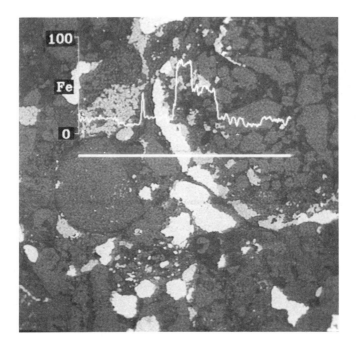

Figure 5.14. Same as Figure 5.13F, the Fe image, but with a line scan through some regions of interest.

"track ball." The histogram procedure sums up the intensity values from all pixels in the outlined region, divides through by the number of pixels, and reports the "average" intensity for the region. Other statistical information can be calculated and reported. A report "summary" can be written to a data file or over part of the image after the calculation and might include the area, circumference, aspect ratio, the mode, the mean, and higher statistical moments, and so on. This information is obviously available for more than one image plane. The actual histograms can also be superposed on the image as shown in Figure 5.15 for two "regions" identified by arrows.

The raw x-ray images of such a "busy" specimen as that in Figure 5.13 clearly demonstrate the difficulty of visualizing which elements coexist in various regions. Primary coloring is an especially effective way to clearly show how any two or three elements in a region of the specimen combine. If more than three elements are of interest, then multiple primary colored images can be created with one (or two) elements common to the images.

To help interpret the following primary color images, it is useful to

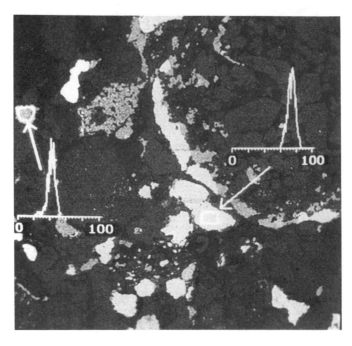

Figure 5.15. Same as Figure 5.14, but quantitative information is obtained from a regional histogram.

be familiar with the colors that result from mixing the three primaries. Figure 5.16 shows this relation. The figure is the so-called color triangle. Since the images are quantitative, it is possible to interpret the resulting colors in quantitative terms. The color triangle serves as a coarse "look-up" table for the relative concentrations of three elements. For example, if we have an alloy consisting of three elements "A," "B," and "C," we could assign pure "A" (represented by a display intensity of 255) to be full red, pure "B," similarly, to be full green, and pure "C" to be full blue. Then any possible phase consisting of a combination of these three displayed elements must lie inside the color triangle. We note that many colors are missing, such as cyan, magenta, yellow, and white. To understand why whole classes of colors are missing from this color triangle, we examine the requirements for pure "yellow." To make pure yellow, we must add together full red and full green—which would correspond to a region of the specimen which contains a phase of 200 wt% in this example. Similarly, "white" would require a region containing all three pure elements, or 300 wt%.

It is, of course, perfectly possible to achieve some, but not all, of the missing colors. An important point is that to achieve some of these "missing" colors we must sacrifice, or make physically unrealistic, other colors already on the color triangle.

Figure 5.17A is a primary color micrograph of the Mg (using Figure 5.13A), Al (using Figure 5.13L), and K (using Figure 5.13H) images. The Mg intensity information is used to modulate the brightness of the red gun in the display monitor, Al the green gun, and K the blue gun. Note the ease with which it is possible to verify how these three elements are distributed with each other and how distinct mineral phases which contain these elements form distinct colors. It should also be noted that none of the colors is fully saturated. That is, if there was a slight change in elemental concentration of any one of the constitutents, the color would vary in those regions where the concentration change occurred.

Figure 5.17B is the same as A except Si is red, Al is again green, and Mg is blue.

Figure 5.17C is intended to highlight the metal and sulfide phases. Fe is red, S is green and Ni is blue.

Figure 5.17D is the same as C but the Fe is Laplacian enhanced. All Fe phases including the mineral phases are visible in this image.

Figure 5.17E is the Si image (Figure 5.13C) pseudocolored. The Si intensity has been "contrast stretched" to fit the full display range of 0–255. The color assignment as a function of the stretched Si intensity is shown at the bottom of the micrograph. It should be noted that while it is possible to easily see a great number of colors—far more than one can see shades of gray—it becomes a chore to tell which color corresponds to a particular intensity. Some sort of assignment chart is essential to display along with the pseudocolored micrograph. In Figure 5.17E this scale is laid across the bottom of the image, the left side corresponds to zero intensity while the right side corresponds to maximum (255) intensity. This scale is the so-called "rainbow" scale and in this example there are 256 "bins" of fully saturated and fully intense colors. In many circumstances, not necessarily in this case, the rainbow scale is inappropriate. This is especially true if there are phases which have similar intensities or phases which contain concentration gradients and the gradients themselves are not of interest. In these cases, a smaller number of "bins" which can be placed in the intensity range where required and colored in such a manner as to produce maximum visibility is to be preferred. Figure 5.17F is the same as E but pseudocolored with nine bins of easily discernible colors. The colors were chosen with control over hue, saturation, and intensity. The bin locations were chosen to delineate all the discrete levels of Si in the scanned area.

We have shown all these images from the same region of a "typical" specimen to demonstrate a number of the topics discussed in this chapter by actually putting them to use. We also wanted to demonstrate that it is possible to obtain a massive amount of chemical and statistical information regarding a region of a specimen in a reasonable time. While long acquisition times (say 1 h all the way up to the life of the filament) may seem ridiculous—at first blush—it is not at all unreasonable when one considers the return. In this case, a 1-mm^2 region has been totally sampled for 11 elements with a sensitivity on the order of several hundred parts per million by weight—with an EDS detector. Not only do we have full quantitative characterization but we can see the distributions of the actual elements as images. We can be confident that nothing has been overlooked. We have all the data in digital form and can come back at any time and reprocess in other ways to extract further information if we so desire. In many cases, only one such "image" is sufficient to completely characterize a nagging problem and convince all concerned. Such is the power of an image over tables of figures and statistical jargon that only statisticians truly understand and the rest of us like to think we do.

Acquisition time is, obviously, arbitrary, and can be reduced considerably in some cases by using shorter time constants in the EDS detector amplifier, or by the use of crystal spectrometers (WDS) coupled with higher electron beam currents.

5.19. Contrast Criteria for Images

We will define contrast to be

$$C = (S_{max} - S_{min})/S_{max} \qquad (5.11)$$

where S_{max} and S_{min} represent the signals detected at any two points or regions in the image for which we wish to determine the "contrast," C. By this definition, C is always positive and assumes values between 0 and 1. Contrast is a quantity which can relate the information in a detected signal to the properties of the specimen which we wish to determine. In discussing contrast, we must consider the specimen and the detector of interest as a closed system. The contrast which we can observe must be initially created by events in the specimen (e.g., backscattered electrons, x-rays). Contrast can be subsequently reduced by the particular detector used. However, the signal leaving the detector contains all the information available for a particular set of imaging conditions employed. Subsequent amplification and signal processing can only serve to control the way in which the information is displayed. The information content in the signal cannot be increased after the detector.

If we assume that a specimen in the SEM can produce a given con-

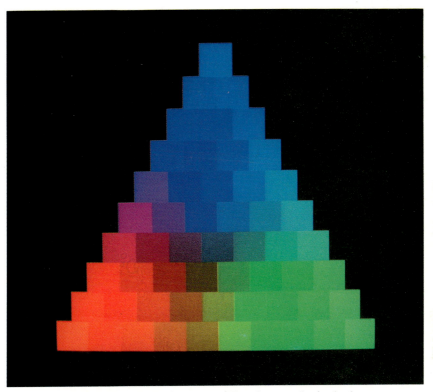

Figure 5.16. The relation between the primary and mixed colors.

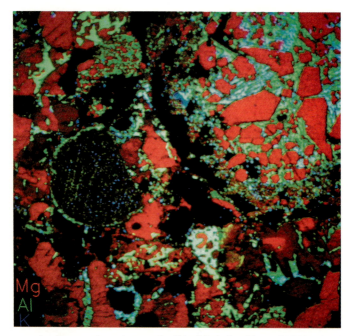

Figure 5.17A. A primary color micrograph of the Mg (using Figure 5.13A), Al (using Figure 5.13L), and K (using Figure 5.13H) images. The Mg intensity information is used to modulate the brightness of the red gun in the display monitor, Al the green gun, and K the blue gun.

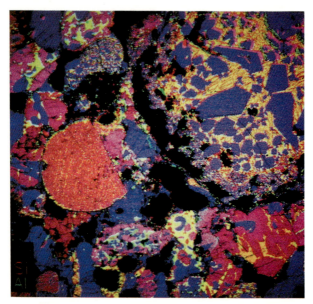

Figure 5.17B. The same as A except Si is red, Al is again green, and Mg is blue.

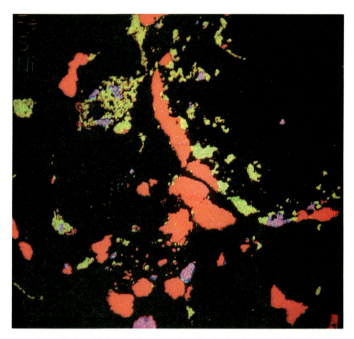

Figure 5.17C. Intended to highlight the metal and sulfide phases. Fe is red, S is green, and Ni is blue.

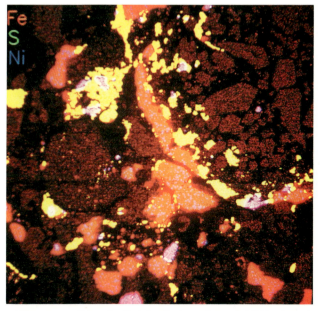

Figure 5.17D. The same as C but the Fe is Laplacian enhanced. All Fe phases including the mineral phases are visible in this image.

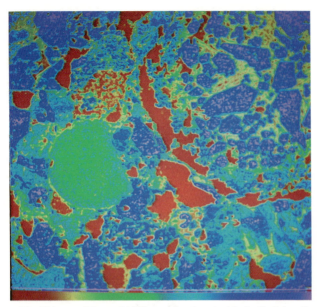

Figure 5.17E. The Si image (Figure 5.13C) pseudocolored with the "rainbow" scale. See text for details.

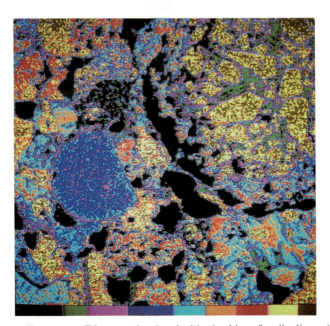

Figure 5.17F. The same as E but pseudocolored with nine bins of easily discernible colors. The bin locations were carefully chosen to delineate all the discrete levels of Si in the scanned area.

trast, we can now consider what criteria must be satisfied to yield a final image on the display tube which conveys the contrast information to the observer.

We are all familiar with the problem of tuning in a distant TV station. If the station's signal is weak, we find the visibility of detail in the picture is obscured by the presence of noise, i.e., random fluctuations in the brightness of the image points which are superposed on the true signal changes we wish to see, the contrast of the image. We note that the first information lost as the noise increases is the fine detail of the image. The presence of randomness or noise as a limitation to the information available in an image is a common theme in all imaging processes.

If a line scan is made across a region of a sample, the signal coming from a detector can be displayed on an oscilloscope, with the scan position along the horizontal axis and the signal plotted on the vertical axis (Figure 5.18). We can identify the signals at any two points of interest, e.g, S_A and S_B, and calculate the contrast from equation (5.11). If the same line scan is repeated, the traces on the oscilloscope will not be found to superpose exactly. If the signal from a single beam location is repeatedly sampled for the picture point time t, the nominally identical signal counts will be found to vary. The SEM imaging process is basically the counting of discrete events, e.g., secondary or backscattered electrons or x-rays arriving with a random distribution in time during a sampling period. Measuring the signal, S involves counting a number of events, n, at the

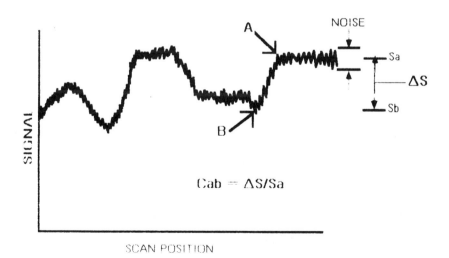

Figure 5.18. Illustration of a scan line across an image; "A" and "B" represent two arbitrarily chosen points of interest.

detector. Because of the random distribution of the events in time, subsequent counts of the same point will vary about the mean value $\bar{n}$ by an amount $\bar{n}^{1/2}$. The signal quality can be expressed by the signal-to-noise ratio S/N:

$$S/N = \overline{N}/\overline{N}^{1/2} = \overline{N}^{1/2} \tag{5.12}$$

As the mean of the counts increases, the S/N ratio improves. The S/N ratio of the SEM image can be estimated from a line scan displayed on an oscilloscope, shown schematically in Figure 5.18.

The noise is estimated from the thickness of the trace, and the signal at the point of interest can be measured directly.

Rose (1948, 1970) made an extensive study of the ability of observers to detect contrast between two very small regions in a scanned TV image in the presence of noise. He found that for the average observer to discern the difference between two such regions, the change in the signal due to the contrast, ΔS, had to exceed the noise N by a factor of 5:

$$\Delta S > 5N \quad \text{(Rose criterion)} \tag{5.13}$$

This visibility criterion can be used to develop the relation between the threshold contrast, that is the minimum level of contrast potentially available in the signal, and the number of signal events. Considering the noise in terms of the number of signal events,

$$\Delta S > 5n^{1/2} \tag{5.14}$$

Equation (5.14) can be converted to a contrast equation by dividing through by the signal, S:

$$\Delta S/S = C > 5n^{1/2}/S = 5n^{1/2}/n \tag{5.15}$$

or

$$C > 5n^{-1/2}$$
$$n > (5/C)^2$$

Equation (5.15) indicates that in order to observe a given level of contrast, C, a mean number of signal carriers, n, given by $(5/C)^2$, must be collected per picture point.

The above discussion develops a contrast criterion for one very small region (comprised of no more than several pixels) in the image compared to another very small region. Frequently, it is more convenient to compare one large region of an image to some other large region. The purpose of the following is to outline a procedure (M. E. Eden, personal communication) which does this for a digital type of display.

We begin by assuming that we have Poisson statistics at each pixel in an image (the mean and variance equal the number of counts in the pixel). We will consider two cases. In each case (image), there will be two approximately uniform intensity areas called P and B (loosely speaking, peak and background, although what we discuss is applicable regardless of the origin of the signal). The "area" of each of these regions is the number of pixels in the region.

I. We let the *average* number of counts in B be 400 and the *average* number of counts in P be 420. Since we are interested in comparing two regions that have nearly the same average intensity, we make the approximation that $N = B^{1/2} = P^{1/2} = 400^{1/2} = 20$ where N is the standard deviation of the mean of both areas. We can then say that $P - B = S$ is the "signal," and then the S/N ratio in this case is 1. We note that P/B = 1.05 or 5% contrast.

We now attempt to improve visibility by subtracting a constant from all pixels in the image. We do not want to subtract a number large enough to "zero" more than a very few pixels. We remember that the display system will "clip" to the minimum gray level "black" any value less than zero. We choose 340 counts in this case which will "zero" only 0.13% of the pixels in the image. Consequently, B = 60 and P = 80 which is a contrast of 25%. Note that the S/N ratio is still 1 as before.

II. Let B = 400 and P = 408, then N = 20 as before, and S/N = 0.4. The contrast is, in this case, 2%. If we again subtract 340, we make B = 60 and P = 68. The contrast is increased to 13.3%, but the S/N ratio remains 0.4 as before.

We now inquire as to how big an area, A, must be to produce a given reduction in the standard error of the noise for the area, Δ_{AREA}. Approximately, but a good approximation, is

$$\Delta_{AREA} = N/A^{1/2} \tag{5.16}$$

Thus, to reduce the standard error of the noise to say $0.4 \times S/N = 0.16$ (for case 2, for example), we have $0.16 \times 20 = 3.2$ counts. Then $20/A^{1/2} = 3.2$ or $A = 3.6$ pixels. This would be about as small an area as one could select as being discrete and trust your visual interpretation.

Visibility criteria valid for all types of images are generally not possible to formulate. If the observer knows what it is he is looking for, and in the best of cases knows the size and orientation of an object in an image, he might very well be able to "see" the object with considerably more noise present as if he knew nothing at all about what he was looking for. Consequently, procedures such as described above can only be considered as rough guidelines which give an idea as to the effect of fundamental statistical limitations but do not and cannot incorporate the pattern-recognizing capability of the human brain.

5.20. Conclusion

The purpose of this chapter was to discuss aspects of imaging in the SEM and x-ray microanalyzer. We have pointed out pros and cons of the various procedures and methods but always in terms of images. We have not forgotten the point mode capabilities of the machines. It was a conscious decision not to make comparisons between the two even when point mode methods would provide a superior result, e.g., trace analysis of an object for which elemental distribution was of no interest. The techniques and equipment discussed in this chapter are just more tools in the bag of the practicing analyst and must be used where appropriate and not used when some other method would work better.

Appendix

The top-hat digital filter described by equation (5.1) can be applied to an x-ray spectrum in a time proportional to the number of channels by calculating the summations in the formula from the difference of two precalculated summations, i.e.:

$$\sum_{j=k}^{h} y_j = \sum_{j=i-M-N}^{h} y_j - \sum_{j=i-M-N}^{k-1} y_j = S_h - S_{k-1} \qquad (A5.1)$$

where S_i is calculated from

$$S_0 = 0 \qquad (A5.2)$$
$$S_i = y_i + S_{i-1}$$

Rewriting (A5.1) in terms of S gives

$$y_i' = \frac{S_{i+M} - S_{i-M-1}}{2M+1} - \frac{S_{i-M-1} - S_{i-M-N-1} + S_{i+M+N} - S_{i+M}}{2N} \qquad (A5.3)$$

Equations (A5.2) and (A5.3) form the basis for the following Pascal procedure (written by K. E. Gorlen, National Institutes of Health):

```
PROCEDURE TopHatFilter(
    VAR  y: ARRAY[yl..yh: INTEGER]  OF  REAL;  { original
spectrum }
    VAR  f: ARRAY[fl..fh: INTEGER]  OF  REAL;  { filtered
spectrum }
    M: INTEGER;  { 2M+1 channels in central section }
    N: INTEGER);  { N channels in side sections }
  VAR
    i, p, q, r: INTEGER;
    S: ARRAY[0..MaxSpectrumChannels] OF REAL;

  BEGIN
    S[0] := 0;
    FOR i := 1 TO yh-yl+1 DO S[i] := y[yl+i-1] + S[i-1];
    p:= N;  q := N+M+M+1;  r:=N+M+M+N+1; {initialize filter
section indices}

    FOR i := 0 TO yh-yl-(N+M+M+N) DO BEGIN
      f[fl+i]:=(S[q]-S[p])/(2*M+1)+
               (S[p]-S[i]+S[r]-S[q])/(2*N);
      p := p+1; q := q+1; r := r+1; { advance filter }
    END;
  END; {TopHatFilter}
```

For x-ray spectra, it is recommended to choose $M = N$. Thus, there are $4N + 1$ channels in the top-hat filter, N in each of the two side sections and $2N + 1$ in the center section. Since the center section should span an energy range approximately equal to the FWHM (full width at half-maximum) of the x-ray peak, then N can be calculated as follows:

$$N = \frac{\text{FWHM}}{2K}$$

where K is the number of electron volts per spectrum channel. The number of channels filtered equals the number of channels in the center section ($2N + 1$), requiring a total of $6N + 1$ channels centered at the peak energy to be sampled and processed.

6

Alternative Microanalytical Techniques

6.1. Introduction

The extraordinary analytical capabilities of combined scanning electron microscopy and x-ray microanalysis (SEM/XM) are not without limitations. Indeed, there exist significant shortcomings of the technique which limit its application to many important problems. Fortunately, a number of alternative microanalysis techniques have been developed, in some cases based on totally different excitation radiations and analytical signals. These alternative microanalysis techniques have often undergone extensive development and possess a large body of literature. A detailed treatment of these techniques is beyond the scope of this chapter. Rather, the general principles of several of the major alternative techniques will be illustrated to show how these techniques can be utilized to augment the information available from SEM/XM. Specifically, the following special forms of microanalysis will be considered: high-spatial-resolution microanalysis, surface microanalysis, trace microanalysis, and molecular microanalysis. To appreciate how these alternative microanalysis techniques can fit into an analytical strategy, the strengths and weaknesses of SEM/XM will be reviewed.

6.2. Strengths and Weaknesses of SEM/XM

The strengths and weaknesses of conventional SEM/XM can best be understood by examining the electron interaction and x-ray generation volumes for a metal target under typical operating conditions. The electron interaction volume and the sites of inner shell ionization for a copper target, as calculated with a Monte Carlo electron trajectory simulation, are shown in Figure 6.1. It is obvious from Figure 6.1 that as an

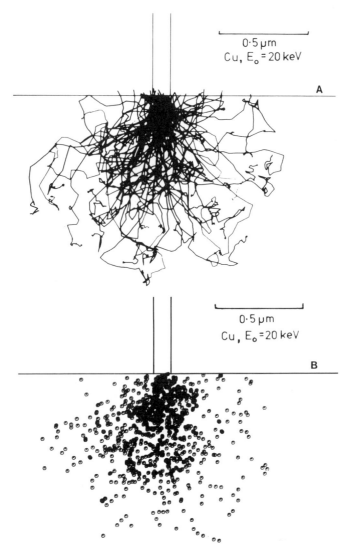

Figure 6.1. Electron interactions in a copper target. (A) Electron trajectories; (B) sites of inner shell ionizations. Beam energy 20 keV.

analytical tool, SEM/XM integrates a compositional measurement over a range of depth of the order of 1 μm or approximately 10,000 atom layers; the lateral spatial resolution is of the same order of magnitude. As such, SEM/XM can be regarded as a bulk analysis as opposed to a surface analysis technique, which would confine the sampled volume to the true surface, i.e., the first two or three atom layers in which the atom properties deviate from bulk behavior. The spreading of the beam electrons from the initial trajectory is caused by elastic scattering, while the finite length of the trajectories is determined by the energy loss which results from inelastic scattering. Another consequence of the development of the interaction volume of finite size is the requirement for complicated corrections to the measured x-ray signals. These corrections must be made to determine the true generated x-ray signals on a properly normalized basis to calculate valid elemental concentrations. Since the analytical signals can be produced throughout a substantial portion of the electron interaction volume, it is a necessary condition for quantitative analysis that the sample must be homogeneous in composition throughout the interaction volume. Compositional gradients or sharp compositional discontinuities which might exist within the interaction volume cannot be directly measured by conventional SEM/XM. In many problems in materials science or biological science, the structures of interest are on the scale of 10 to 100 nm, which is well below the spatial resolution of conventional SEM/XM. Thus, analytical methods with a spatial resolution one to two orders of magnitude smaller in scale are needed.

The properties of the characteristic x-rays which are used to identify and quantify the elemental constituents set limits to the elements which are accessible to qualitative and quantitative analysis. Qualitative analysis is restricted to elements with atomic numbers greater than or equal to 5 (boron). Hydrogen and helium do not produce an x-ray, while the x-rays of lithium and beryllium are so long in wavelength and low in energy that they are absorbed in the specimen and spectrometer components. In the case of the energy-dispersive x-ray spectrometer, these x-rays do not produce charge pulses of sufficient magnitude to exceed the fundamental noise of the detector/amplifier system. The x-rays of the elements boron through fluorine can be detected with both wavelength-dispersive and energy-dispersive spectrometers, but again because of their low energy, the sensitivity limit will be of the order of 1–10%, depending on the matrix in which the element resides.

A great strength of electron probe microanalysis is the capability to achieve a high degree of accuracy in a quantitative analysis, typically better than 5% relative, with a very simple standards suite consisting of pure elements or simple compounds. This capability provides a great degree of flexibility in dealing with unknowns of arbitrary composition. However, accurate quantitative analysis by means of ZAF matrix correction procedures is limited to elements with atomic numbers of 11 (sodium) or higher. While progress is being made in extending the matrix correction technique to light elements, the paucity of accurate mass absorption coefficients for the x-rays of these elements severely limits the extent of application (Brown *et al.,* 1980). Moreover, the poor detection limits are an even greater and insurmountable barrier to application of SEM/XM to the analysis of light elements. Even for heavier elements with atomic numbers of 11 or more, the practical detection limits are of the order of 100 to 1000 parts per million (ppm), a direct result of the inherently poor peak-to-background of electron excited x-rays caused by the existence of a significant background at all x-ray energies due to the x-ray bremsstrahlung process.

While the term "trace analysis" is somewhat ambiguous as to the specific concentration level which constitutes "trace," a useful concentration scale of "major," "minor," and "trace" might be defined as follows:

major constituent: $C > 10\%$ (0.1 mass fraction)
minor constituent: $0.1\% < C < 10\%$ (0.001 to 0.1 mass fraction)
trace constituent: $C < 0.1\%$ (0.001 mass fraction or 1000 ppm)

By these arbitrary and modest definitions, SEM/XM analysis barely penetrates into the trace analysis regime, and even that level of detection is only achievable with wavelength-dispersive spectrometry. Moreover, analyses of concentration levels near the limit of detection are only practical at individual points or at best with line scans. The preparation of an x-ray area scan, which might be thought of as a qualitative compositional map, requires an extremely long time for constituents at a trace level if statistically meaningful results are to be obtained. Thus, x-ray area scans on a trace level are only practical in certain cases, and alternative "trace microanalysis" techniques, particularly those which can obtain qualitative and quantitative compositional maps, are desirable.

SEM/XM can provide information on the elements which are present within the sample, subject to the limitations on sensitivity and elemental coverage noted above. However, it is often of interest to know the chemical state of the elements in the sample. In many SEM/XM analyses, this speciation is inferred in the solution for a constituent such as in the case of indirectly determining oxygen by means of stoichiometric calculations. However, in those cases where the valence of an element can take on multiple values, stoichiometric calculations are subject to uncertainty. When low-energy x-rays in the range 0.2–2 keV are measured, small shifts are observed in the wavelength of the peak position. These shifts from the ideal value are observed when the element of interest is chemically bonded so that the energy levels of the outer shell electrons are altered by the chemical state of the element. While these chemical shifts can be used to derive molecular (compound) information about a sample, the magnitude of the chemical shifts is small and requires high-resolution wavelength spectrometry to make reliable measurements. Chemical speciation studies by x-ray spectrometry in a microanalysis mode are thus practical in special cases only. Alternative microanalysis techniques which provide direct information on molecular constituents would usefully augment the mostly elemental information of SEM/XM.

6.3. General Observations on Analysis Methods

6.3.1. Quantitative Analysis Procedures

A measure of the maturity of an analysis technique is the level of sophistication which has been achieved in the quantification of spectral data, i.e., the conversion of measured intensities into the concentrations of the various constituents. In general, the measured intensity, i_m, is a function of the intensity generated within the sample, i_g. The functional dependence of i_m on i_g involves the concentration of the constituent of interest, C_i, matrix effects, M, which depend on the concentrations of the other constituents in the excited volume, C_j, and instrumental effects, I, which have to do with the efficiency with which signal carriers, e.g., photons, are converted into individual recorded counts:

$$i_m = f[i_g, C_i, M(C_j), I] \tag{6.1}$$

Quantitative analysis involves measuring i_m and determining the corresponding value of C_i. Clearly, a quantitative analysis procedure must be capable of calculating or otherwise compensating for the matrix and instrumental effects. Several different levels of sophistication exist for the quantitative analysis process: working curves, sensitivity factors, matrix correction procedures for sensitivity factors, and first principles analysis.

In addition to the obvious questions of accuracy and reproducibility, we are also interested in the "analytical flexibility" of a method, i.e., the capability of dealing with an unknown of arbitrary composition. It is this factor which determines the ability to respond to new analytical problems.

6.3.1.1. Working Curves

In the simplest form of quantification procedure, an empirical relation called a "working curve" is determined between the spectral intensity and the concentration of the constituent(s) of interest as measured in a suite of standards whose composition has been determined by independent analysis techniques. An example of a working curve is illustrated in Figure 6.2 for a minor alloying species in a steel as measured by the tech-

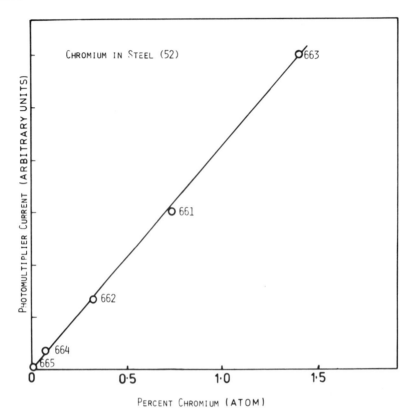

Figure 6.2. Working curve for secondary ion intensity as a function of concentration for a minor constituent in an iron matrix.

nique of secondary ion mass spectrometry. In this case, the signal is the secondary ion intensity for the elemental ion species as measured by a photomultiplier, and the concentrations have been provided for the suite of steel standards by independent bulk chemical analysis techniques. For the particular working curve shown in Figure 6.2, a simple linear relation is observed. While linearity is usually observed for dilute constituents at levels below approximately 10%, at higher concentrations the working curve is often found to be nonlinear as a result of matrix effects. Matrix effects can change substantially as the relative concentrations of the solute and matrix elements become comparable levels in the sample. Although the working curve may be nonlinear over higher concentrations, it is still useful for quantitative analysis providing the spectral intensity shows a monotonic increase with concentration and sufficient standards are available to fully define the working curve.

The working curve directly incorporates the effects of the matrix in which the constituent is dispersed as well as instrumental factors which determine the efficiency of signal conversion in the measuring system. As such, the working curve method of quantitative analysis suffers from two severe limitations which limit its applicability as a flexible analysis procedure. (1) The same instrument operating conditions, such as beam energy, beam current, spectrometer gain, specimen orientation relative to the beam and spectrometer, and so on, must be employed for any subsequent analysis with the working curve. In fact, working curves are usually valid only for the particular instrument on which they were measured. Because of local operating technique, even nominally identical instruments will produce different working curves from the same standards suite. (2) The unknowns for analysis must have similar concentrations of major constituents as those of the standards, if the matrix effects are to be sufficiently similar to make the working curve applicable. When these conditions are satisfied, the working curve approach can produce analyses whose accuracy is limited only by the uncertainty in the concentrations in the standards. If the constituent for which the working curve has been measured appears in an unknown with a different matrix composition, then a new working curve appropriate to that new matrix must be determined, an expensive and time-consuming process since a new set of standards is required.

6.3.1.2. Relative Sensitivity Factors

The next level of sophistication in analysis methods is that of relative sensitivity factors. A relative sensitivity factor, denoted $S_{x/R}$, can be defined as:

$$S_{x/R} = (i_x/C_x)/(i_R/C_R) \tag{6.2}$$

where i is the measured instrument response (signal), C is the concentration (mass fraction or atomic fraction can be used, providing consistency is maintained), the subscript x denotes the constituent of interest while R is a reference constituent which coexists in the same standards and unknowns as constituent x. The reference constituent is usually chosen from the major constituents of the sample. In order to determine a suite of relative sensitivity factors, suitable multiconstituent standards must be available, where the composition of the standards has been independently determined. Like working curves, relative sensitivity factors incorporate the response characteristics of the instrument upon which they are measured. The sensitivity factors should thus be redetermined if the instrument operating conditions are changed or if a different instrument is used.

After the relative sensitivity factors have been measured with a particular analytical instrument, these factors can be used to determine the composition of an unknown as follows. The intensity ratios for constituents x and R measured in the unknown are converted to concentration ratios by rearranging equation (6.2):

$$C_x/C_R = (i_x/i_R)/S_{x/R} \tag{6.3}$$

The concentration for each constituent x can thus be expressed in terms of the concentration of the reference contituent:

$$C_x = (i_x/i_R)(C_R/S_{x/R}) \tag{6.4}$$

If all of the constituents of the sample can be measured directly in the spectrum, then

$$\sum_j C_x + C_R = 1 \tag{6.5}$$

The value of C_x from equation (6.4) can be substituted in equation (6.5):

$$\sum_j (i_x/i_R)(C_R/S_{x/R}) + C_R = 1 \tag{6.6}$$

Since (i_x/i_R) is a quantity measured from the spectrum of the unknown and the relative sensitivity factors have been previously determined from standards, equation (6.6) is clearly an equation in one unknown, C_R, which can therefore be solved directly. This value of C_R can then be substituted in equation (6.4) to obtain values for all of the other constituents, C_x. For elemental analysis, if a constituent such as oxygen cannot be measured directly by the spectroscopic technique but can be calculated indirectly by stoichiometry, such calculations can be incorporated in equation (6.6):

$$\sum_j (i_x/i_R)(C_R/S_{x/R}) + \sum_j (i_x/i_R)(C_R/S_{x/R}) f_{O/x} + C_R + C_R f_{O/R} = 1 \tag{6.7}$$

where $f_{O/x}$ is the oxygen/element ratio appropriate to the stoichiometry of each element.

The utility of the sensitivity factor method of analysis arises from the increased analytical flexibility which is obtained. First, since one constituent is measured relative to another in the same sample volume, those factors which similarly affect both the measured element and the reference element, such as beam current and sample thickness, are effectively eliminated from the analytical expression. Thus, fluctuations in these factors are less significant. Second, the number of standards necessary can be kept small if several constituents can be dispersed in a homogeneous multiconstituent mixture, such as an alloy or glass. Third, to a lesser degree, the sensitivity factor method also confers some independence from matrix effects if the signals from the constituent of interest and the reference constituent are similarly affected by changes in composition. An example of the reduction of matrix effects observed with relative sensitivity factors as compared to absolute measurements is shown in Figure 6.3 for the technique of secondary ion mass spectrometry. This figure shows relative sensitivity factors calculated from measurements made of intensities from pure elements with actual relative sensitivity factors measured in a multielement mixture. The factors calculated from absolute measurements show a range of approximately four orders of magnitude and no noticeable trends are observed with atomic number. When relative sensitivity factors are measured in a common matrix consisting of a silicate glass, the range is reduced to one order of magnitude, and the behavior as a function of atomic number is found to be much more regular.

6.3.1.3. Matrix Correction Factors

The third stage in the development of quantitative analysis methods is the direct treatment of matrix effects through physical modeling. Thus, if the factors which influence the generated and measured intensities can be described physically and/or modeled mathematically, calculated cor-

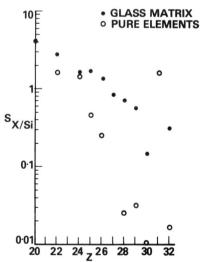

Figure 6.3. Relative sensitivity factors as measured by secondary ion mass spectrometry for elements in the first transition series. Open circles: relative sensitivity factors calculated from absolute secondary ion yield data of Andersen and Hinthorne (1973). Solid circles: relative sensitivity factors directly measured in a silicate glass matrix.

rections can be applied to the measured intensities to compensate for matrix effects in order to derive accurate values of the concentrations. An outstanding example of this analytical approach is the "ZAF" method used in electron probe microanalysis. The ZAF method makes calculations for each of the matrix effects which modify the intensity generated in the sample:

$$C_x = C_S k \, Z \, A \, F \qquad (6.8)$$

where C_x is the concentration of element x in the unknown, C_S is the concentration of x in the standard, k is the ratio of measured intensities from the unknown and the standard, Z is the atomic number correction, A is the absorption correction, and F is the fluorescence correction due to characteristic and continuum induced fluorescence. The ZAF factors are each a ratio of calculations for the sample composition and the standard composition. A great benefit of expressing each factor as a ratio is the degree of independence which this procedure offers from needing exact knowledge of the physical parameters such as cross sections.

While matrix effects are calculated from a physical model of electron and x-ray interactions with matter in the ZAF method, the measurement of the k ratio used in equation (6.8) serves to eliminate instrumental effects. The k ratio is a relative intensity ratio for the same radiation from the same element measured in the sample and the standard. Instrumental effects such as the absolute value of the electron dose and the spectrometer efficiency are effectively canceled from further consideration since these factors must be identical for radiation from the sample and the standard and thus they cancel from the numerator and denominator of the k ratio. However, it is clear that while knowledge of the absolute value of the instrumental parameters is not needed, it is necessary that these conditions must be maintained constant. Such a condition is easy to fulfill and confirm if the standards and samples are measured sequentially. If stored standard spectra are employed which were recorded at some time in the past, then errors are likely to be introduced unless meticulous attention is paid to reestablishing identical operating conditions.

The ZAF method allows the analyst to use a simple standards suite, in the form of pure elements or simple compounds, for the analysis of complex multielement unknowns. The ZAF method thus conveys a large measure of analytical flexibility, i.e., the ability to deal with an unknown of arbitrary composition.

6.3.1.4. ''First Principles'' Analysis

The highest level of analytical sophistication is the development of an analysis method based on "first principles." In such a method, all quantities necessary in equation (6.1) to relate the measured intensity to the actual number or fraction of atoms in the sample can be directly calculated from prior knowledge of the physics which describe the interaction of the primary (exciting) and secondary (analyzing) radiations with the atoms of the sample. A first principles method provides the ultimate in analytical flexibility, since no standards would be needed regardless of the composition of the unknown.

A current example of a microanalysis technique which comes close to achieving first principles analysis is the "standardless" analysis method of electron probe microanalysis (Russ, 1980). In this procedure, the x-ray intensities for the elements are calculated on a relative basis from the x-ray generation equation for solid specimens. Note that the so-called "standardless" procedures are not truly standardless. Generally, the intensity of a single pure element standard must be measured in such a "standardless" procedure in order to establish the local instrumental response. While matrix effects can be calculated, instrumental factors are often poorly defined and difficult to specify and calculate. The standardless method can only be used effectively with the energy-dispersive x-ray spectrometer for which the spectrometer efficiency is relatively constant with time and which can be calculated with reasonable accuracy over the x-ray range from 1 to 15 keV. For wavelength spectrometers, the relative efficiency varies in a complicated fashion which depends on the x-ray wavelength and the characteristics of the diffracting crystal, making a first principles calculation of relative elemental efficiency quite difficult.

While highly flexible, standardless or first principles analysis is often subject to the largest analytical errors. There are usually considerable uncertainties in the cross sections and energy loss models which are inherent in the models, and physical parameters such as fluorescence yields are often not known with high accuracy.

6.3.1.5. Looking at Errors

When an arbitrarily chosen unknown is analyzed, it is generally not possible to make detailed statements about the uncertainty in the quantitative analysis which results from the particular analysis procedure being employed unless a previous body of analytical experience has been accumulated through the analysis of known materials. The analyst should be wary of published analytical schemes which provide a limited set of test analyses. Often, the examples chosen are those which represent ideal cases for which the model in question works well. In fact, a distribution of errors can be expected from the application of an analytical model to a wide range of specimen compositions which test its assumptions and data base of parameters. It is important to know, if possible, the form of this distribution of errors and the maximum credible error which might be encountered in practice. Depending on the form of the distribution, statements can be made about the expected magnitude of the error in the analysis and the maximum error which might be encountered. A rare example of an error distribution for a quantitative microanalysis technique is shown in Figure 6.4, which gives the relative errors encountered in quantitative analysis by the ZAF method. This error distribution is symmetric about zero relative error, and is well described by a normal distribution with a standard deviation of 3.5% relative. The maximum relative errors encountered are of the order of 10% relative. Such an error distribution is invaluable in supporting claims for the estimated uncertainty in a reported analysis of an unknown. However, in using such an error distribution, the analyst must be aware of the analytical technique used in preparing the error distribution and the assumptions behind it. Thus, an error distribution for quantitative EPMA analysis by the ZAF technique should not be applied to analysis by a standardless technique, since the use of standards in the ZAF technique is important in minimizing errors.

6.3.2. Detection Limits

An important characteristic of an analysis technique is the limit of detection for a constituent of interest. The limit of detection can be expressed in various ways: two of the most useful concepts are the minimum detectable mass, which is the smallest absolute quantity of mass of a particular constituent which can be detected, and the minimum mass fraction, which is the minimum amount of a constituent which can be detected normalized to the mass of total sample which must be excited to make the measurement. Note that these two concepts are fundamentally different in nature. A microbeam analysis technique may have the capability of isolating an extremely small mass of sample as far as excitation is considered. In solid samples, useful x-ray spectra can be obtained from a sample volume which typically contains a mass of 10^{-12}g, a limit which is determined by the physics of electron scattering within the target. For isolated particles and thin foils where electron scattering is limited by the physical dimensions of the sample, the minimum mass excited may be as small as 10^{-16} g or even less. Thus, in terms of minimum detectable mass, electron probe analysis appears to be a technique of high sensitivity and might even appear to be capable of trace analysis. "Trace," however, properly describes a fractional quantity rather than an absolute quantity. When we consider instead the minimum mass fraction which can be detected by electron probe analysis, the sensitivity is found to be substantially less, typically 0.1% (1000 ppm) for energy-dispersive x-ray spectrometry and 100 ppm for wavelength-dispersive x-ray spectrometry in the most favorable cases.

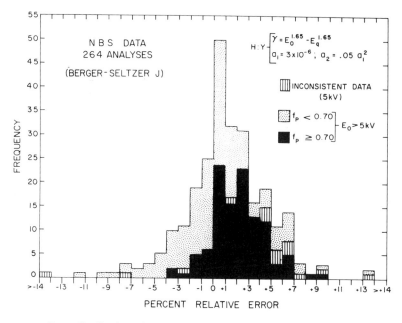

Figure 6.4. Error distribution histogram observed for quantitative electron probe microanalysis with ZAF data analysis performed on known materials. (From Myklebust *et al.*, 1973.)

The following argument, due to Wittry (1980), is useful in understanding the factors that determine the minimum mass fraction (concentration) which can be detected. For a statistically valid characteristic signal to be detected against a background signal at the same energy, the signal, S_x, must be greater than three times the root mean square (rms) statistical fluctuation of the background, B_x:

$$S_x > 3(B_x)^{1/2} \qquad (6.9)$$

The concentration of constituent "x" is related to the signal measured from the unknown, S_x, and that measured on a pure standard, S_s, by a proportionality factor, f:

$$C_x = f(S_x/S_s) \qquad (6.10)$$

For electron probe analysis, the factor f is the product of the ZAF factors. Substituting for S_x from equation (6.9) gives the minimum detectable concentration, $C_{md} = C_x$:

$$C_{md} > (3f/S_s)(B_x)^{1/2} \qquad (6.11)$$

The signal-to-background ratio (S_s/B_s) on a pure standard, which can serve as a convenient characteristic of the sensitivity of a technique, can be introduced into equation (6.11) as follows:

$$C_{md} > (3f/S_s)[B_x(B_s^2/B_s^2)]^{1/2} = 3f(B_x/B_s^2)^{1/2}/(S_s/B_s) \quad (6.12)$$

If the background on the unknown and the background on the standard are similar, $B_x \sim B_s$, then equation (6.12) can be reduced to the expression

$$C_{md} > 3f(1/B_s)^{1/2}/(S_s/B_s) \quad (6.13)$$

Another useful form of the equation for the minimum detectable concentration incorporates the efficiency of signal generation, Q (events/incident particle per unit area), the efficiency of collection, ϵ (events detected/events produced), the brightness of the source β (incident particles/unit time per unit area), and the counting time t (Wittry, 1980). Assuming $B_x \sim B_s$,

$$C_{md} > 3f(1/Q\epsilon\beta t)^{1/2}/(S_s/B_s) \quad (6.14)$$

Equation (6.14) reveals that the signal-to-background ratio obtained at the output of the spectrometer has a very strong influence on the minimum detectable concentration. The influence of generation and collection efficiency, brightness, and measurement time is reduced because of their inclusion within the square root term in equation (6.14). The minimum detectable concentration is thus strongly dependent on the signal-to-background ratio in the measurement; the higher S_s/B_s as measured on a pure standard, the lower the value of C_{md} which can be achieved. The S/B ratio depends on two main factors: (1) the physics of the interaction of the primary and secondary radiation with the sample, and (2) the physics of the spectrometer used to measure the radiation. Thus, in the case of electron probe microanalysis of solid samples, the characteristic-to-bremsstrahlung x-ray ratio in a 10-eV window centered on the characteristic energy can be as high as 1000, depending on the element. The effect of the spectrometer is to degrade this natural S/B ratio by spreading the characteristic radiation over adjacent bremsstrahlung channels. For a wavelength spectrometer, the S/B ratio is typically in the range of 100 to 1000, while for an energy-dispersive spectrometer, this value falls to 10 to 100; the difference in S/B ratios between WDS and EDS results in the differences in detection limits noted above.

The minimum detectable mass, MDM, in absolute terms can be

determined by multiplying the minimum detectable concentration, C_{md}, by the mass of the sample which is excited by the beam, M_x:

$$MDM = C_{md}M_x \qquad (6.15)$$

For a simple specimen geometry such as a thin foil, M_x, is given by

$$M_x = (\pi d^2/4)\, \rho t \qquad (6.16)$$

where d is the beam diameter, t is the specimen thickness, and ρ is the density.

6.4. High-Spatial-Resolution Microanalysis

The limitation to spatial resolution in conventional electron probe analysis of solid samples which is imposed by elastic and inelastic scattering can be substantially reduced by employing two different techniques: (1) analysis of thin (100 nm thick) specimens at high beam energies (> 100 keV) or (2) analysis of bulk samples at low beam energies (< 5 keV).

6.4.1. Thin Specimens: Analytical Electron Microscopy

The elastic scattering cross section is a strong inverse function of the beam energy, varying as the inverse square. Thus, the rate of elastic scattering per unit of path length rapidly decreases as the beam energy is increased. This reduction in the elastic scattering cross section with increasing beam energy is of no value when bulk specimens are considered. The increased energy simply leads to a much greater electron range, which increases approximately as the 1.7 power of the incident energy. Although scattering near the surface of the specimen is reduced, the increase in the total range serves to severely degrade the spatial resolution. However, if the sample is analyzed in the form of a thin foil as opposed to a bulk solid, the opportunity for elastic scattering is greatly reduced if the thickness dimension is comparable to the mean free path for elastic scattering. In such foils, there is a great reduction, compared to a bulk specimen analyzed under conventional beam energies (e.g., 20 keV), in large-angle elastic scattering events as well as multiple small-angle events, which scatter the electron out of its initial direction and degrade the spatial resolution. The technique which has been developed based upon this approach has become known as analytical electron microscopy (AEM) (Hren *et al.*, 1979).

Table 6.1. Beam Broadening in Thin Foils
(100 nm Thick)[a]

Material (Z)	Beam energy (keV)		
	100	200	400
C (6)	4.7	2.3	1.2
Al (13)	8.1	4.1	2.0
Fe (26)	19.3	9.6	4.8
Au (79)	48.8	24.4	12.2

[a]Broadening expressed in nm.

As an indication of the improvement in spatial resolution which can be realized by operating with thin foils at high beam energies, consider a series of Monte Carlo electron trajectory plots for 100-nm-thick copper with beam energies of 100, 200, and 400 keV, as shown in Figure 6.5. The interaction volume of the primary electrons is a cone with the apex placed at the beam impact point. As an approximation, the base diameter of the cone which contains 90% of the trajectories after single elastic scattering is described by an analytical expression of the form (Goldstein *et al.*, 1977)

$$b = 6.25 \times 10^2 (Z/E_0)(\rho/A)^{1/2} t^{3/2} \tag{6.17}$$

where b is the broadening in cm, Z is the atomic number, E_0 is the beam energy in keV, ρ is the density, A is the atomic weight, and t is the thickness in cm. Equation (6.17) describes the broadening from a point incident beam; the effect of finite beam size can be taken into account by addition in quadrature. Table 6.1 contains calculations of the broadening as described by equation (6.17) for a number of materials over the range of beam energies generally in use. Spatial resolution of the order of 10 nm can be achieved for even the heaviest targets at the highest beam energy.

The values in Table 6.1 can be compared in Table 6.2 to calculations of the Kanaya–Okayama range for bulk targets of the same materials analyzed at 20 keV (Kanaya and Okayama, 1972). An improvement in spa-

Table 6.2. Kanaya–Okayama Range in
Bulk Materials at 20 keV

Material	K–O range (nm)
C	5330
Al	4200
Fe	1610
Au	860

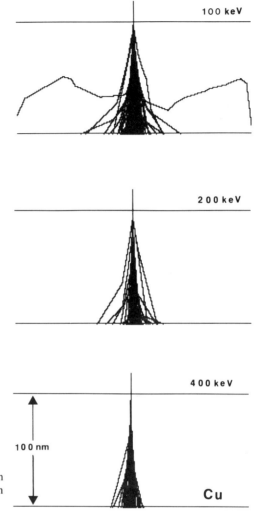

Figure 6.5. Interaction volume in 100-nm-thick copper foils at beam energies of 100, 200, and 400 keV.

tial resolution of about two orders of magnitude can be realized by analyzing thin foils at high beam energies compared to conventional bulk specimen analysis. As an example of the dramatic improvement in spatial resolution which can be achieved, consider the compositional profile shown in Figure 6.6. In this example, the spatial resolution across an alpha–gamma phase boundary in a uranium–6 wt % niobium alloy is of the order of 50 nm, which can be compared with a spatial resolution of the order of 1 μm which can be achieved with conventional analysis of bulk materials (Romig *et al.*, 1982).

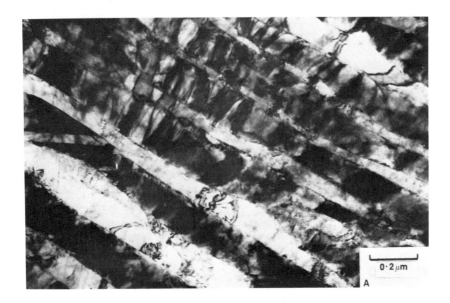

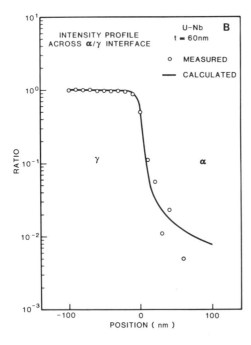

Figure 6.6. Compositional profile across an alpha–gamma interface in a uranium–6 wt% niobium alloy as determined by analytical electron microscope. (A) Transmission electron microscope image of lamellar structure; (B) Intensity profile across interface. (From Romig *et al.*, 1982.)

In order to take advantage of the greatly improved spatial resolution available by analyzing thin foils at high beam energy, a whole new class of instrumentation has arisen, the so-called "analytical electron microscope" (AEM) (Hren *et al.*, 1979; Williams, 1984). The AEM combines the functions of a conventional transmission electron microscope, scanning transmission electron microscope, and scanning electron microscope. With high-brightness lanthanum hexaboride electron sources, probes containing useful beam current for analysis as small as 5- to 10-nm diameter can be formed so that the beam contribution to the degradation of spatial resolution is of the same order or smaller than the contribution due to elastic scattering. If specimens can be made thin enough, 10–20 nm depending on the material, so that elastic scattering is insignificant, then the analytical performance will eventually be limited by the brightness of the electron source. In the AEM form known as a "dedicated STEM" or "field emission STEM," a high-brightness field emission electron source is incorporated to produce probes as small as 1nm which can carry 1 nA of electron current, and at reduced beam current, probe diameters as small as 0.3 nm can be obtained.

The strengths of the AEM (Williams, 1984) include the capabilities of high resolution imaging in both the conventional fixed beam and scanning beam modes, with lattice resolution of 0.2 nm or finer achievable in the TEM mode in the most sophisticated instruments, and 1-nm resolution in the scanning modes. A wide variety of electron diffraction techniques is also available, with selected area diffraction routinely achieved from 10-nm-diameter areas, extendable to 3-nm-diameter areas with special techniques. With the special technique of convergent beam diffraction, highly accurate and precise lattice parameter and structure information is available. Finally, analytical information can be obtained by x-ray spectrometry using the energy-dispersive x-ray spectrometer. With ultrathin window or windowless spectrometers, the elemental coverage can extend from boron to uranium. Moreover, an alternative spectrometry, electron energy loss spectrometry (EELS), is available providing the specimen is thin enough compared to the inelastic mean free path so that a condition of single or plural scattering exists. EELS can examine the energy levels of an atom as revealed by characteristic energy losses suffered by the beam electron while passing through the sample. The energy loss for inner shell ionization is one of the processes which can be detected, thus providing direct measurement of the lightest elements, including Li, Be, and B.

A significant strength of the AEM technique arises from the applicability of a simple approach to quantitative analysis based upon the method of relative sensitivity factors. To a first approximation, the effects of electron scattering, x-ray absorption, and x-ray-induced fluorescence can be neglected for most elements in extremely thin foils, less than 50 nm in thickness. In such foils, relative sensitivity factors measured on standards can be used to determine quantitative values of elemental ratios from unknowns. The thickness of most practical specimens is, however, typically 100 nm or more. For such specimens the effects of x-ray absorption and, in a few cases, x-ray-induced fluorescence, cannot be neglected if high accuracy is to be achieved. Correction factors for these effects closely resembling the familiar ZAF factors for bulk specimens have been developed by various workers and demonstrated to yield accurate results from thick foils involving heavy elements (Goldstein *et al.*, 1977; Romig, 1981).

The principal disadvantage of the AEM approach to high-spatial-resolution microanalysis lies in the necessity of compromising the specimen in order to prepare a thin foil. In some cases, the use of chemical or ion beam thinning can lead to alteration of the composition, especially at the surfaces of the foil, due to preferential dissolution or sputtering of one or more elemental components.

6.4.2. Analysis at Atomic Resolution

6.4.2.1. Analysis of Individual Atoms

The ultimate analytical tool for high spatial resolution is an instrument which measures the individual atoms of the sample. Such an instrument is the atom probe, an analytical field ion microscope first described by Muller *et al.* (1968). In the field ion microscope, the atoms at the tip of a voltage-biased, highly pointed specimen are imaged by point projection through the imaging medium of inert gas atoms which are field ionized at the tip (for a recent review, see Panitz, 1982b). In the atom probe, a voltage pulse of short (ns) duration, or alternately, an externally applied laser pulse, is applied to the tip and a layer of atoms at the tip can be desorbed as ions. These specimen ions follow the same point projection paths as the imaging inert gas ions followed, and hence the specimen ions arrive at the imaging plane in the same geometric arrangement in which they existed on the sample surface. In the initial arrangement, an aperture in the image plane allowed the passage of the ion into a time-of-flight mass spectrometer, where the velocity dispersion of the ions, which are all accelerated to the same kinetic energy, was converted into a time dispersion to identify the mass of the single atom. In later instruments, time gating techniques allowed the recording of elemental maps for the whole surface of the tip simultaneously (Panitz, 1974), and the use of laser desorption gave access to high-resistance materials such as intrinsic silicon (Kellogg and Tsong, 1980). Comparisons between analysis with the atom probe and the field emission STEM have revealed generally good agreement (Smith *et al.,* 1981).

The field emission STEM is also capable of directly imaging atoms (for a review, see Isaacson *et al.,* 1979). The specimen requirements for the FE-STEM are less rigid than those needed for the field ion microscope. The arrangement of atoms on a surface of a thin foil has been directly observed by FE-STEM, and diffusion can be followed in dynamic experiments. The ratio of elastic and inelastic scattering can be used to selectively enhance the contrast of heavy atoms against the light atoms of the support film.

6.4.2.2. Analysis of Individual Molecules

The imaging and analysis of individual molecules is an area of continuing development. Molecules which have been stained by heavy atoms can be directly imaged by high-resolution TEM (see review by Koller *et al.,* 1973). The details of the selective staining can be used to deduce the nature of specific sites on macromolecules if the staining reagents can be reliably recognized. The combined techniques of FE-STEM and EELS may eventually provide the capability of identifying individual atoms at specific sites on a molecule (Isaacson *et al.,* 1979; Johnson, 1984; Shuman, 1982). Finally, alternative imaging and analysis methods which do not utilize electrons can be applied to individual molecules. Panitz (1982a) has demonstrated that the details of individual molecules can be viewed in the point projection field ion microscope.

6.4.3. Analysis of Bulk Samples

In a number of materials analysis problems, it is not possible to modify the specimen by preparing a thin foil; the specimen must be analyzed as a bulk target which precludes the use of the AEM as a means of achieving high spatial resolution. Two alternative methods now exist for improving the spatial resolution of analysis of bulk specimens to resolution values significantly below 1 μm. These methods are (1) low-energy electron beam analysis and (2) ion beam analysis.

6.4.3.1. Low-Energy Electron Beam Analysis

An alternative to high-beam-energy analysis of thin foils is the analysis of solid specimens with low beam energies. The advantage of low-beam-energy analysis can be readily appreciated by considering the electron range at low beam energy listed in Table 6.3, as calculated with the

Table 6.3. Electron Range in Solid
Specimens at Low Beam Energy

Material	K–O range (nm) 5 keV	2.5 keV
C	530	165
Al	414	130
Fe	159	50
Au	85	27

Kanaya–Okayama formula. At low beam energies, the electron range decreases dramatically compared to the range at conventional analysis energies, which is given in Table 6.2. While the improvement in spatial resolution is not as great as the two orders of magnitude which can be achieved by AEM, the improvement by operating at low beam energy is quite substantial, approximately one order of magnitude.

This improvement in spatial resolution at low beam energies is not obtained without significant sacrifices. Under conventional analysis conditions, e.g., at 20-keV beam energy, an overvoltage factor of $U = 2$ or more is considered necessary in order to obtain adequate x-ray generation. In order to operate at low beam energy and still have access to an analytical x-ray line for each element, it is necessary to relax this condition to allow operation with an overvoltage factor as low as $U = 1.25$. At an incident energy of 5 keV, it is possible to obtain this overvoltage of 1.25 for an analytical line of all elements from atomic number 4 to 92, as shown in Table 6.4.

It should be recognized, however, that an overvoltage of 1.25 will greatly reduce the rate of x-ray generation so that with practical counting times, e.g., 200 s, detection limits will be as much as an order of magnitude poorer than those obtained under conventional analysis conditions and will be in the range 1–5%.

6.4.3.2. Ion Beam Analysis

The factor which limits the spatial resolution of analysis by means of electron beams is the lateral motion of electrons out of the ideal exci-

Table 6.4. Analytical Lines for Low-Beam-Energy Analysis

$E_0 = 5$ keV ($U_{min} = 1.25$)
K-lines: Be ($Z = 4$; $K_{ab} = 0.116$ keV) to Ca ($Z = 20$; $K_{ab} = 4.038$ keV)
L-lines: K ($Z = 19$; $LIII_{ab} = 0.294$ keV) to Sn ($Z = 50$; $LIII_{ab} = 3.928$ keV)
M-lines: In ($Z = 49$; $MV_{ab} = 0.443$ keV) to U ($Z = 92$; $MV_{ab} = 3.552$)

tation cylinder, whose area is defined by the cross-sectional area of the incident beam and whose altitude is the electron range in the solid. This lateral motion is a direct result of the process of elastic scattering, which acts to change the trajectory of the incident electrons. Ion beams offer an attractive alternative to electron beams to achieve high-spatial-resolution analysis in bulk specimens. The advantage of bombarding with energetic ions is that ion scattering by target atoms is greatly dominated by inelastic scattering processes compared to elastic processes so that relatively little lateral scattering of ions occurs. Thus, the ion beam excitation volume more closely approximates the ideal excitation cylinder.

The lateral spatial resolution attainable with ion beams is chiefly limited by the focusing of the high-energy beams. Typical beam diameters which can be achieved with megaelectron volt proton beams are of the order of 1–3 μm (Legge, 1980; Nobiling *et al.*, 1977). For beam energies in the range of 10 to 100 keV, the development of high-brightness liquid metal (e.g., gallium) ion sources based on field ionization has led to the realization of beam diameters as small as 20 nm. Imaging by means of scanning ion microscopy with secondary electron detection has demonstrated images containing topographic and crystallographic information (Levi-Setti, 1983). The analytical signals which are accessible with focused ion beams include characteristic x-rays and secondary ions.

The cross section for K-shell ionization for protons and electrons is compared in Figure 6.7. Because particle velocity is an important parameter in determining ionization, for a given kinetic energy above the edge energy, an electron is more efficient than an ion in ionization processes. Note that in Figure 6.7, the overvoltage factor $U' = (m/M)(E/E_k)$ is modified by the inclusion of the ratio m/M, where m is the electron mass and M is the proton mass, a ratio of 1/1836. Thus, if the required K-edge ionization energy is 1 keV, the proton energy to obtain the same value of U' as the electron must be about 1800 times greater, or 18 MeV. An important point to note from Figure 6.7 is that although the ionization cross section for electrons falls to zero at $U = 1$, the ionization cross section by proton bombardment is still substantial down to values of U' as

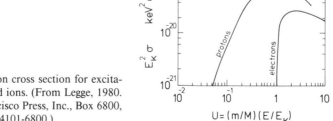

Figure 6.7. Ionization cross section for excitation by electrons and ions. (From Legge, 1980. ©1980 by San Francisco Press, Inc., Box 6800, San Francisco, CA 94101-6800.)

low as $U' = 0.05$. Thus, proton beams of 3 MeV still produce a useful cross section for K-shell ionization.

Secondary ions produced by sputtering the sample with a low-energy ion beam provide a useful signal which is surface sensitive, trace sensitive, and capable of detecting all elemental constituents. Several aspects of secondary ion mass spectrometry will be discussed below.

6.4.4. Surfaces

While we normally think of lateral resolution as being the important spatial dimension of interest in applying microanalysis techniques, there is a broad class of analysis problems for which the important analytical spatial resolution also involves the depth dimension. Techniques which have sufficient depth sensitivity to restrict the analysis to approximately the first nanometer in depth are considered "surface analysis techniques." The surface of a sample is that region over which the atoms of the sample are perturbed from their bulk behavior, and this layer extends only a few atom layers into the sample. The topic of surface analysis is itself a separate discipline of tremendous activity, involving a wide range of techniques based on combinations of a variety of primary exciting radiations and secondary analytical radiations. We shall briefly consider two techniques which are capable of high spatial resolution in both the lateral and depth dimensions and which can thus be considered "surface microanalysis."

6.4.4.1. Auger Microanalysis

The interaction of a beam of energetic electrons with the sample can result in the process of inner shell ionization, providing the energy of the beam electrons exceeds the critical ionization energy of the atomic shell(s) of the sample atoms. The sites of inner shell ionization events are distributed throughout virtually the entire interaction volume, as shown in Figure 6.1b. These excited ionized atoms can undergo electron transitions which result in the emission of a characteristic x-ray, the basis for x-ray spectrometry in electron probe microanalysis. However, the deexcitation can follow another path which involves an electron transition to fill the primary inner shell vacancy with the excess energy transferred to another outer shell electron, which is subsequently emitted with a characteristic energy, the so-called Auger electron. Auger electrons can arise at any site of a primary ionization event in the interaction volume. Thus, the generation volume for Auger electrons is the same as for characteristic x-rays of similar energy. However, the sampling volumes for the two analytical signals is greatly different. While passing through the sample on a

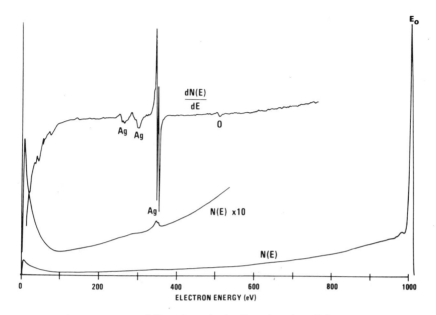

Figure 6.8. Auger spectrum of silver shown in the direct (number of electrons versus energy) and derivative (dN/dE versus energy) forms.

path toward the detector, the characteristic x-rays are not significantly affected by inelastic scattering processes. The x-rays are either totally absorbed by photoelectric capture or they escape the specimen with the same characteristic energy with which they were initially created. Auger electrons, on the other hand, can undergo continuous energy loss through the same inelastic scattering processes which affect the high-energy beam electrons. Passage through a few nanometers of the sample will result in a sufficient energy loss so that the Auger electron no longer retains the characteristic energy with which it was created. Thus, despite the fact that Auger electrons are generated throughout the interaction volume, the Auger electron signal represents a surface-sensitive signal by virtue of energy loss processes. An example of an Auger spectrum is shown in Figure 6.8.

Auger electron spectrometry has several important features in addition to its surface sensitivity which make it an attractive analytical technique:

1. The yield of Auger electrons is complementary to the yield of characteristic x-rays. The Auger yield a and the fluorescence yield ω of characteristic x-rays are related by the equation

$$a = 1 - \omega \qquad (6.18)$$

When the yield of characteristic x-rays is low, the Auger yield is high, and vice versa. Thus, Auger electron spectroscopy is particularly well-suited to the analysis of light elements such as carbon for which the fluorescence yield of x-rays is low, of the order of 0.001.

2. Auger electron formation frequently occurs with electron transitions which involve the outer electron shells of the atom. The energy levels of these shells are likely to be perturbed as a result of chemical bonding of the atom in the formation of chemical compounds. Thus, chemical shifts can be recognized in Auger peak position and shape which can be used to determine speciation.

3. Since the Auger signal is constrained both laterally and in depth, scanning Auger maps can be obtained which are effectively surface images with a depth resolution of 1 nm and a lateral resolution which is a convolution of the beam size and the backscattered electron distribution, since backscattering electrons can generate Auger electrons while exiting the sample at a point remote from the beam impact. The effective limitation to lateral resolution imposed by this backscattering effect is of the order of 100–500 nm. An example of Auger mapping of the surface of a graphitized iron is shown in Figure 6.9. The Auger maps reveal that the oxygen coverage of the surface is not uniform, existing only on the iron and not on the graphite regions.

4. Since the Auger signal is confined to originate from the first few atom layers, it is possible to obtain an in-depth profile of the distribution of elemental constituents by progressively removing atom layers by ion beam sputtering. Since the Auger signal can be confined laterally by the extent of the scan of the electron beam, Auger depth profiles can be recorded with high spatial resolution in all three dimensions, micrometer resolution laterally and nanometer resolution in depth.

Auger electron spectroscopy suffers from a number of significant limitations:

1. A consequence of the surface sensitivity is the loss of most of the signal generated by the primary electron beam, since the Auger generation takes place below the surface. Moreover, the Auger electrons which have lost energy through inelastic scattering contribute to the background along with the continuous spectrum of backscattered beam electrons and secondary electrons generated by the beam electrons in direct electron–electron collisions. The signal-to-background in the Auger spectrum is much lower than that which is encountered with the characteristic x-ray spectrum. As a result, the detection limit in analytical Auger spectrometry is of the order of 1%.

2. The Auger signal is very strongly absorbed, thus leading to significant uncertainty in the matrix corrections which must be applied to the spectral data to obtain a quantitative analysis. The most reliable and accurate analyses are based upon a relative sensitivity factor approach.

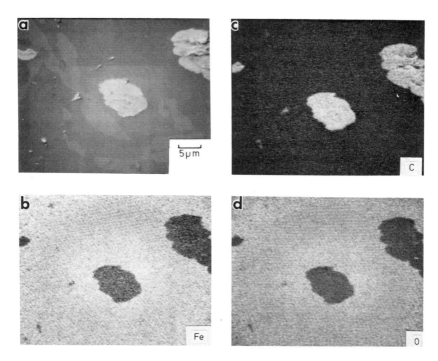

Figure 6.9. Auger electron emission map of the surface distribution of elements in a graphitized cast iron. (a) Total secondary electron image; (b) iron distribution; (c) carbon distribution; (d) oxygen distribution.

3. Because the useful Auger signal is obtained exclusively from the surface of the sample, it is necessary to provide *in situ* surface cleaning capabilities by means of ion sputtering in order to remove surface contamination layers which might exist on the sample. In order to keep the surface clean for the period of the analysis, ultrahigh clean vacuum conditions must be obtained in the microscope, with a vacuum level of 10^{-8} Pa desirable. Since vacua of this level are difficult to achieve in ordinary SEMs, purpose-built ultrahigh-vacuum scanning Auger microscopes have been constructed.

6.4.4.2. Secondary Ion Mass Spectrometry

The technique of secondary ion mass spectrometry (SIMS) is based on the process of sputtering, which is the ejection of atoms of the sample induced by the impact of the energetic primary ions, typically in the energy range of 1–25 keV. The process is illustrated schematically in Figure 6.10, which shows the ejection of neutral and ionized atoms and molecules. The ionized particles, which form a fraction of the order of 0.1–1% of the total sputtered particles, can be attracted by means of electro-

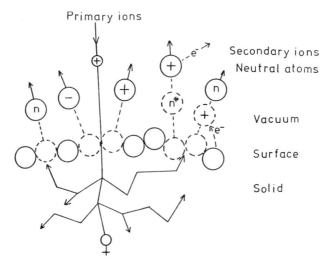

Figure 6.10. Schematic diagram of the origin of secondary ions through the process of sputtering.

static fields into a mass analyzer of either the electrostatic (quadrupole) or electrostatic/magnetic variety.

The SIMS technique can provide a wide range of information about the sample, including all elemental and isotopic constituents, and molecular constituents under certain special circumstances. These special attributes will be considered in subsequent sections, but in the context of this section on surface microanalysis, it is useful to note that the SIMS signal is derived from the first few atom layers of the sample and is thus capable of providing surface-sensitive information. As a surface analysis tool when high lateral resolution is also of interest, SIMS offers a number of advantages:

1. It is the only surface analysis tool which offers access to the entire periodic table, including all isotopes.

2. As discussed in Section 6.5, the sensitivity of SIMS is such that major, minor, and trace constituents can be detected in most instances. By using ion multipliers, a dynamic measurement range of six orders of magnitude can be achieved, making the wide sensitivity range accessible in the measurement of a single spectrum.

3. The spatial resolution of the focused primary ion beam can be realized without any significant degradation due to the primary ion–specimen interaction. Inelastic scattering dominates the interaction of the primary ions with the sample, so that relatively little lateral scattering of ions occurs.

4. Since sputtering must be used to generate the secondary ions, the progressive removal of material from the sample can be used to clean the surface *in situ,* eliminating contamination which may obscure the surface of interest.

5. By measuring the signal as a function of sputtering depth, elemental depth distributions can be determined with a wide dynamic range, as illustrated in Figure 6.15 which shows a depth distribution measurement of an ion-implanted species in silicon. By preparing a series of secondary ion distribution maps as a function of sputtering depth, a three-dimensional representation of the distribution can be achieved.

6. SIMS measures the sample atoms emitted from the surface rather than those left behind. The sputtering process often tends to cause preferential accumulation of one species on the surface, which would be detected by an analytical technique which measures the outer atom layers, such as Auger microanalysis. Once the sample has been sputtered to a depth equal to the range of the primary ions in the sample, a condition of "dynamic sputtering equilibrium" is achieved in which the atoms emitted from the sample are representative of the bulk composition. SIMS can still measure the true "bulk" composition of the sample despite such surface composition changes.

The principal disadvantage of SIMS as a surface analysis tool is the destructive nature of the sputtering process. Since it is a necessity to sputter the sample in order to measure it, it is not possible to repeat a measurement on exactly the same volume of material. Moreover, since virtually all SIMS instruments are single-channel measuring systems capable of detecting only one mass-to-charge value at any time, it is not possible to measure several species from exactly the same region of the sample. For magnetic spectrometers, rapid (100–1000 Hz) electrostatic peak switching can be used over a narrow mass range of the order of 5% of the nominal mass, but peak switching over a wider range typically requires time periods of seconds, so that true simultaneity of data collection cannot in general be achieved. Unless the sputtering rate is kept very low, a significant offset of several nanometers in the depth sampled may exist between data sets for different elements. However, because of the sensitivity of SIMS, sample consumption to obtain a measurement is low, so that major and minor constituents can usually be determined within a total sputtering depth of a few nanometers. The important concept in determining the extent of the surface sensitivity of a SIMS measurement is the useful yield, τ, which is the fraction of ions detected $[N_i(M^+)]$ relative to atoms of that species sputtered from the sample $[N(M)]$:

$$\tau = N_i(M^+)/N(M) \qquad (6.19)$$

In order to sputter $N(M)$ atoms of species M, a volume V of sample must be removed, where $V = 1/nC(M)$, with n the number of atoms per unit volume and $C(M)$ the concentration of species M. If the desired precision of the measurement is a fraction p (e.g., $p = 0.01$ or 1%), then the number of ions of type M which must be counted is $N_i(M^+) = 1/p^2$. Combining these conditions gives the volume of material which must be sputtered in order to realize a certain level of precision for a certain useful yield:

$$V = 1/nC \, \tau p^2 \qquad (6.20)$$

The volume V which must be sputtered to achieve detection at a specific precision can be configured in various ways depending on the selection of the primary beam. Thus, while a shallow depth can be sampled with a large beam diameter, the use of a microanalysis beam with fine lateral resolution may necessitate sputtering to a greater depth than can be accepted for surface analysis. Table 6.5 lists calculations of the depth sensitivity which can be achieved with a primary ion beam of various diameters for different values of the concentration. Depending on the choice of primary beam diameter and the required sensitivity, SIMS can serve as a surface analysis technique, subject analysis technique, subject to the limitations noted above. An example of a SIMS image of the surface distribution of chromium on an integrated circuit is shown in Figure 6.11.

6.5. Trace Microanalysis

6.5.1. X-Ray Analysis Techniques

In the discussion of limits of detection, it was noted that a major factor which determines the minimum mass fraction which can be detected is the peak-to-background ratio, P/B. With electron excitation, a significant background process exists, that of bremsstrahlung or "deceleration radiation," which produces a continuum of x-ray energies includ-

Table 6.5. Surface Sensitivity of SIMS[a]

Beam diameter	Concentration 0.5 (50%)	Concentration 0.01 (1%)
0.1 μm	2 nm	100 nm
1	0.02	1
10	0.0002	0.01

[a]Thickness (nm) of a layer which must be removed to detect a constituent with a precision of 0.05 (5%) and a useful yield of 0.001 (0.1%).

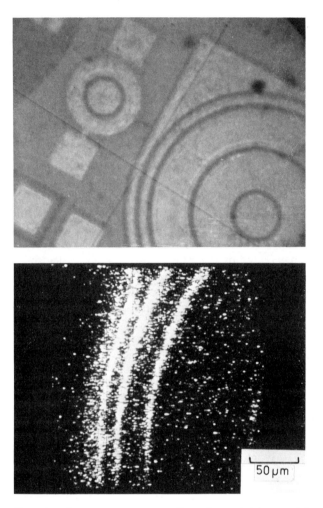

Figure 6.11. Secondary ion mass spectrometry (ion microprobe) image of the surface distribution of chromium on an integrated circuit.

ing those of the characteristic peaks of interest. For a wavelength spectrometer, the useful P/B ratio with electron excitation of pure element targets is typically of the order of 100 to 1000, which results in detection limits of the order of 0.1% (1000 ppm) to 0.01% (100 ppm). Inner shell ionization by means of x-rays and high-energy ions can significantly lower the background, resulting in higher P/B ratios and much reduced detection limits.

The use of x-rays to induce inner shell ionization with subsequent emission of characteristic x-rays of the target is the analytical technique known as "x-ray fluorescence." In order for a primary x-ray to be absorbed by photoelectric capture with the ejection of a photoelectron, the primary x-ray must have an energy greater than the energy of the shell to be ionized. The maximum efficiency for photoelectric capture occurs for those x-ray energies just above the edge excitation energy, with the efficiency falling rapidly as the primary energy is increased above the edge energy of interest. Thus, if a monochromatic primary x-ray beam is employed, high-sensitivity analysis is only achieved for a limited range of elements. To extend the sensitivity to more analytical lines, continuum excitation is often employed. In continuum excitation, the complete spectrum derived from a high-atomic-number target such as tungsten bombarded with a high-energy electron beam, ~ 50 keV, is used to excite the specimen, providing x-rays near an excitation edge of virtually all elements. The background in x-ray fluorescence analysis arises primarily from elastic and inelastic scattering of the incident x-ray flux and from bremsstrahlung created by the scattering of the photoelectrons and Auger electrons generated through the ionization process. The P/B which can be realized is typically two orders of magnitude better than the direct electron excitation case, resulting in detection limits in the ppm range.

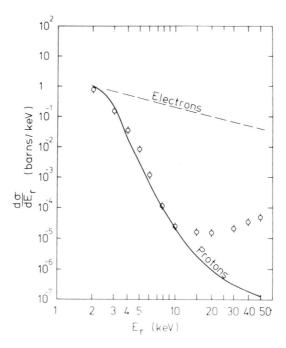

Figure 6.12. Bremsstrahlung in the energy range 1–50 keV as generated by electrons and by ions. (From Legge, 1980. © 1980 by San Francisco Press, Inc., Box 6800, San Francisco, CA 94101-6800.)

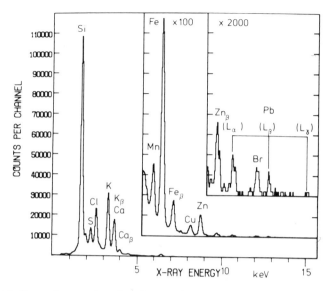

Figure 6.13. Trace element detection from a single cell in wheat leaf epidermis. (From Legge, 1980. © 1980 by San Francisco Press, Inc., Box 6800, San Francisco, CA 94101-6800.)

Classical x-ray fluorescence analysis is carried out with large beam diameters, typically centimeters in size, and is thus properly thought of as bulk analysis technique. Recently, the development of high-brightness, tunable-energy x-ray sources from synchrotron particle accelerator rings has made possible the development of the x-ray fluorescence microprobe. In such a system, beam dimensions of the order of micrometers can be achieved, yielding an analytical volume in a bulk specimen which can have lateral dimensions of 1–3 μm and a depth dimension of 10 μm or more, determined by the range of the primary and secondary x-rays in the matrix of interest.

X-ray generation by ion beams provides an enormous reduction in the bremsstrahlung produced by ions as compared to electrons. Figure 6.12 compares the production of 1- to 50-keV bremsstrahlung by electrons and protons with sufficient energy to also ionize inner shells in this energy range. At low energies, e.g., 1 keV, the production is similar, while at 10 keV the proton bremsstrahlung is five orders of magnitude below that produced by electrons. The improvement in peak-to-background with ion bombardment results in detection limits in the ppm to ppb range. Beam focusing to produce microprobes with 3-MeV ion beams has been devised. Trace element detection from a single cell in wheat leaf epidermis with such a microprobe is illustrated in Figure 6.13 (Legge, 1980).

6.5.2. Secondary Ion Mass Spectrometry

The analysis of a sample by means of mass spectrometry, in which the atoms are directly measured, brings, in principle, the distinct advantage of eliminating the background entirely. Examination of a SIMS spectrum, Figure 6.14, reveals that P/B ratios of 1,000,000/1 or more can be achieved for at least some elements. With such high P/B ratios, detection limits in the ppm or ppb range can be realized. A demonstration of this sensitivity in a microanalysis experiment is shown in Figure 6.15, which is a depth profile of ion-implanted boron in silicon. This profile, which was recorded from a 60-μm-diameter area, shows a dynamic measurement range of six orders of magnitude, from a level of 10% boron to 100 ppb at the background. The background in this case arises from the sputtering process itself, since the nature of the sputtered crater is such that the high concentration regions, once passed during sputtering, are continually exposed on the crater walls. Sputtered material from the walls can redeposit on the crater floor, eventually forming a background. In fact, if the peak concentration of the depth profile is lower, the detection limit determined by the resputtering phenomenon is proportionally lower, leading to detection limits of 10 to 100 ppb.

One of the most impressive aspects of SIMS for trace analysis is the

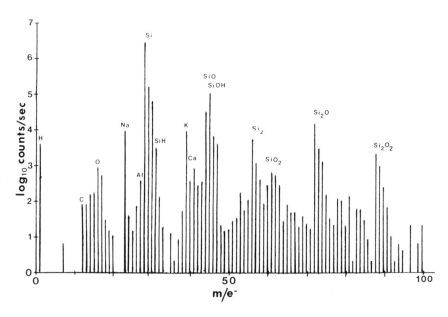

Figure 6.14. Secondary ion mass spectrum of high-purity silicon showing elemental and molecular ion peaks.

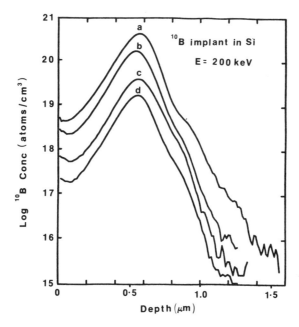

Figure 6.15. Secondary ion mass spectrometry depth profile of boron which was ion-implanted into silicon. Doses: d, 4×10^{14} atoms/cm³; c, 10^{15}; b, 4×10^{15}; a, 10^{16} (courtesy of David Simons).

capability of mapping the distribution of trace elements in the specimen. Whereas with EPMA an x-ray area scan for a constituent at the 1% level might require in excess of 6h of accumulation time to obtain adequate statistics for the image, a SIMS image at trace level can be accumulated in seconds. This is a direct result of the great difference in the efficiency of the characteristic signal generation and in the peak-to-background between the EPMA and SIMS. Both the scanning and direct imaging SIMS instruments are capable of trace element imaging. Figure 6.16 contains examples of SIMS imaging of trace constituents in samples. Figure 6.16a is a scanning ion microprobe image of the distribution of boron in steel where the total boron concentration in the bulk material is only 50 ppm. Figure 6.16b is an ion microscope image of the distribution of aluminum in reaction-bonded silicon carbide where the bulk concentration of aluminum was approximately 100 ppm. In both cases, the accumulation time was less than 30 s, which can be compared to 6 h for a WDS area scan at the 1 wt% concentration level.

Even in the absence of the resputtering phenomenon, the background may not be negligible. Two main sources of background are encountered in SIMS analysis. First, the possibility of the formation of molecular ions and multiply charged atomic ions can lead to the exis-

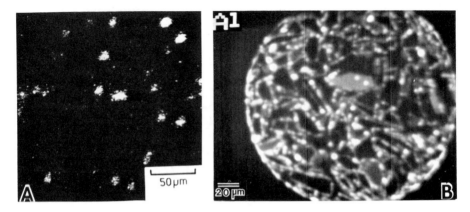

Figure 6.16. Secondary ion mass spectrometry images of trace constituents in materials. (A) Scanning ion microprobe image of the boron distribution in a steel which contains 50 ppm total in the bulk. (B) Ion microscope image of aluminum in reaction-bonded silicon carbide at a level of approximately 100 ppm in the bulk.

tence of interfering species at the nominal mass of the species of interest. For example, in the analysis of silicon, the production of Si-dimer, Si_2, at mass-to-charge 56 causes a strong interference with the principal isotope for iron, while the formation of doubly charged Si^{2+} at mass-to-charge 14 creates an interference with the principal isotope of nitrogen. Some interference situations can be avoided by switching to an alternative isotope, such as Fe-54 in the case of the silicon dimer interference on iron, or by selectively filtering the ions according to their initial kinetic energy, which discriminates selectively against the molecular ions due to their narrow energy distribution. The second source of background occurs as a result of the high intensity associated with the peak of a major or minor constituent. In the vicinity of a high-intensity peak, the local background may be higher than expected due to the effect of scattering of the ions due to collisions with gas molecules in the mass spectrometer, thus raising the background on nearby peaks which may represent trace constituents.

One alternative which is being explored in order to avoid limitations which arise from the presence of high-intensity matrix peaks in the spectrum involves the use of selective ionization of the species of interest. Laser beams tuned to specific wavelengths provide extremely selective "resonance ionization" such that only one species can be ionized at a time, thus eliminating the possibility of collisions between the ions and gas molecules in the mass spectrometer. This sputter-initiated resonance ionization spectrometry (SIRIS) has demonstrated ppb sensitivity with the possibility of reaching ppt sensitivity (Parks *et al.*, 1983). As an added bonus, since the ionization occurs after sputtering and therefore external to the specimen, matrix effects are greatly reduced, to the degree that the intensity for a solute element dispersed in matrices as different as metallic iron and semiconductor silicon lie on the same working curve.

6.5.3. Laser Microprobe Mass Analysis

Another approach to trace microanalysis is that of the laser micro-probe mass analysis (LAMMA) (Hillenkamp *et al.,* 1975; Kaufmann *et al.,* 1979). In the LAMMA technique, which is illustrated schematically in Figure 6.17, a pulsed photon beam is focused to a probe of micrometer dimensions. The power density in the probe is of the order of 10^8 to 10^{11} W/cm^2, which is sufficient to thermally evaporate a small volume of the sample. A fraction of the order of 0.1% of the evaporated atoms is ionized by thermal and nonresonant photon absorption. The ions are then accelerated through a 3-kV potential, imparting to all ions the same kinetic energy. Since the laser ionization pulse duration is short, approximately 10 ns, the ions are created essentially at the same instant, and since all

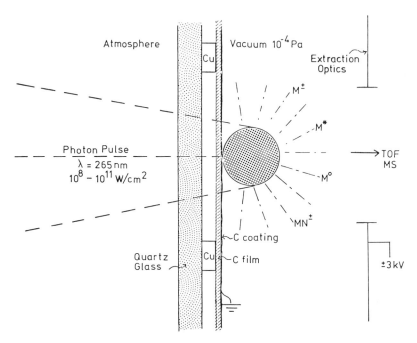

Figure 6.17. Schematic diagram illustrating laser microprobe mass analyzer (LAMMA). M^+, M^-: atomic ions; M^0: neutral atoms; M^*: excited neutrals; MN^+, MN^-: molecular ions; TOF MS: time-of-flight mass spectrometer.

are given the same kinetic energy, a velocity distribution results according to mass. The LAMMA ion source is thus well suited to measurement by the technique of time-of-flight mass spectrometry. The ions pass through a field-free drift tube and are detected by ion-to-electron conversion at the first dynode of an electron multiplier. The current output of the multiplier is recorded by means of a 100-MHz digital transient recorder, which divides the signal into 10-ns channels digitized to 8-bit resolution. Two separate transient recorders are employed at different gains, which provides an effective dynamic range of 14 bits (16,000), allowing for overlap of the two scales. Thus, from a single micrometer-sized volume of the sample, a complete mass spectrum can be obtained which contains all constituents from hydrogen to the actinides. Such a spectrum is illustrated in Figure 6.18, as measured from a single micrometer-sized chip of NBS SRM 610 glass, which contains many elements at a concentration of 500 ppm. The strong signals which can be detected from these constituents confirm the utility of the LAMMA technique for trace microanalysis. Measurements have shown that it is possible to obtain a useful mass spectrum from a sample mass as low as 10 fg, and mass fraction levels of 1–10 ppm have been successfully detected.

The great strength of the LAMMA technique comes from the effective parallel detection which is achieved by the time-of-flight mass spectrometry. Thus, from a single micrometer-sized particle, a complete mass

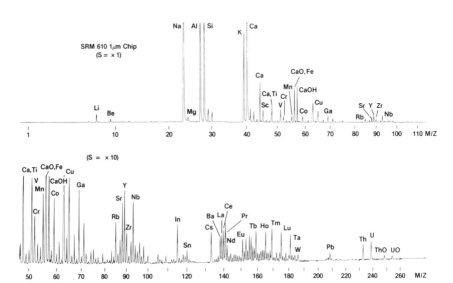

Figure 6.18. Laser microprobe mass analyzer (LAMMA) spectrum of NBS Standard Reference Material 610 glass, showing complete spanning of the periodic table from a single 1-μm particle (courtesy of David Simons).

spectrum can be measured, whereas in a single-channel instrument typically used in SIMS or other forms of mass spectrometry, the entire micrometer-sized particle might have to be consumed in order to detect a single trace constituent. The major limitation of LAMMA arises from the presence of a background due to molecular ions, although this source of possible interference can be reduced by using sufficiently high power densities to reduce all evaporated particles to atomic species. A second problem is the limited dynamic range of the detector system, which limits the detection to trace/minor or minor/major constituents on a single shot because of the tendency of the detector to saturate at high signal levels.

6.6. Molecular Microanalysis

In many instances in applying microanalysis to real problems, we are confronted with the need to determine how the elements we measure are combined into chemical compounds. Often the presence of these compounds can be inferred, such as the coincident measurement of iron and sulfur suggesting the presence of FeS_2 in the sample. However, when multiple valence states can exist, the confidence in an inferred chemical analysis may be low. What is needed is a technique(s) which can directly measure and characterize the compounds present in the sampled region. The analysis at high spatial resolution of the molecular (chemical) composition can be accomplished by two broad categories of analytical techniques:

1. Mass spectrometry techniques, in which the molecular constituents are directly observed as the ionized parent molecular ions as well as associated fragment ions which serve to reveal the details of the molecular structure.

2. Photon techniques, in which photons in the ultraviolet (UV), visible (V), or infrared (IR) interact with the specific energy levels associated with vibrations and rotations of the bonds of the molecules, with subsequent detection by means by absorption, fluorescence, and scattering techniques.

6.6.1. Mass Spectrometry Techniques

6.6.1.1. Desorption-Mode LAMMA

At the high power densities typically used in LAMMA analysis, the molecular constituents are very effectively broken down into atomic species or simple two- or three-component molecular ions. However, if the power density is reduced to 10^6 W/cm^2, a condition of laser desorption can be achieved in which a surface layer of molecules can be selectively desorbed without perforation of the underlying substrate or particle (Kaufmann *et al.,* 1979). Despite the low power density, the spatial resolution can still be better than 5 μm in the desorption mode, which provides a rare example of spatially resolved organic mass spectrometry. An

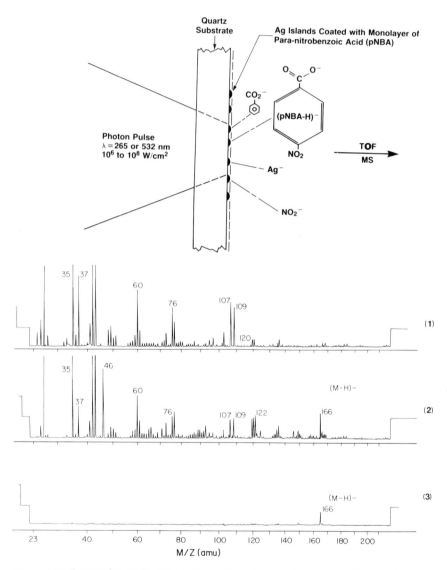

Figure 6.19. Laser microprobe mass analyzer desorption-mode spectrum of a monolayer of *para*-nitrobenzoic acid applied to a silver film. (From Fletcher *et al.,* 1984.)

example of a laser-desorption spectrum of an organic compound applied as a monolayer to a silver film is shown in Figure 6.19. The parent ion and a few peaks arising from various daughter ions are indicated.

6.6.1.2. Static SIMS

Under the usual primary ion bombardment conditions of high ion beam energy (5–20 keV) and current density (1 A/cm^2) used in conventional SIMS, the sample surface is quickly disrupted by the high-density ion beam. This disruption breaks bonds of chemical compounds so that after the initial bombardment of a few seconds' duration, subsequent primary ions can only sputter atomic ions or simple molecular ions for subsequent detection in the spectrum. These bombardment conditions are generally referred to as constituting "dynamic SIMS," since the specimen is constantly changing during the measurement process.

An alternative bombardment condition which can be established is that of "static SIMS," in which the current density is kept low (10^{-6} to 10^{-9} A/cm^2) (Benninghoven, 1973, 1979). With this condition, any primary ion incident during the time period necessary to record a spectrum has a high probability of striking unperturbed molecules, so that the specimen remains essentially unchanged or static during the measurement process. The ion energy is also kept low (0.5–3 keV) to minimize the damage area involved with each impact. Under static SIMS conditions, complex organic molecular ions, including those of nucleic acids, sugars, fatty acids, and many others, have been successfully analyzed. In order to achieve a static SIMS condition, the beam size is normally made quite large, of the order of millimeters, so that lateral spatial resolution is greatly diminished. The resolution in depth, however, corresponds to the single outermost molecular layer. An example of a static SIMS spectrum of the compound methionine is shown in Figure 6.20.

As a compromise between the static and dynamic SIMS conditions, useful molecular spectra can be obtained with primary ion beams focused as small as 20 μm with a current density of 10^{-4} A/cm^2, which gives a bombardment condition intermediate between the static and dynamic conditions and provides at least some level of spatial resolution.

6.6.1.3. Laser-Induced Desorption-Mode Ion Imaging

The use of a laser to desorb atomic and molecular constituents from a surface has been combined with the secondary ion imaging optics of the ion microscope (Furman and Evans, 1981) to provide desorption-mode ion imaging. The high collection efficiency of the ion microscope optics is valuable in deriving the maximum utility from the limited ion signal

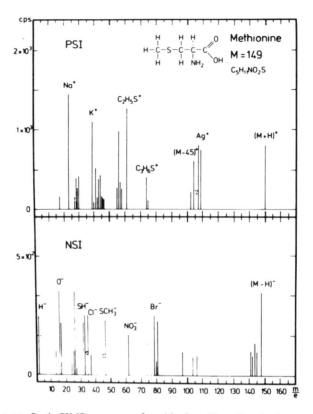

Figure 6.20. Static SIMS spectrum of methionine. (From Benninghoven, 1979.)

produced by the laser beam. An example of a spectrum of arginine obtained in the desorption mode is shown in Figure 6.21, and a desorption-mode ion image of rubidium in glass particles is shown in Figure 6.22.

The laser-induced desorption mode holds promise for compositional mapping at high spatial resolution of delicate molecular constituents on surfaces. This capacity will augment the high-spatial-resolution point analyses which can be made by the LAMMA technique.

6.6.2. Photon Beam Microanalysis

The use of photon beams to probe the chemical structure of matter of micrometer spatial resolution is the oldest of the microanalysis techniques, extending in some cases back into the 19th century. The physical basis for the analysis is the interaction of the incident photons with the

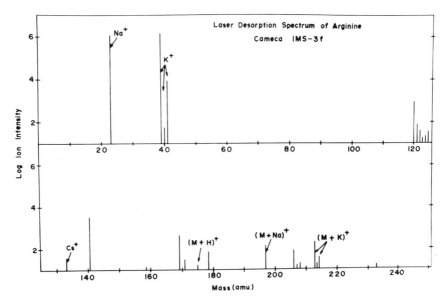

Figure 6.21. Laser-desorption spectra of arginine obtained in the ion microscope. (From Furman and Evans, 1981. © 1981 by San Francisco Press, Inc., Box 6800, San Francisco, CA 94101-6800.)

atomic electrons whose energy levels are involved in chemical bonding. In general, radiation of a particular energy interacts most strongly with electrons at a similar energy. Since bonding generally involves electrons with an energy level of a fraction of an electron volt to several electron volts, the ideal probes of these levels are photons in the UV (E = 5 eV at 250 nm), V (E = 2.5 eV at 500 nm), and IR (E = 1.2 eV at 1000 nm).

Detection of the interaction of the photons with atomic electrons can take place in several possible ways: absorption, fluorescence, and scattering. A variety of techniques are based on these excitation and detection modes. Only the general categories of microspectroscopy will be considered below, based on the review of Hirschfeld (1982). In considering these methods, it must be remembered that in virtually all cases, the analysis can be coupled with high-quality optical imaging in spatial resolutions from 20 μm to 250 nm, depending on the wavelength of the radiation involved.

6.6.2.1. Absorption

When the wavelength (energy) of incident beam is varied and its intensity is measured after passage through the sample, decreased intensity is observed at characteristic absorption energies, which represent effi-

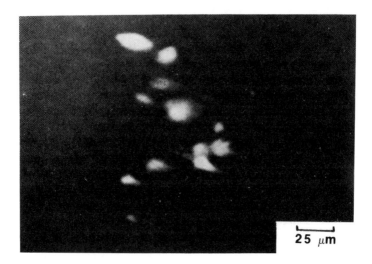

Figure 6.22. Laser-desorption ion image of rubidium distribution in NBS SRM 661 glass particles. (From Furman and Evans, 1981. ©1981 by San Francisco Press, Inc., Box 6800, San Francisco, CA 94101-6800.)

cient coupling of the incident beam energy with an excitation in a molecular electron energy state such as a rotation or vibration of a specific molecular bond.

In the UV–V range of excitation, most materials are quite transparent to the radiation. As a result, in order to generate adequate signals for detection, a suitable chemical dye must be added to selectively stain the sample. By using dyes with appropriate discrimination, minor differences in chemical, structural, and steric properties can be detected. Extreme selectivity can be achieved through the use of specific enzymatic or immunochemical reactions which serve to either generate dyes at specific sites in the sample or to bind the dyes to those sites. Absorption differences of 0.3% can correspond to a constituent at a mass concentration of 100 ppm or an absolute mass of 10^{-17} g. Localization can be restricted to a volume 250 nm in diameter and 100 nm thick.

An example of micro-IR spectrometry applied to the analysis of a contaminant particle found in a semiconductor process is shown in Figure 6.23 (Scott and Ramsey, 1982). In this case, based on the observation of CO stretch bands at 1270 and 1100 cm^{-1} and the match to a reference spectrum, the particle was found to be polyethylene terphthlate polymer debris from laboratory gloves.

6.6.2.2. Fluorescence

Upon absorbing a photon, an atom or molecule will be raised in energy above the ground state to some characteristic excited state. After

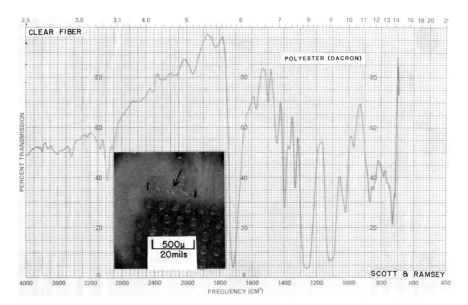

Figure 6.23. Detection of polyethylene terphthlate contamination by micro-infrared analyses. (From Scott and Ramsey, 1982. © 1982 by San Francisco Press, Inc., Box 6800, San Francisco, CA 94101-6800.)

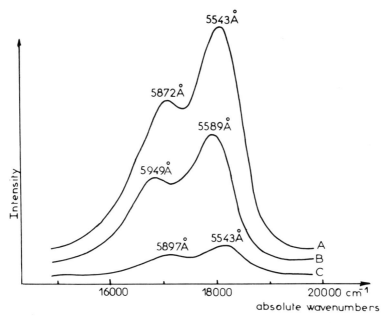

Figure 6.24. Application of microspectrofluorimetry to the detection of adriamycin in human leukemia cells. (From Dhamelincourt, 1982. © 1982 by San Francisco Press, Inc., Box 6800, San Francisco, CA 94101-6800.) Spectrum A: free adriamycin; spectrum B: leukemia cell nucleus; C: cytoplasm of leukemia cell.

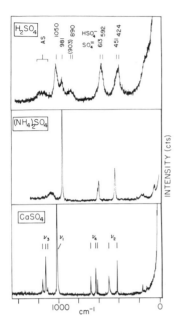

Figure 6.25. Raman microprobe spectrum of various sulfates with identification of various modes of vibration characteristic of the sulfate group within the different compounds. (From Etz, 1979.)

a short period, typically of the order of nanoseconds, this excited state will decay via electron transitions between characteristic energy levels, and a photon will be emitted from the atom or molecule. This fluorescence radiation can be described by a number of specific properties, including wavelength (energy), intensity, polarization, emission lifetime, and efficiency, all of which may vary with the wavelength and polarization of the exciting radiation.

Fluorescence has the distinct advantage of being absent from the background of a sample, whereas in the absorption case, the background around the sample is bright due to the illumination field. The shot noise of the dark background is so much lower than in the case of a bright background that the fluorescence detection limit may be as much as a factor of 1000 lower than the absorption detection limit. Concentrations as low as 1 ppb can be detected, with the minimum detectable mass as low as 10^{-21} g. The limiting spatial resolution is approximately 350 nm, but because of the high sensitivity, well-separated discrete objects as small as 10 nm can be detected. The principal limitation of the technique arises because many samples will not show fluorescence. In such cases, a reagent tag may be necessary to create a detectable signal. However, the reagent must be purposely developed for each problem, and the specimen must be permeable to the reagent, which may be difficult in the case of solid examples.

An example of microspectrofluorimetry applied to the study of individual human leukemia cells is shown in Figure 6.24 (Dhamelincourt, 1982). A chemotherapeutic agent, adriamycin, is detected in the nucleus and cytoplasm of a single leukemia cell. The frequency and intensity shifts relative to the reference adriamycin spectrum are attributed to interaction of the adriamycin with the DNA in the nucleus.

6.6.2.3. Raman Scattering

The third general type of microspectrometry to consider is based upon Raman scattering. The Raman phenomenon involves the scattering

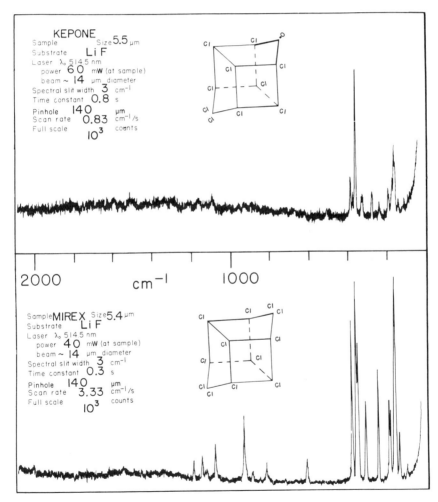

Figure 6.26. Raman microprobe spectra of particles of kepone and mirex, showing specificity in identification. (From Etz, 1979.)

of the incident photon by a molecule which causes a shift in the wavelength (energy) of the photon due to interactions with the various vibrational modes of the molecule. The Raman spectrum which results is a complex pattern which can be used to identify the detailed structure of the molecule. Examples from the work of Etz (1979) of Raman spectra

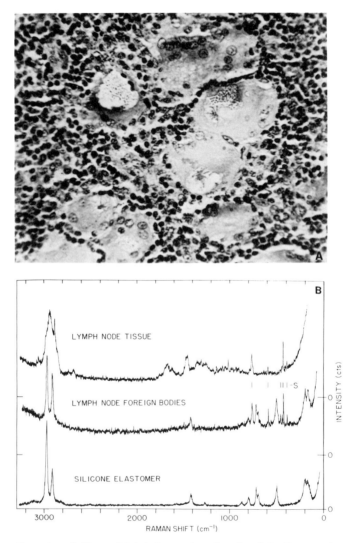

Figure 6.27. Detection of silicone debris in human lymph node cells by Raman microprobe. (A) micrograph showing debris in unstained cells; (B) spectra of particles and reference materials. (From Abrahams and Etz, 1979. © 1979 by the AAAS.)

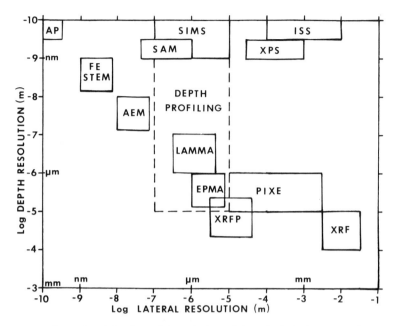

Figure 6.28. Lateral and depth spatial resolution of the principal elemental microanalysis methods. Abbreviations: AP, atom probe; SIMS, secondary ion mass spectrometry; LAMMA, laser microprobe mass analysis; SAM, scanning Auger microscopy; ISS, ion scattering spectrometry; XPS, x-ray photoelectron spectroscopy; FE STEM, field-emission scanning transmission electron microscopy; AEM, analytical electron microscopy; EPMA, electron probe microanalyzer; PIXE, proton-induced x-ray emission; XRF, x-ray fluorescence; XRFP, x-ray fluorescence probe.

for the sulfate compound are shown in Figure 6.25 with the various peaks assigned to different bonds and groups within the molecule. The specificity of the technique can be judged by the comparison of the Raman spectra for the nearly identical structures of kepone and mirex shown in Figure 6.26; the spectra are sufficiently different to unambiguously identify the two compounds.

The chief limitation of the Raman technique arises from the fundamental weakness of Raman scattering. In order to collect a useful signal at all from a microscopic sample, Raman microprobes must be designed with high-intensity focused laser sources, which bring to bear an extremely high power density, typically MW/cm^2, onto the sample, and a high-efficiency collector for the scattered Raman light must also be employed. The high power density may lead to beam-induced damage of the sample; indeed, if the sample is highly absorbing, the beam may cause total destruction of the sample. Also, fluorescence emission, if it occurs, will generally be more intense than the Raman emission and may swamp it in the recorded spectrum. Beam damage effects have been reduced to some extent by the use of high-efficiency multichannel Raman detectors, so that useful spectra can now be obtained from sensitive materials, such as trinitrotoluene (Steinbach *et al.,* 1982). Despite these improvements, Raman microanalysis is limited to concentrations greater than 0.1% and minimum detectable masses of 10^{-13} g.

An example of the utility of the Raman microprobe, especially when used in conjunction with other microanalysis techniques, is shown in Figure 6.27, (Abrahams and Etz, 1979). Figure 6.27a is a tissue section of lymph node from a patient who showed the formation of unusual large cells. The anomalous cells were associated with foreign debris, which when analyzed with an electron probe showed the presence of the element silicon. Raman microanalysis revealed that the chemical state of the silicon in the foreign debris was that of silicone elastomer (Figure 6.27b). The silicone elastomer was deposited in the lymph node from a synthetic finger joint replacement which underwent wear erosion in service.

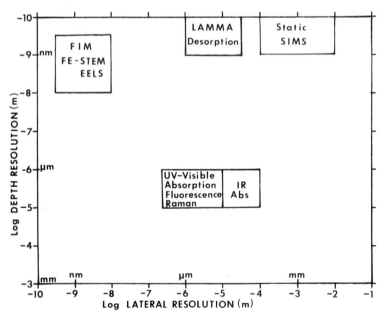

Figure 6.29. Lateral and depth spatial resolution of the principal molecular microanalysis methods. Abbreviations: SIMS, secondary ion mass spectrometry; LAMMA desorption, laser microprobe mass analyzer, desorption mode; FIM, field ion microscope; FE-STEM EELS, field-emission scanning transmission electron microscopy with electron energy loss spectrometry; UV, ultraviolet; IR, infrared.

Table 6.6. Principal Characteristics of the Elemental Microanalysis Techniques

Technique[a]	Primary radiation	Secondary radiation	Constituents measured	Detection limits	Quantitation technique	Relative accuracy
EPMA	Electrons	X-rays	Z > 4 (WDS, UTW EDS)	100 ppm	ZAF	1–5%
			Z > 11 (EDS)	0.1%		
AEM, FE-STEM	Electrons	X-rays	Z > 4 (UTW EDS)	0.1% (EDS)	Sx/m	5–10%
			Z > 3 (EELS)	1% (EELS)		
SAM	Electrons	Electrons	Z > 3	0.1–1%	Sx/m	10–25%
SIMS	Ions	Ions	All Z	10 ppb–10 ppm	Sx/m	10–25%
LAMMA	Photons	Ions	All Z	10–100 ppm	Sx/m	10–50%
PIXE	Ions	X-rays	Z > 4 (EDS)	10 ppb–100 ppm	Working curve	1–10%
AP	None	Ions	All Z	0.1–1%	Internal calibration	5–25%
XPS	X-rays	Electrons	Z > 3	0.1–1%	Working curve	5–25%
ISS	Ions	Ions	Z > 3	1%	Working curve	10%
XRF (bulk)	X-rays	X-rays	Z > 4 (WDS)	1–10 ppm	Working curve	1–5%
			Z > 11 (EDS)			

[a]Abbreviations: AP, atom probe; SIMS, secondary ion mass spectrometry; LAMMA, laser microprobe mass analysis; SAM, scanning Auger microscopy; ISS, ion scattering spectrometry; XPS, x-ray photoelectron spectroscopy; FE-STEM, field-emission scanning transmission electron microscopy; AEM, analytical electron microscopy; EPMA, electron probe microanalyzer; PIXE, proton-induced x-ray emission; XRF, x-ray fluorescence.

Table 6.7. Principal Characteristics of the Molecular Microanalysis Techniques

Technique[a]	Primary radiation	Secondary radiation	Detection limits	Specificity	Structural information	Relative accuracy
Static SIMS	Ions	Ions	1–5%	High	Yes	Qualitative
LAMMA desorption	Photons	Ions	1–5%	High	Yes	Qualitative
UV–visible Absorption	Photons	Photons	10–100 ppm	With reagents	Yes	1%
Fluorescence			1 ppb	Good	Yes	1%
Raman			1%	High	Yes	1–5%
IR absorption	Photons	Photons	1%	High	Yes	1%
FE-STEM EELS	Electrons	Electrons	10%	Good	No	Qualitative
FIM	None	Ions	10%	Good	Yes	Qualitative

[a]Abbreviations: SIMS, secondary ion mass spectrometry; LAMMA desorption, laser microprobe mass analyzer, desorption mode; FIM, field ion microscope; FE-STEM EELS, field-emission scanning transmission electron microscopy with electron energy loss spectrometry; UV, ultraviolet; IR, infrared.

6.7. Summary

The spatially resolved analysis techniques considered in this chapter can be compared by means of Figures 6.28 and 6.29, which graphically represent the lateral and depth resolution of techniques which provide primarily elemental microanalysis information (Figure 6.28) or molecular microanalysis information (Figure 6.29). A number of the major characteristics of these techniques are summarized in Tables 6.6 and 6.7. Such a comparison is somewhat cursory, and somewhat uneven, since the requirements on the specimen are far from equal in the techniques. These figures and tables nevertheless provide a useful impression of the broad capabilities of the analytical techniques. Examination of Figures 6.28 and 6.29 reveals that, while there is some overlap among the techniques, in general the variety of associated microanalysis techniques are highly complementary to each other. A comprehensive approach to the solution of many problems will often require the use of a variety of these tools to maximize the information obtained from the sample (Newbury, 1979; Anderson and Ramsey, 1979; Etz et al., 1985).

7

Specimen Coating

7.1. Introduction

It is the purpose of this chapter to review the advances in coating techniques for nonconducting samples which are necessary to eliminate problems of surface charging. The ways by which one may hope to improve the bulk conductivity of such samples are discussed elsewhere in this book. It is not our intent to discuss the optimal parameters of standard coating procedures such as thermal evaporation and diode sputtering, which are designed to increase the secondary electron emission and surface conductivity of samples. Such details may be found in *SEMXM*. There is now considerable overlap between the high-resolution coating techniques which were once used exclusively for transmission electron microscopy and the current refinements of the methods routinely used for scanning electron microscopy. This overlap is an inevitable consequence of the improving resolution of the conventional SEM, the increasing use of STEMs, and the appearance of hybrid machines, which allow a conventional TEM to be used as an SEM. It is generally accepted that the increased resolution available on most electron beam instruments necessitates much more attention being paid to the ways by which the coating layers are applied to samples. It should be remembered that the two main reasons for coating nonconductive samples are to eliminate the artifacts brought about by electrical charging and by thermal loading. Whereas a thin (1–3 nm) continuous layer of metal is a reasonably good electrical conductor, at least double that thickness of metal is needed to conduct away the heat which can readily build up in the specimen.

The general trend in the recent work has been aimed at decreasing both the final thickness and grain size of the film. Small grain size is favored by low total deposition, low rate of deposition, low substrate temperature, high (i.e., normal) angle between source and sample, and low rate of contamination. High-melting-point metals are better than low-melting-point metals as they condense more rapidly. Alloys of metals, provided they are deposited congruently, reduce aggregate size by increasing the distance over which an atom has to move to find a place in the crystal lattice. The primary energy of the emitted particles (or atoms) has little effect on the final grain size, which is related more to the nature of the metal, the mobility of its atoms, and the amount of secondary energy transfer by particles such as photons, ions, and electrons. With these factors in mind, a number of workers have sought to design instrumentation and techniques to improve the quality of the coating layers applied to nonconductive specimens.

The discussions will center on the recent advances in coating techniques and will cover the following topics:

- Diode sputter coating
- Diode sputter coating at low voltages
- Penning sputter coating
- Ion-beam sputter coating
- Thermal evaporation
- Coating at low specimen temperature
- High-resolution coating
- Coating thickness measurements
- Artifacts
- Non-thin-film coating methods

7.2. Diode Sputter Coating

Diode sputter coating, with or without substrate cooling, still remains the most popular way of applying a coating layer to a nonconducting sample. Although the basic instrumentation has remained unchanged for the past 10 years, there is a tendency to automate the coating procedure. One can only view this as a mixed blessing. For the novice and for a laboratory with a high throughput of standard samples, it is a distinct advantage as it allows relatively inexperienced operators to obtain reasonably good and, more important, reproducible results. But for someone interested in using the full capabilities of the SEM, fully automated coaters do not allow very much leeway in varying the basic coating parameters.

There has been little attempt to diminish the high contamination rates of some sputter coaters although it could be argued that for routine SEM at low magnifications, a small amount of contamination is of little consequence. Nevertheless, it is important to use pump oils with a low back-streaming coefficient, to use rotary pumps with sufficient capacity to enable an activated alumina trap to be placed in the backing line, and to use high-purity (low hydrocarbon) argon as the sputtering gas. The studies carried out by Echlin *et al.* (1980a) have shown that provided attention is paid to minimizing contamination, it is better to work at lower accelerating voltages and sputter for a longer time at a lower sputtering rate, e.g., for the noble metals about 4 nm/min as shown in Table 7.1. This will provide thin continuous films suitable for medium-resolution SEM. Kemmenoe and Bullock (1983) carried out a comparative structure analysis of diode and ion-beam sputter-coated films and concluded that for low-resolution SEM where thicker films can be tolerated, it is probably best to diode-sputter noble metals at a high deposition rate, provided the specimens are not heat sensitive. They concluded that the small increase in grain size is outweighed by the marked improvement in film structure. Kemmenoe and Bullock found that the average grain size of the thinnest gold and platinum films were more or less independent of the mode or rate of deposition. However, as the film thickness increased, there were significant changes in the size of both the grains and the gross appearance of the film structure. The effects of lowering substrate temperature will be discussed elsewhere in this section, but this too increases the resolution of the film layer. Nockolds *et al.* (1982) have developed a planar magnetron sputter coater which gives a high sputtering rate without generating excessive amounts of heat in the specimen. Noble metals can be sputtered at a rate of 1.0 nm/s with a temperature rise of 0.15 K/s. These workers also found that the gas pressure had a significant effect on thin film formation. At high pressures, i.e., 10^{-1} Torr, severe cracking in the film was observed, which disappeared at 10^{-2} Torr. Nockolds *et al.* considered this effect to be due to the development of tensile stresses in the film. Care must also be taken to minimize the secondary energy transfer from high-energy gas atoms during the coating process. Colquhoun (1984) has recently presented details of a process called sputter shadowing. By placing a horizontal circular shield a few millimeters above the sample surface, it is possible to restrict the coating to a cone of vertical deposition. The distance between the shield and the surface and the diameter of the shield with respect to the surface will determine the angle of shadowing at each point on the specimen surface. These dimensions are near or below the minimum free path of the sputtered atoms which minimizes multiple scattering and gives a directionality to the sputter deposition. The specimens are thus coated in a manner analogous to rotary shadowing. Colquhoun has successfully applied this technique to shadow strands of DNA. The results are comparable to those obtained by unidirectional metal evaporation shadowing and rotary shadowing with, it is claimed, minimal radiant and metal deposition heating of the sample. It has the added advantage of providing on a single grid a spectrum of contrasts with a heavy deposition at the periphery ranging to a light deposition at the center. The simple device is easy to make and may be placed at the anode of any sputter coater.

7.3. Low-Voltage Sputter Coating

Films for conventional SEM generally need to be 10–12 nm thick and are currently best being produced by ion-beam sputtering. However, this procedure is time-consuming and also requires complex and expensive equipment; it thus appeared appropriate to seek a less complicated method of coating nonconducting samples for conventional SEM. Preliminary experiments by Echlin *et al.* (1980a, 1985) and Echlin (1981) have shown that diode sputter coating at low voltages gives thin films with a grain size nearly as small as that obtained by ion-beam sputtering.

Echlin *et al.* (1980a) found a reduction in particle size when the coating was carried out at 1.8 keV compared to 2.4 keV. In a later study (Echlin, 1981), sputter coating was carried out at between 400 and 1000 eV. Using gold as a target, there was a diminution in particle size as the voltage was decreased. Robards *et al.* (1981) have also described a low-voltage sputter-coating system which uses 250 eV at 12–15 mA and a pressure of 20 Pa and is capable of depositing a 15-nm gold film within 2–3 min.

A newly designed cathode head has been constructed for the Polaron E5400 high-resolution sputter coater. With the exception of the new cathode head, the sputter coater is identical to the Polaron Series II cool sputter coater which allows the specimen table to be cooled to 268 K. The new cathode head consists of an interchangeable disk target, surrounded by a matched pair of curved ceramic magnets within an aluminum shroud. The matched pair of magnets are placed at 180° to each other, with the north and south poles of the two magnets opposite. The maximum magnetic field is 0.08 T (800 G). A 35-mm-deep circular magnetic shield surrounds the target, and the whole cathode assembly can be moved vertically in relation to the specimen table. This configuration of magnet–target–shield molds the shape of the plasma flux between the anode (specimen table) and the cathode, maximizing the sputtering efficiency of the target while at the same time causing minimal thermal input onto the specimen. Using this newly designed cathode head and with the target 50 mm from the specimen, thin films of gold, gold/palladium (80:20), and platinum were deposited onto carbon-coated electron microscope grids using argon as the plasma-forming gas. The results of these studies are found in Echlin *et al.* (1982a) and a brief summary is given below (see Figure 7.1 and Table 7.1). The difference in particle size between the TEM and SEM observation (Table 7.1) is due to the fact that one is able to measure the smallest particles in the TEM whereas the SEM with its lower resolution can only give an average value.

7.3.1. Gold/Palladium

There is a clear decrease in the average size of the particles with a decrease in accelerating voltage in films examined in both the TEM and

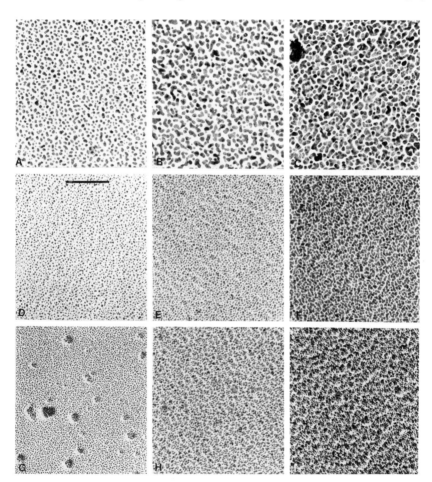

Figure 7.1. Low-voltage sputter-coated films. (A–C) Gold; A = 400 eV, B = 600 eV, C = 800 eV. (D–F) Gold/palladium; D = 400 eV, E = 600 eV, F = 800 eV. (G–I) Platinum; G = 400 eV, H = 600 eV, I = 800 eV. All sputter coated at 20 mA in argon. Bar = 100 nm. (From Echlin *et al.*, 1982a.)

Table 7.1. Sputtering Conditions and Resulting Film Characteristics[a]

Target (eV)	Voltage (eV)	Plasma current (mA)	Thick-ness (nm)	Coating rate (nm/min)	Temp. (K)	Pres-sure (Pa)	Particle size (nm) TEM	Particle size (nm) SEM
Au/								
Pd	800	20	15	1.5	268	4	4.9 ± 0.12	11.5 ± 0.2
	600	20	15	0.7	268	4	3.6 ± 0.10	9.5 ± 0.15
	400	20	10	0.25	268	4	2.3 ± 0.10	6.7 ± 0.14
Au	800	20	15	2.2	268	4	12.5 ± 0.37	14.3 ± 0.3
	600	20	15	1.4	268	4	8.7 ± 0.35	11.0 ± 0.5
	400	20	10	0.4	268	4	7.2 ± 0.32	9.3 ± 0.2
Pt	800	20	15	1.4	268	4	3.0 ± 0.09	7.5 ± 0.1
	600	20	15	0.9	268	4	2.4 ± 0.10	3.5 ± 0.15
	400	20	10	0.18	268	4	2.0 ± 0.08	2.3 ± 0.1

[a]From Echlin *et al.*, 1981.

the SEM (Table 7.1). At a nominal film thickness of 15 nm, the gold/palladium forms a continuous layer. The average size of particles measured in the SEM is about three times larger than the size of the same particles measured in the TEM.

7.3.2. Gold

Although there is a similar decrease in the average size of the particles with a decrease in accelerating voltage, the gold particles are larger than the gold/palladium particles deposited under the same conditions.

7.3.3. Platinum

The platinum target provided the smallest particle sizes in films produced using low-voltage sputter coating. There is a decrease in particle size with accelerating voltage. In the film deposited at 800 eV, the particle size as measured on the SEM image is more than twice the size of the particles measured on the TEM image. In the films deposited at 400 and 600 eV, the particle sizes are almost the same. These results indicate that low-voltage sputter coating can produce films with particle sizes that are smaller than those in films produced at higher voltages. Although low-voltage sputter-coated films have a finer grain size compared to films produced at higher accelerating voltages, i.e., 1.5–2.5 kV, such films do not approach the very-fine-grain films which may be produced using ion-beam sputtering. There are several reasons why this should be so, and these reasons merit some discussion.

The final vacuum pressure in the ion-beam sputter coater (20 mPa) is 200 times better than the vacuum pressure used in low-voltage sputter coating (4 Pa). High vacuum favors a cleaner surface, one consequence of this being that the film is built up from many small particles coalescing, rather than fewer larger particles growing to form the final film. This effect is dramatically evident in the papers by Clay and Peace (1981) and Kemmenoe and Bullock (1983) who sectioned metal coatings and showed that the sputter-coated film was distinctly granular compared to the smooth appearance of the ion-beam sputtered film.

Another consequence of the poorer vacuum is that the argon ions act as nucleating sites for crystalline growth of the coating metal while it is in transit in the plasma. A further reason for the smaller particle size in ion-beam sputtered material compared to low-voltage sputter-coated material is probably related to the difference in energy used to sputter away the target.

Although it is unlikely that low-voltage sputter coating will ever produce the fine-grain films which may be obtained by using ion-beam sputtering, the films which can be formed by diode-sputtering at 400–800 eV have an important place among the preparative techniques for SEM. The technique can be used to deposit a nominal 15-nm-thick film of either Au/Pd or Pt onto bulk nonconducting specimens with a grain size between 2 and 4 nm and within 10–25 min.

The earlier studies on coating at reduced temperature (Echlin, 1981) showed that reduced grain size could also be obtained by cooling the specimen.

7.4. Very-Low-Voltage Sputter Coating

Recent studies by Echlin *et al.* (1985) have shown that it is possible to sputter-coat noble metals and refractory metals at voltages as low as

Table 7.2. Gold/Palladium (80:20) Films Applied at Different Voltages[a]

Film thickness (nm)	Cathode voltage (V)	Plasma current (mA)	Deposition rate (nm/ min)	Temp. rise (K)	Particle size (nm)
15	175	5	1.2	1	0.9
15	200	8	1.4	3	1.0
15	225	17	7.4	7	1.3
15	250	27	12.6	12	1.5
15	275	43	16.8	19	1.7
15	300	56	19.4	19	1.7

[a]Argon pressure 13 Pa; initial temperature of specimen 283 K; specimen–target distance 50 mm. From Echlin *et al.*, 1985.

Table 7.3. Refractory Metals Deposited at Different Thicknesses[a]

Metal	Film thickness (nm)	Cathode voltage (V)	Plasma current (Ma)	Deposition rate (nm/ min)	Temp. rise (K)	Particle size (nm)
Ta	15	250	45	0.35	28	2.2
	1.5	250	40	0.37	11	2.0
W	15	250	55	3.0	20	1.8
	1.5	250	49	0.25	12	1.5
Nb	15	250	40	0.72	40	1.8
	1.5	250	40	0.25	11	1.5
Mo	15	250	50	3.0	28	1.8
	1.5	250	40	0.23	11	1.7

[a]Argon pressure 3–5 Pa; specimen temperature initially at 273 K; specimen–target distance 50 mm. From Echlin *et al.,* 1985.

100 V. A newly designed cathode head has been fitted on the Polaron E5400 high-resolution sputter coater. It consists of a high-flux rare earth ceramic magnet placed behind a disk-shaped metal target. This configuration molds the shape of the plasma flux into a 2- to 3-mm-wide intense band in the immediate vicinity of the target, maximizing the sputtering efficiency of the target while minimizing the thermal input into the specimen. This system has been used to sputter-coat thin (5–15 nm) films of noble metals in less than 1 min with a grain size of between 1.5 and 2.0 nm, and a temperature rise of no more than 20 K above ambient (see Table 7.3). The sputtering rate was much slower and thin (1.5–15 nm) films were deposited in 5–25 min, with a grain size between 1.5 and 2.0 nm, and a temperature rise of up to 313 K. Figure 7.2 shows typical results using noble and refractory metals. It has also been possible to sputter-coat aluminum using this system although the rates (0.5–1.0 nm/ min) are rather slow and the temperature rise (40 K) in the sample is too high for delicate samples. By using more powerful magnets and high-purity argon, i.e., O_2 2 ppm, H_2O 3 ppm, we can sputter aluminum at 10– 15 nm/min with a negligible heat load into the sample. Very-low-voltage sputter coating may be used to produce finely structured metal films for use in high-resolution SEM. The times taken to produce such films are shorter than those taken to produce similar films by Penning and ion-beam sputtering and except at ultrahigh resolution, i.e., below 1.0 nm, the quality of the films produced at very-low-voltage sputter coating is comparable to those produced by other methods.

7.5. Penning Sputtering

Peters (1980) gives details of Penning sputtering which can be used to make very thin metal coatings for both high-resolution SEM and TEM.

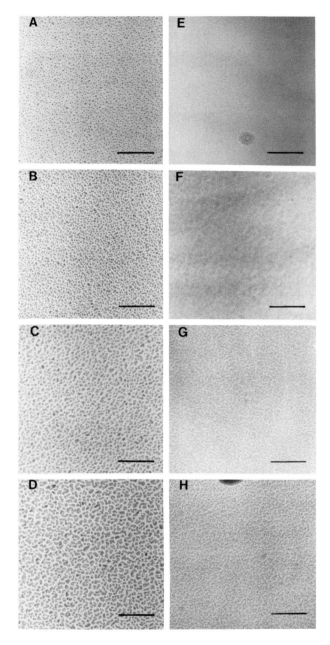

Figure 7.2. Transmission electron micrographs of metal films on a carbon substrate. (A–D) Thin films of gold/palladium sputtered at varying voltages (A = 175 V; B = 200 V; C = 225 V; D = 250 V). Notice the increase in particle size with the increase in voltage. (E) Thin film of niobium. (F) Thin film of tungsten. (G) Thin film of molybdenum. (H) Thin film of tantalum. Bars = 100 nm. (From Echlin *et al.*, 1985.)

In the earlier stages of this work, the equipment was homemade. It is now commercially available (Penning sputter coater PSC 1a, from Zentrum für Elektronenmikroskopie, Graz, Austria). Penning sputtering (or more correctly "Penning discharge") is a form of ion-beam sputtering in which the target is placed inside the discharge where the ions are generated. The specimen is shielded from the target by a small aperture, and the gun assembly is arranged to focus the argon ions on the target in a very narrow spot. The actual vacuum in the sputter head is only a few millipascals and the specimen is held at approximately 15 μPa during coating. This means that the vacuum pressure during coating is one order of magnitude lower than that used during ion-beam sputtering. Even when an ion current of 10 mA is applied, virtually no argon atoms leave the chamber. The absence of argon ions among the target atoms is an important feature of this form of sputtering. The positive ions and electrons which are generated in the plasma are deflected by large electrodes immediately outside the chamber with the result that virtually a pure stream of target atoms is directed onto the specimen. The mean free energy of the target atoms is an order of magnitude greater than can be obtained by thermal evaporation, and unlike diode sputtering systems, this primary energy is not reduced by scattering with residual gas atoms in the atmosphere. The high primary energy of the target atoms coupled with a low deposition rate means that metal is deposited onto the substrate with little lateral movement and that these anchored atoms act as nucleation centers establishing a horizontal crystal growth with a minimum vertical growth. Peters (1984b) has found that the continuity of metal films depends on the mobility of the metal atoms. Increased substrate heating, applied as secondary energy during metal deposition, increased surface diffusion. Low surface mobility allowed extensive surface covering with coalesced small crystals. Increased surface mobility prevented coalescence and resulted in large crystallites. Peters also found that the thickness required to achieve film continuity increased with higher atom mobility. Penning sputtering can thus produce very thin films which are well suited for high-resolution SEM. Although the Penning sputtering head works at 1–2 mPa, the specimen may be held at 50 μPa without a cold trap and 5μPa with a cold trap. The high vacuum conditions and the presence of a large liquid nitrogen-cooled trap very close to the specimen result in very low contamination rates, another prerequisite for high-resolution film formation.

Because the mean free path of the target atoms is many times larger than the target–substrate distance, the multiple scattering advantage of diode coating is lost and it is necessary to rotate and tilt complexly sculptured specimens during coating. By conventional sputter coating standards, the deposition rates are slow: for the noble metals, about

2 nm/min; for high-melting-point refractory metals, about 0.5 nm/min. But Penning sputtering is not a conventional sputter coating technique, and there would be little advantage gained in using it for preparing specimens for conventional low-resolution SEM. The technique is designed for high-resolution microscopy and has been successfully used to apply ultrathin (about 1.0 nm) films of molybdenum, tantalum, and tungsten to tubulin filaments and ferritin macromolecules. In a recent study on retinal rod cells (Peters *et al.*, 1983), 3–5 nm of gold is used for routine survey micrographs, whereas 1–2 nm of niobium or chromium is used for high-resolution observations. Examples of the technique are given in Fig. 7.3.

Although individual metal atoms and monoatomic layers may be imaged in STEM instruments, it is necessary to make thin films several atomic layers thick in order to have sufficient contrast to be imaged by other modes of electron microscopy. Topographic resolution on organic specimens with conventional secondary electron imaging is rather low, because of the multiple scattering within the specimen. Backscattered electrons (BSE) give rise to secondaries which degrade the resolution of the final image. Peters (1982a, b) showed that these backscattered effects could be virtually eliminated from the secondary signal by shielding the final polepiece with a carbon-coated aluminum plate. Peters considered that since the true secondary electrons are generated in the probe cross section at the specimen surface, this BSE absorption plate should give an improvement in the topographic resolution. The use of the BSE absorption plate coupled with thin (2.0 nm) layers of low-atomic-number metals such as niobium or chromium enabled Peters *et al.* (1983) to obtain ultra-high-resolution images from organic samples.

There is still some discussion regarding the minimum thickness of metal which is necessary for different modes. Peters considers 0.5–1.0 nm to be sufficient for conventional TEM in the brightfield mode, 2–4 nm for the low-loss SEM mode, and 1–2 nm for the secondary-emission SEM mode. Although such thin films are discontinuous, they are effective in reducing charging and provide sufficient contrast for imaging. It is doubtful whether such a thin layer would be effective in reducing the thermal effects which may be brought about by irradiation with a high-energy beam of electrons. As a result, it would be useful to have the specimen on a cold stage.

7.6. Ion-Beam Sputtering

A series of recent papers has confirmed the earlier work of Grasenick *et al.* (1972) and Kanaya *et al.* (1974) that ion-beam sputtering is an effective technique for applying high-resolution films. The method employs a

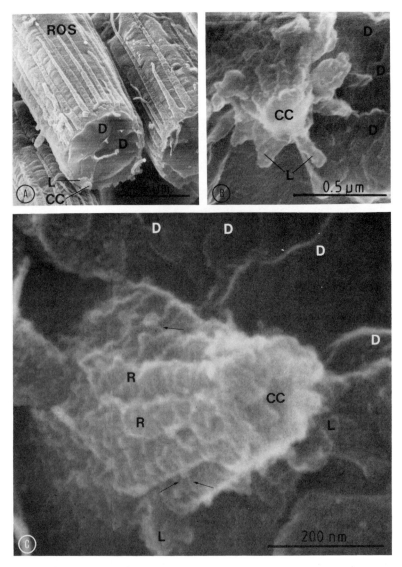

Figure 7.3. Fine structures of rod outer segments (ROS) from frog retina imaged with high-resolution SEM in SE-I image mode. (A) Low-magnification image of ROS gold decorated with 3.0-nm (average mass) thickness. A lip (L) and disks (D) of progressively larger diameter expand from the connecting cilium (CC) at the basal surface of the ROS. (B) Medium-magnification image of lip protrusions at the distal end of the CC. Retina prepared from a frog which spent ½ h in the light part of a 12-h light cycle. Specimen coated with a fine crystalline niobium film of 2.0-nm thickness. (C) High-magnification image of the CC. Specimen coated with a fine crystalline chromium film of ~ 1-nm thickness. Longitudinal ribs (R) cover peripheral microtubule doublets. Arrows point to fine fibrils of diameter 1.0–1.5 nm. (From Peters *et al.*, 1983.)

collimated argon ion beam at 7 kV and an ion current of 300–500 μA. The ion source is a cold cathode saddle-field source in which the plasma is contained within the source and only ions and neutrals escape through a hole in the cathode. The vertical target holder, which can be carbon, a noble metal, or one of the refractory metals, is set at an angle of 30° from glancing incidence to the horizontal ion beam, 40 mm from the ion source. The target is rotated normal to the beam to ensure even erosion. The specimen is placed 20–25 mm from the target, and is simultaneously rotated in an axial direction and rocked between 0 and 90° to ensure omnidirectional coating. The coating chamber is maintained at 20–30 mPa, thus minimizing the contamination rate.

The coating rates are comparatively slow, although there is some confusion over the actual rate of coating. Franks *et al.* (1980), using optical absorption techniques, quote a figure of between 3 and 7 nm/min for noble metals and this is within the same order of magnitude for cool diode sputter coating. The figure for carbon is much slower between 0.5 and 1.0 nm/min. This rate is approximately 20 times faster than the rate reported by Kemmenoe and Bullock (1983) and Clay and Peace (1981) using the same equipment, who state that typical coating times for gold are between 20 and 60 min. If the Franks *et al.* figure is correct, it would mean that Clay and Peace and Kemmenoe and Bullock have been coating specimens with up to 0.4 μm of gold. An examination of their micrographs suggests that the actual coating layer is much thinner. The answer to this discrepancy probably lies in the inaccuracy of the quartz thin-film monitor used to measure the film thickness. The papers by Flood (1980) and Peters (1980) detail the reasons for this inaccuracy. Most workers are now aware of this inaccuracy and experiments suggest a five- to tenfold error. Another reason for this discrepancy lies in the fact that it is necessary to rotate and tilt the specimens during coating to ensure an even coating. As a general principle, assuming minimal sample irradiation with electrons, ions, and photons, high deposition rates and low substrate temperatures are recommended for smooth continuous films of minimum thickness, whereas low deposition rates and low substrate temperatures favor the formation of very thin films which are unlikely to be continuous. On the available evidence, it appears that ion-beam sputtering is slower than diode sputtering, occurs at about the same rate as Penning sputtering, and takes less time to adequately coat a flat specimen than one with a rough surface. Ion-beam sputtered films have the advantage of being more uniform and of a finer grain size than diode sputtered films.

Franks *et al.,* Kemmenoe and Bullock, and Clay and Peace provide a convincing series of pictures in which they compare specimens coated by diode sputtering, ion-beam sputtering, and thermal evaporation. In all instances, the ion-beam coated material has the finest grain size, which in some cases is below the resolving power of the microscope. Figure 7.4 shows examples of the type of images which may be obtained by these coating methods. In addition, ion-beam sputter coating is better than diode sputter coating for the production of thick films for use in routine SEM. Kemmenoe and Bullock (1983) have examined 15-nm-thick ion-beam sputtered films and find they are continuous and without significant grain size. Films produced by ion-beam sputter deposition are initiated on a high density of nucleation sites as very fine equiaxial crystals, although the actual density of nucleation and crystallite sizes is very dependent on substrate and target materials.

Because the ion source operates at a high vacuum, it can be used to preclean substrates before coating, thus minimizing substrate surface contamination, although it must be appreciated that this precleaning also causes a small amount of surface etching. This surface cleaning can also be used in conjunction with thermal evaporation procedures and it is usual to continue surface cleaning during the early phases of thermal evaporation to ensure the production of fine-grain films with better adhesion characteristics. Boone (1984) has modified a commercial ion-milling machine to deposit fine-grain films for electron microscopy. An ion-milling machine usually consists of two ion guns which simultaneously ion etch two surfaces of a specimen. In the system described by Boone, only one surface is milled and the other is coated with a thin film. Another advantage of the technique is that the specimen is not exposed to high-energy electrons or ions, and thus there are little or no heating artifacts. Because the coating is carried out at a much higher vacuum than that used for diode coating, there is virtually no multiple scattering. This means the specimen must be rotated or tilted during the coating procedure. Care must be taken with measurements of film thickness as Kemmenoe and Bullock have shown an eightfold increase in the deposition rate on a stationary compared to a rotating specimen.

In spite of the apparent disadvantage of extended coating times, ion-beam sputtering appears to be the answer to many of the problems associated with diode sputter coating. The ability to use carbon as a target material is most useful, and the high-resolution images which have been obtained, even with gold as a target material, suggest this technique will find a wide range of applications from conventional SEM to high-resolution STEM. The studies of Kemmenoe and Bullock (1983) show that for medium- and high-resolution SEM, ion-beam sputtered films of platinum give the best result. This technique produced very-fine-grain films (1–2nm) relatively independent of film thickness, at least in the range of thickness one would normally use in SEM. Alternatively, 1- to 5-nm-thick films of ion-beam sputtered tungsten had a slightly smaller grain

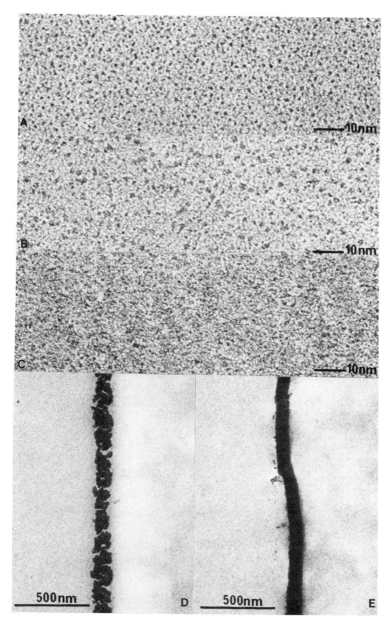

Figure 7.4. (A–C) Shadowed metal particles: (A) ion-beam sputtered platinum, average particle size 1.2 nm; (B) evaporated carbon platinum, average particle size 1.2 nm; (C) electron beam-deposited tungsten, average particle size 0.9 nm; $\times 1,000,000$. (D,E) Sectioned metal coatings: (D) diode-sputtered gold/palladium showing granular nature of coat; (E) ion-beam sputtered gold; $\times 50,000$. (From Clay and Peace, 1981.)

size, and would also provide films for high-resolution SEM where contrast is less important than resolution. Figures 7.5 and 7.6 show the high quality of the thin films which may be obtained using this method of thin-film formation.

The success of ion-beam sputtering and Penning sputtering can be attributed to a number of factors. When compared to diode sputter coating, the deposition rate is slower, the environment and substrate surfaces are cleaner, and the specimen is not exposed to high-energy electrons and ions. These three factors all favor the formation of thin films with smaller grain size and should be encouraging to the majority of us who own and

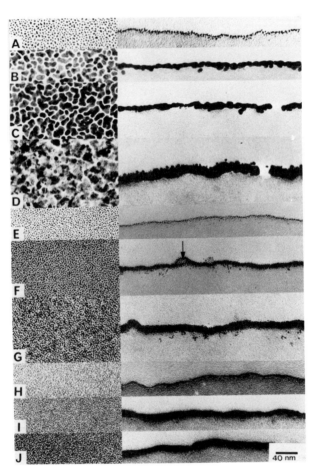

Figure 7.5 Ion-beam sputter-coated films (5 mA, 8kV). (A) 4-nm gold; (B) 9-nm gold; (C) 10-nm gold; (D) 15-nm gold; (E) 3-nm platinum; (F) 6-nm platinum; (G) 14-nm platinum; (H) 3-nm tungsten; (I) 8-nm tungsten; (J) 12-nm tungsten. Arrow marks an area of oblique sectioning due to uneven topography. ×250,000. (From Kemmenoe and Bullock, 1983.)

use diode sputter coaters, as it is relatively easy to reduce contamination, lower coating rates, and minimize specimen exposure to high-energy electrons and ions. But for high-resolution SEM and STEM, ion-beam sputtering and Penning sputtering should be the methods of choice.

7.7. Thermal Evaporation

Slayter (1980) discusses some of the advances which have been made in thermal evaporation coating techniques. Shadow casting by thermal

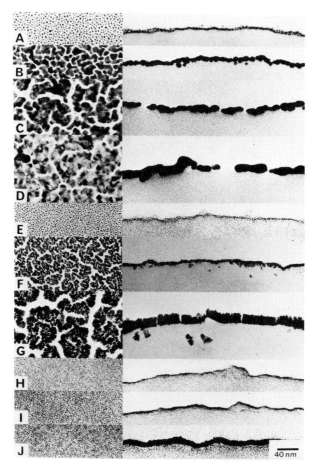

Figure 7.6. Diode sputter-coated films (8 mA, 450 V). (A) 4-nm gold; (B) 8-nm gold; (C) 11-nm gold; (D) 15-nm gold; (E) 3-nm platinum; (F) 6-nm platinum; (G) 17-nm platinum; (H 3-nm tungsten; (I) 5-nm tungsten; (J) 9-nm tungsten. ×250,000. (From Kemmenoe and Bullock, 1983.)

evaporation at grazing incidence has been widely used for contrast enhancement of topographical features. However, the condensation of a metal vapor into discontinuous microcrystalline aggregates rarely produces films with a grain size smaller than 3 nm. Slayter (1980) describes techniques for producing very thin films, in which the grain size is considerably reduced. He finds, for example, that the number of crystallites per unit area for platinum and tungsten is at a maximum in films 0.5 nm thick. High-melting-point metals form more crystallites per unit area, and although the scattering power of such films is diminished, they have sufficient contrast to be used in high-resolution STEM and TEM instruments. The effect is enhanced at low substrate temperatures and in clean environments. There still remains some uncertainty as to how much damage thermal evaporation can cause an organic sample. The momentum of an atom evaporated at between 2300 and 4800 K is quite considerable and this energy is dissipated in the sample. Colquhoun (1984) has calculated that the energy of a vaporized platinum atom is about 13 kcal/mol which would be about enough to disrupt intermolecular forces but not enough to break bonds. Colquhoun considers 13 to be a median value and that some of the evaporated atoms would be traveling at much higher speeds with energies approaching 40–50 kcal/mol. Such energies would be sufficient to break bonds in molecules. Colquhoun has calculated that a substantial proportion of the radiant flux from evaporating platinum consists of UV radiation which would also disrupt chemical bonds. Although some of these problems may be overcome by cooling the specimen, there is still some doubt as to whether metal evaporation methods favorably reproduce the structure of heat-sensitive samples.

A large number of interacting factors influence the formation of high-resolution small-grain-size films. The melting point, crystallographic lattice, purity, and reactivity of the metal evaporant, the surface temperature and energy input into the specimen during coating, and the rate and amount of metal deposited, all influence the final appearance of the thin film. The thinnest films with the finest grain size have been produced in 0.2- to 2.0-nm films of tungsten thermally evaporated from an electron gun onto a substrate cooled to 77 K. Co-evaporation of tungsten/tantalum mixtures seemed to have little advantage and there is still some uncertainty regarding the relationship between final grain size and rate of evaporation. Slayter uses a platinum deposition rate of 1.2 nm/min and a tungsten deposition rate of 0.9 nm/min and concludes that a 0.5- to 1.0-nm layer of platinum would be the best coating for high-resolution secondary electron imaging as it combines fine grain size and high crystallite density with good secondary emission properties. A 1.0-nm layer of paltinum would be the best coating for low-loss backscattered imaging and a 0.5- to 1.0-nm layer of tungsten would be useful for STEM applications where the highest resolution is necessary and secondary electron emission is less important. Slayter favors a much increased target—specimen distance, i.e., 60 cm for optimal evaporation of tungsten, in order to minimize the photon radiation on the sample; Peters (1980) has shown this radiation can cause an increase in crystallite size. Provided a number of precautions are taken, thermal evaporation of tungsten onto relatively flat specimens such as thinly spread macromolecules, can provide high-resolution (1–2 nm) information. A thin layer of evaporated carbon applied to the specimen after coating appears to stabilize the coating layer and diminishes recrystallization of the thin film layer under the influence of the electron beam. An interesting corollary to the studies of Peters and Slayter is the observation by Pulker (1980) that other heavy metals are an excellent prenucleation material before applying a layer of gold. This finding is in line with the well-established procedure of precoating samples with a thin layer of carbon before applying a second coat of one of the noble metals. It remains to be shown whether this initial layer provides a clean surface and/or sites for high nucleation density. A recent study by Peters (1984b) describes a simple method of obtaining reproducible thin and ultrathin carbon films using a flash evaporation method with carbon fiber as the source material. Films of any thickness up to 20 nm can be produced with a minimum of photon radiation into the sample. In addition, the flash-evaporated films have less background structure than films produced by evaporation from carbon rods. Such films will have a wide application in both microscopy and analysis and will be particularly useful for heat-sensitive samples.

7.8. Coating at Low Specimen Temperatures

There is general agreement that low specimen surface temperature favors high nucleation density resulting in finer-grain films. Low specimen surface temperatures also favor thinner film thickness, and smaller dimensional changes on specimens which are being coated from an angle to emphasize small changes in relief. Slayter (1980) showed that the number of nucleation sites is inversely proportional to the substrate temperature, and that twice as many crystallites developed per unit area on a sample held at 77 K when coated with platinum than one held at 300 K. This temperature effect is only seen when all other parameters have been optimized, and it is of paramount importance that the surface to be coated is clean and free of contamination. This is particularly important when frozen-hydrated tissue surfaces are being coated as for example when a replica is made of a frozen-fractured cell. Haggis (1985) has shown that if the specimen temperature is too high, it is impossible to make a good replica because of the stream of water molecules leaving the frozen surface.

The grain size in cool-diode sputtered films generally becomes smaller as the substrate temperature is lowered in the range 303–203 K. In all instances, the particle size was smaller whether examined by SEM, TEM, or low-loss imaging. These studies have been extended to the 203–103 K range. Full details of the experiments may be found in the studies by Echlin (1981). The coating was carried out in a Polaron E5100 Series II liquid nitrogen-cooled diode sputter coater using annular targets of gold/palladium and platinum. Care was taken to minimize contamination, and samples were only transferred to and from the specimen chamber at ambient temperatures. Half-masked carbon film-coated electron microscope grids were coated at various temperatures with a nominal 15 nm of gold/palladium 80:20 and platinum at a rate of 4 nm/min using high-purity agron at 2.0 kV, 15 mA plasma current, and a chamber pressure of 4 Pa.

Gold/palladium films. At 303 K there is evidence of crystal growth and the particle size is quite large. At 273 and 223 K there is little difference in the appearance of the film, and the average size of the interlocking granules, which form the islands, is 6–7 nm. At 173 K the islands of metal are less continuous and there are small granules in the clear space between the islands. At 110 K the individual islands are somewhat larger but the particles between the islands are smaller. The smallest particles are 1.5 nm.

Platinum films. Although there is no evidence of extensive crystal growth at 303 K, the intergranular spaces are large and devoid of fine particles. The films deposited at 273 and 223 K are made up of a series of discontinuous islands similar to the Au/Pd films deposited at the same temperature. The discontinuous islands are still present at 173 K but are absent from the film deposited at 110 K.

At lower temperatures there is less surface migration and an increased sticking coefficient for metal to metal than for metal to substrate. This means that at a lower temperature, there are fewer larger islands, more smaller islands and smaller inter-island particles. The films deposited at 303 K have a definite granularity (~9–11 nm) when viewed at high magnification in the SEM. It might just be possible to resolve the granules (~5–7 nm) in films produced at 273 and 223 K, and the larger islands (~11–13 nm) would certainly be resolved in films deposited at 173 and 110 K.

There seems to be little advantage in depositing 10- to 15-nm films at really low temperatures although there are advantages to lowering the temperature to about 220 K. If thin (i.e., 1–5 nm) films are to be deposited, then there are advantages in working at lower temperature. For ultrathin films (1–3 nm), there is every advantage in working at really low temperatures and obtaining very small particle size. In addition to the advantages of decreased grain size in films deposited at low temperatures, but examined at ambient temperatures, it is also possible to coat frozen-hydrated samples maintained below the recrystallization temperature of ice. Echlin *et al.* (1982a) describe how evaporated films may be deposited, and Robards *et al.* (1981) describe procedures for sputter coating at low temperatures. The only precautions needed in coating samples held at low temperature are to minimize the thermal input into the sample, to prevent transient melting and sublimation of the surface water, and to make sure the entire operation is carried out in a clean environment. One particular problem arises in specimens which are freeze-dried after the coating has been applied. There are sufficient dimensional changes from shrinkage during drying to cause the films to buckle and crack (Hook *et al.*, 1980). It is usually necessary either to apply a second coating layer after freeze-drying, or to delay the whole coating process until after drying is complete.

7.9. Coating Thickness Measurements

Although there have been no new significant developments in the techniques for measuring the thickness of thin films, serious doubts have been cast on the accuracy of measurements made using quartz crystal thin-film monitors. Flood (1980) has written an excellent review of the general methods of thin-film thickness measurement, and it is apparent that accurate measurement of thin-film thickness requires rigorous attention to detail. Peters (1980) has calculated that temperature fluctuations of the quartz crystal thin-film monitor must be held to within ±0.06 K for carbon measurements to be within ±0.1 nm, and must be within ±0.13 K for metal measurements to be within ±0.02 nm. The influence of temperature is variable and is related to the angle at which the quartz disk is cut relative to the main axes of the crystal. Most disks are cut along an axis where the frequency response is stable between 273 and 333 K (Flood, 1980). This is within the temperature range normally experienced in cooled diode, Penning, and ion-beam sputter coaters, and in thermal evaporation units. Slayter (1980) carefully cross-checked measurements of thin-film thickness, using quartz thin-film monitors, interferometry, and direct-weight microbalance, and found the accuracy to be within 15% for carbon films in the range 10–70 nm.

It is evident that accurate measurement of thin-film thickness can be made using quartz thin-film monitors provided sophisticated (and expensive!) equipment is used. But as Slayter (1980) is at pains to point out, these monitors do not produce an absolute measurement as they average out discontinuous thin metal coats. Crystallites within the film could easily have thicknesses greater than the average coat thickness. Quartz crystal monitors measure the *average mass thickness,* which, if the film is discontinuous, is much less than the *average metric thickness.* There does not appear to be a simple relationship between the two methods of measurement. Kemmenoe and Bullock (1983) have calculated that a 4 nm average metric thickness gold film would be about 1 nm average mass thickness. As the film thickness increases and becomes less discontinuous, the two forms of measurement come closer to giving the same value. It would be naive to equate a film thickness measurement given on a planar quartz crystal monitor with that on a complexly sculptured specimen which is being rotated and rocked during the coating process. Peters (1980) has calculated that using a tooling factor of 50% to correct for differences in location of monitor and specimen, only 12.5% of the coating thickness measured on the thin-film monitor actually lands on a tumbling specimen. This is due, in part, to differences in the surface roughness of the quartz crystal and the sample to be coated and to inaccuracy in the method of measurement. Slayter considers that there may be as much as a tenfold increase in film thickness on topographical features presented at normal irradiance to the beam. Clay and Peace (1981) find that sections of embedded ion-beam and diode sputtered films are 5–10 times thicker than the reading given on the thin-film monitor. The range of inaccuracy is quite large: in a specimen which is being rotated and tilted, the thickness is underestimated by a factor of 8; in a stationary specimen normal to the beam, the coating thickness may be overestimated by a factor of 10. The accuracy of thin-film measurement is also a function of the method by which the film is deposited. Because of energy transfer to the quartz crystal monitor, measurements in evaporative and diode coaters may be off by $\pm 100\%$. This is less of a problem with ion-beam and Penning sputter coaters.

What do these discrepancies mean to the practicing microscopist who is concerned with providing a reasonable coating thickness to ensure maximum specimen-image information transfer? For thick continuous films, i.e., more than 15 nm, the average mass thickness given by a quartz thin-film monitor is fairly close to the average metric thickness which may be measured on a planar surface. If accurate measurements are required on films less than 10 nm in thickness, the indicated average mass thickness given by the thin-film monitor should be checked by some independent means (for details see Flood, 1980). Provided standardized conditions are used for coating, i.e., set target/substrate distance, residual gas pressure, source and substrate temperature, and so on, it should be possible to achieve reproducibility to within $\pm 20\%$ (Flood, 1980). Alternatively, if a standard coating procedure is to be repeatedly used on more or less the same type of specimen, a coating thickness should be applied which results in an optimal image in the microscope. This thickness is measured during coating by a quartz thin-film monitor positioned at a fixed place relative to the specimen and it is this thickness which is applied each time to the specimen. The actual thickness on the specimen is probably irrelevant because on a complexly sculptured sample, there may be a 20-fold variation in thickness, depending on the topography of the specimen and whether it is stationary or moving. It is nevertheless necessary to calibrate the thin-film monitor, especially if it is of the less expensive variety, in order to have some idea of its accuracy. A novel method of calibration which requires no special equipment has recently been described by Johansen and Namork (1984). Using transmission electron micrographs, these workers measured the thickness of thin platinum films sputter coated on 20-nm colloidal gold particles, which protruded from the edge of torn rolled-up carbon films. Up to a platinum film thickness of 10 nm, there was a 17% increase in metric thickness over mass thickness. This method of calibration is particularly useful for films less than 10 nm thick where the inaccuracy of measurement is greatest. An example of their technique is shown in Figure 7.7.

Broers and Spiller (1980) have provided some interesting new information on measuring the roughness of thin metal films. The roughness measurements are made using the variations in the scatter of incident soft x-ray radiation on the film surface. The method has been used on films in the 0.2- to 1.5-nm range and the results correlate well with measurements made on low-loss image micrographs of the same films. Broers and Spiller find the smoothest surfaces are on thin (0.75 nm) films of tungsten and a rhenium/tungsten alloy (68% Re). The noble metals give a film surface roughness 2–5 times more coarse than the refractory metals. It is hoped that further studies will lead to the provision of standard reference surfaces of known roughness. Such standards would be invaluable in studies which try to relate the film thickness on a quartz crystal with that actually landing on a rough specimen.

7.10. Artifacts

Leaving aside the inaccuracies which may occur during the measurement of film thickness, coating artifacts may be considered under two headings, contamination and decoration effects. Contamination can occur during coating by trapping gas atoms and/or hydrocarbons, or after coating as a result of gas absorption and dust deposits on the surface. At a gross level, contamination in coating systems can be recognized as a

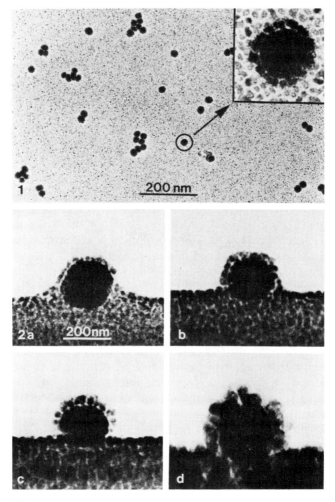

Figure 7.7. Platinum-sputtered colloidal gold particles imaged at the periphery of a rolled-up carbon film. ×1,000,000. The thickness in 2a–d is represented by the four frequency changes, 240, 480, 720, and 1440 Hz, respectively. (From Johansen and Namork, 1984.)

yellow–brown layer on a white background, and as a blue–black tarnish on metal surfaces. Other more subtle signs of contamination are the large cracks on the surface of thin layers of films which have been deposited over a long period of time. A reexamination of some of our own micrographs of cool diode sputter-coated tantalum prepared over a 15-min period (Echlin and Kaye, 1979) has revealed such contamination-related cracks. Once the sputter coater was cleaned (for details see Echlin *et al.,* 1980a), this artifact was no longer a problem. Provided the few simple housekeeping measures which are given in *SEMXM* are followed, contamination with the standard cooled diode sputter coater should not be a problem in the production of coating layers for conventional SEM. Contamination may also be practically eliminated in diode sputter coaters by operating the systems at very low voltages. Peters (personal communication) has calculated that operating voltages of 100–200 V are insufficient for generating contamination products from hydrocarbons. Under these conditions, much longer coating times are necessary and it is important to diminish the thermal input into the specimen to prevent the accumulation of recrystallization effects. High-resolution thin films (i.e., 1–2 nm) can only be produced under high vacuum conditions. There is no doubt from the studies made by Peters (1980) and Slayter (1980) that a high, clean vacuum favors the formation of ultrathin, low-grain-size films.

Decoration effects are more insidious, for they may be either a delicate reflection of a true inhomogeneity on the specimen surface, or a result of contamination and/or uneven coating. A good example of "natural" decoration effect occurs where a very thin layer of metal is deposited onto alkali halide crystals, i.e., NaCl (Willison and Rowe, 1980, p. 10). A "natural" decoration effect is a real substructural feature whose appearance is enhanced by a thin metal coating. Such decoration effects must be distinguished from artifacts due to an initial random event which enhances the sticking power of the incoming molecule and in turn gives a decoration artifact. Monomolecular steps between crystal lattices can be demonstrated provided the step heights are sufficient to catch and hold onto the absorbed atoms. The images appear as long lines of oriented particles which correspond to the crystal planes. This molecular level effect disappears once the film layer becomes more than a few nanometers thick. Walzthony *et al.* (1984) found that different heavy metals and carbon displayed distinctive banding patterns on a series of elongated helical macromolecules which had been rotary shadowed at low elevation angle. They considered that diffusion, nucleation, and coalescence of heavy metals were different among the molecules examined. The differences in grain patterns reflected differences in the physico-chemical properties of the underlying molecules such as surface relief and charge distributions. Thus, Ta and W, which probably carry a positive charge, will preferentially decorate clusters of negative charges along the myosin macromolecule. A preliminary coating with C masks these effects, presumably by neutralizing some of the surface charges. Walzthony *et al.* consider that positive "staining" with heavy metals which condense and coalesce at specific sites along macromolecules could be used to provide information about the structure of these specimens. Haggis (1985) has found an analogous phenomenon in platinum-coated actin with surface temperatures playing an important role in regulating the effect. A similar, molecular decoration artifact can be seen in some high-resolution freeze-etched surfaces contaminated with water vapor. The water vapor shows a preferential affinity for hydrophilic sites and can give rise to some quite misleading images. "Natural decoration effect" may also occur at the SEM resolution level. If there are surface features which favor condensation and nucleation, they will accrete more of the metal coating and increase the topographic contrast. Thus, Rosowski *et al.* (1984) found that the surfaces of diatom frustules coated with a thin metal film showed a granular matrix which was not present on the supporting glass surface. The authors consider that minute surface irregularities on the silica frustule favored the formation of fine granules. This same general effect may be seen on surfaces which are contaminated. The presence of contaminants causes an unequal distribution of surface forces and the migrating atoms/molecules settle at places with the highest binding energy. This would be considered an "unnatural effect" and the difficulty comes in separating these "unnatural effects" from "natural effects." The only sure way is to ensure that the coating is carried out in as clean a vacuum as possible, and the finer the resolution required from the specimen, the higher the vacuum conditions under which the coating should be carried out. Consideration must be given to the way the thin films are applied as it is possible to relate some decoration effects to the mode of application. Pashley *et al.* (1964) were able to demonstrate that the radiation from an evaporation source can melt nucleation centers, giving rise to roundish drops and a delay in continuous film formation. Peters (1980) has shown that the excessive photon radiation which usually occurs during thermal evaporation may generate crystallites which in turn give the film a resolvable structure. This is not a feature of ion-beam and Penning sputtering. Flood (1980) has demonstrated that it is possible to suppress the coalescence and growth of islands, and diminish crystal growth, in films which are sputtered rather than thermally evaporated. One type of decoration artifact, which may be found in specimens coated unidirectionally from an angle, usually referred to as shadowing, is the appearance of lines running normal to the shadowing direction. The self-shadowing occurs when there is diminished grain development in the shadow of a developing grain. A closely related artifact, called capping, is the exaggeration of specimen dimensions by accumulation of shadowing material. Neugebauer and Zingsheim (1979) showed that misapplication of the rotary shadowing method can produce images in which known solid spherical particles appear to be penetrated with holes. These kinds of artifacts are uncommon in SEM preparations which are usually omnidirectionally coated but they are a problem in high-resolution coating for SEM/STEM, in freeze-etch replicas, and in macromolecule shadowing techniques; the excellent book by Willison and Rowe (1980) considers these matters in some detail.

It would be wrong to think that once the coating layer has been deposited that no further effects can occur. Pulker (1980) showed that the number of gold particles decreased and their relative size increased after a thin layer of gold had been heated to 603 K. Peters (1980) showed the same effects at 293 K. These temperature rises can readily be achieved in electron beam instruments. A thin layer of carbon (5 nm) evaporated on top of a carefully applied ultra-thin layer of metal (0.5 nm Ta/W) reduced recrystallization in the film. Rosowski *et al.* (1981) have found that an initial thermal evaporation with Au/Pd can protect delicate structures from the thermal damage which can occur with diode sputter coating. Unless high-resolution films are going to be examined immediately after application, it is advisable to coat the sample with an additional layer of carbon. This precaution is probably not necessary for specimens to be examined by conventional SEM.

One coating effect which is now fortunately relatively easy to recognize is that where the coating layer is so thick that it falsifies the surface morphology of the specimen. Blaschke (1980) gives a nice example of this effect together with a good example of the decoration of crystal edges with gold spheres—a result of injudicious coating.

7.11. Coating Techniques for X-Ray Microanalysis

A discussion of the general principles to be followed when coating samples which are to be analyzed by x-ray microanalysis is given in *SEMXM*. It is important that the coating layer should neither mask the elements being analyzed nor give rise to spectral overlaps which might prove difficult to deconvolute. The thin film should be thick enough to provide a good thermal and electrical pathway, but not so thick as to attenuate the incoming primary electrons and the radiated x-ray photons. The coating becomes more of a problem with light-element analysis and one is left with only three alternatives, carbon, beryllium, and chromium. The high thermal radiation flux from carbon evaporation can easily damage delicate specimens; the procedure of flash evaporation of carbon fiber suggested by Peters (1984a) overcomes many of these problems. The extreme toxicity of beryllium has led most workers to avoid using this metal. Marshall and Carde (1984) give details of a procedure for using this toxic material, but potential users are warned of the hazards associated with this material. Marshall and Zercher (1982) describe a method of using sputter-coated thin films as accurate standards for TEM x-ray microanalysis. Such standards are easy to prepare, have negligible absorption and fluorescence effects, and can give reproducible k values. Chromium is relatively easy to use and has no toxic effects. Although the characteristic peaks of chromium are sufficiently far away from most light elements of common interest not to cause any interference, the background associated with these chromium peaks may contribute to the background of the light elements. It is necessary to strip the chromium spectrum from the spectrum of the biological material in order to obtain quantitative data. A recent paper by Echlin and Taylor (1986) discusses these procedures in some detail.

7.12. Non-Thin-Film Coating Methods

There are a number of techniques which increase the surface conductivity but do not utilize either sputtering or thermal evaporation methods. Antistatic agents, e.g., Duron (a polyamine), have limited usefulness with SEM sepcimens examined at low resolution. Katoh and Matsumoto (1979) have used Denkil-SEM (sodium-alkyl-benzene sulfonate, Hodogaya Chemical Company, Japan) either as a 5% solution in water, or as a 3% solution in ethanol, in the SEM examination of plant material. The image quality is quite good, but, on their own report, much improved after coating with gold. Kubotsu and Veda (1980) give details of a conductive treatment called vapor phase impregnation which involves brief exposure (10–20 min) of the specimen to osmium tetroxide vapor followed by exposure to hydrazine hydrate vapor which reduces the OsO_4 to metallic osmium. It has been successfully applied to a wide range of organic specimens at magnifications up to $100,000 \times$ and the only precaution which appears to be necessary is to remove the deposits of unabsorbed OsO_4. Although the final image quality is not as good as can be achieved with a properly coated specimen, it does provide a coating method which avoids the use of high vacuum. An alternative approach is to prevent the charge buildup in the first place. Crawford (1980) describes a low-energy ion charge neutralization technique which can stabilize the surface potential and allow insulators to be examined without the benefit of a coating layer. A similar approach has been adopted by Kotorman (1980) for the examination of FET wafers. The accelerating voltage was adjusted under 1 kV in an attempt to eliminate trapped charges. Muranaka *et al.* (1982) found that uncoated biological specimens bombarded with an argon beam (50–100 μA, 1–5 kV) for 30 min prior to examination in the microscope showed no surface charging effects, even when examined at 25 kV. It is clear that such an argon beam dosage would erode the specimen surface and could remove surface contaminants which might favor charging. However, Muranaka *et al.* consider that the elimination of surface charging is caused by a neutralization between negative charges of electrons and positive charges on ions trapped within the specimen. A similar effect has been observed by Kanaya *et al.* (1982). Prebombardment of biological and organic material with an argon beam allows such samples to be observed at up to 20 keV in an SEM without metal coating. The suppression of the negative charge was thought to be due to positive ions being trapped in the porous surface. An ion beam dose of between 0.75 and 1.25 mA/min appeared to be the optimal condition for limiting specimen charge-up without any sample etching. Lametschwandtner *et al.* (1980) have devised a simple method of preventing highly porous nonconducting specimens from charging. It is usually very difficult to attach such specimens to the specimen stub using conductive paints as the capillary nature of the specimens results in complete infiltration with the paint and a consequent disappearance of the surface detail. These workers found that it was possible to attach their vascular corrosion cast specimens to the substrate using small pieces of copper wire which had previously been attached to the stub with colloidal silver paint. The specimen is pressed onto these conductive projections and may be examined in the SEM without any coating. A paper by Jeszka *et al.* (1981), while not directly concerned with coating, has interesting implications for the reduction in specimen charging of nonconductors. Jeszka *et al.* investigated the properties of conductive polymers made by growing microcrystalline complexes of tetracyanoquinodimethane (TCNQ) and tetrathiotetracene (TTT) in cast films of polycarbonate polymer. At a concentration of 1% TCNQ/TTT, the dark resistivity of 15-μm-thick films is 3×10^{-2} Ω-cm at room temperature. These so-called organic metals do not contain any of the metallic elements associated with high conductivity. Such polymer films may provide the basis for an inexpensive conductive support to be used in connection with x-ray microanalysis of light elements. A recent review by Bryce and Murphy (1984) gives details of the unusual properties and technological potential of these interesting materials.

7.13. Conclusions

In concluding this chapter on specimen coating, it would be appropriate to make some recommendations on coating methods for practicing microscopists.

1. For high-resolution SEM and STEM (spatial resolutions 1–5 nm) where one is attempting to push the instrumental capabilities to their limit, Penning and ion-beam sputtering must be the methods of choice. The coating material and final thickness of the film must be dictated by

the exigencies of the experiment. For high-resolution STEM studies, heavy metals such as tantalum and tungsten which have a low specific mobility appear to be the best choice. For high-resolution SEM where one can be sure only to be collecting the primary secondary electrons, then chromium or niobium is the material of choice. Where this is not the case, the noble metals and their alloys should be used. In all instances, a film thickness of 1–3 nm appears to give the best result. In situations where one wishes to achieve high-resolution spatial decoration, Peters (1984b) recommends fast evaporation of a small amount of metal with high specific surface mobility. The crystallites round up as a result of vertical growth and give the best contrast with the smallest amount of metal. Increased spatial resolution can be obtained with metals with lower mobilities, i.e., platinum, rhodium, and tungsten.

2. For medium-resolution SEM (spatial resolutions 4–8 nm), low-voltage sputter coating with either gold/palladium or platinum gives the best result. Alternatively, ion-beam or Penning sputtering gives an equally good coating layer. The final film thickness should be in the range 5–10 nm.

3. For routine scanning microscopy on coated specimens (spatial resolutions greater than 10 nm), a diode sputter coater using Au/Pd working at a relatively high deposition rate gives good even films. However, care must be taken with thermolabile samples. The final film thickness should be in the range 8–12 nm.

Advances in Specimen Preparation for Biological SEM

8.1. Introduction

This chapter should be read in conjunction with the chapters on the same subject in *SEMXM,* where we attempted to enunciate some of the general principles of specimen preparation. Here we will deal with the new methods which have been developed specifically for use in the SEM as distinct from electron microscopy generally. This is a rapidly developing topic in microscopy and it will not be possible to deal in depth with all new developments. Frequent reference will be made to specialist papers which give detailed instructions on how to carry out a particular technique. Much of what will be discussed here will apply to biological and organic samples, for it is with these samples that the problems are most exacting. As well as providing an updated guide to the general problems of specimen preparation, emphasis will be placed on the techniques which permit an analysis of the chemical properties of specimens.

8.2. General Methods of Specimen Preparation

The general methods for preparing biological specimens for SEM are explained in some detail in our earlier book. The major problem centers around the conversion of a normally wet sample to a dry state while still preserving its three-dimensional shape, to allow it to be examined in the high vacuum of the microscope. This conversion, which, by and large, involves changing the organic matrix of the cells and tissues to an inorganic form with a concomitant loss of water, can be separated into three distinct phases: (1) fixation, which involves stabilizing, either by cross-linking, denaturation, and/or precipitation, the labile organic molecules present in the cells and tissues; (2) dehydration, the removal of water; (3) coating, which involves the application of a thin layer of conducting material to an otherwise nonconducting surface. This latter phase is more or less unique to SEM and is the subject of Chapter 7 in this book. The procedures of fixation and dehydration are common to all methods which are used to prepare hydrated materials for examination in electron beam instruments. There is, unfortunately, no single book which covers all these methods as applied to SEM. The recent book by Hayat (1982), although a general text for electron microscopy, contains much useful information on specimen handling procedures. The recent compendium edited by Revel *et al.* (1984) also contains a number of useful papers which provide a rigorous explanation of the assumptions which are made in choosing the most appropriate technique for biological specimen preparation.

Before considering some of the more specialized methods for preparing specimens for morphological and chemical analysis in the SEM, it is appropriate to consider some of the well-proven general methods of specimen preparation. Nowell and Pawley (1980), while not providing a series of all-embracing recipes, have attempted to standardize the preparative techniques for the examination of experimental animal tissue in the SEM. One of the problems this paper tackles successfully is to distinguish the surface changes inherent in any preparative protocol for the preparation of bulk tissue blocks from those changes produced by experimentation and disease. The authors describe a wide range of methods for the handling of specimens, stabilization, dehydration, drying, and exposing the surface of interest in a variety of experimental animals. This paper is a particularly useful introduction to the specialized techniques used with animal tissue because it has gathered together methods of proven usefulness. In addition, it emphasizes the potential problems which can occur at the various stages of preparation and offers practical suggestions how they may be avoided.

A similar approach has been taken in the review paper by Falk (1980) which considers the problems associated with the preparation of plant material. The methods of fixation he describes are identical to those used in TEM preparations except for the recommendation that the fixatives should as far as possible be isotonic with fluid in the living cells. A wide range of buffer systems is available for plant cells, although there is general agreement that the best results are obtained when the buffer and fixative are at or around, a neutral pH. The review by Falk covers a wide range of plant materials and it should be consulted for specific preparative recipes for particular plant and fungal specimens.

The preparation of microbial, hematological, and unicellular aquatic organisms present their own set of problems and Watson *et al.* (1980). Wouters *et al.* (1984), and Maugel *et al.* (1980) provide a number of useful suggestions on how these specimens may best be preserved. Paradoxically, the main problem is the small size of the specimens. Although the fixation, and dehydration times can be very short owing to the small specimen size, problems are created in handling the specimens. The usual procedures are either to collect and handle the samples by centrifugation from an aqueous suspension (Wouters *et al.*, 1984) or fix the specimens firmly to a large solid support such as a filter pad or glass substrate. Walz *et al.* (1984) have used polylysine-coated polyacrylamide beads as a means for attaching intact cells. The cells remain attached throughout processing, and can be released at the end of preparation. Similar problems are experienced with cultured mammalian cells, and the papers by Allen (1983) and Evers *et al.* (1983) provide a number of useful methods which can be applied to these specimens.

8.3. Fixation

Much of the success of specimen preparation centers on the initial stabilization of the specimen. If this step is performed correctly, the sample can usually withstand the subsequent steps of dehydration, exteriorizaton, and coating.

In the past two or three years, chemical fixation of cells and tissues has moved away from morphological preservation alone to a situation where the chemical constitution of the sample is of equal importance. In some cases, this retention of chemical activity as revealed by cytochemistry, immunocytochemistry, or autoradiography comprises the optimal preservation of ultrastructure. This more informed approach of combining good morphology and biological activity has led to the development of new fixatives as well as to a better understanding of the existing methods. In a seminal paper on the subject, Bullock (1984) has taken a careful look at the current state of fixation for electron microscopy. While not offering a panacea for all tissue types, the suggestions in the paper do allow a more intelligent approach to fixation. A number of examples will suffice to demonstrate this new approach.

Glutaraldehyde still remains the fixative of choice for the structural and enzymatic component of cells. Despite its slow rate of entry, it is still widely used and at much lower concentrations than originally suggested. A recent study by Coetzee and van der Merwe (1984) has shown that although fixation in glutaraldehyde invariably leads to more or less extraction of a variety of elements, compounds, and macromolecules, the amount of material actually extracted is also very dependent on the buffer used to make up the fixature. Least extraction was found in phosphate-buffered 2–3% glutaraldehyde.

In a later paper, Coetzee and van der Merwe (1985) showed that the rate of fixative penetration, as measured by bovine serum albumin cross-linking, is dependent on the composition of the buffer vehicle as well as the fixative concentration. They recommend a sodium phosphate buffer for use with plant material.

The move to lower concentrations also applies to osmium tetroxide where new data (Luftig and McMillan, 1981; Aoki and Tavassoli, 1981; Bendayan and Zollinger, 1983) indicate that brief exposure to a low concentration of osmium tetroxide both preesrves protein structure and retains antigenicity. The work of Aoki and Tavassoli (1981) is of particular interest because these workers found that brief exposure to osmium tetroxide followed by thiocarbohydrazide, and then a second exposure to osmium tetroxide, adequately preserved actin filaments. Such a technique would have an immediate appeal for high-resolution SEM.

The lipid component of cells is notoriously difficult to fix and retain *in situ*. Here the aldehydes are less useful, and it is necessary to use osmium tetroxide at a concentration somewhat higher than would give optimal preservation of proteins. Wolf-Ingo *et al.* (1982) have found that a complex of (1) palladium–tungsten, (2) lead–iron, and cobalt–molybdenum salts helps to preserve phospholipids, cholesterol, and lipoprotein particles for subsequent examination in the SEM. The other two major chemical components of cells, nucleic acids and carbohydrates, appear best perserved after glutaraldehyde and formaldehyde fixation.

Bullock (1984) discusses at some length the various additives which may be included in a fixative. These include calcium and lithium ions, ferri- and ferrocyanides, tannic and picric acids. While each in its own way enhances fixation in a particular case, there does not seem to be any reason to use them in all fixatives. Tannic acid should be of interest to scanning microscopists, as its mordanting action allows an increased loading of metal salts to biological tissue (see later).

Bullock raises the question of the newer fixatives, such as the imidoesters and the carbodiimides which have been suggested as replacements for some of the aldehydes. The advantage of these new materials appears to be not so much in morphological preservation but rather, in combination with glutaraldehyde, of retaining chemical activity for subsequent identification by immunocytochemical methods.

Because of the increased interest in retaining biological activity as well as structure, there has been a move away from the traditional phosphate and cacodylate buffers to organic buffers such as PIPES [piperazine-N,N'-bis-(2-ethanesulfonic acid)]. Such buffers avoid the precipitation of inorganic ions and effectively contribute to the osmolality and pH balance of the fixative. An alternative to extended wet-chemical fixation is suggested in a recent paper by Chew *et al.* (1983). These workers found that animal tissue cells mixed with dilute glutaraldehyde and then immediately subjected to 4 s microwave radiation (2450 MHz) appeared to be satisfactorily fixed. It remains to be seen whether this type of fixation is any better than conventional methods and whether the short period of intense radiation did no more than speed up a long diffusion process.

8.4. Dehydration

This still remains a problem with scanning microscopy although Chapter 9 on cryomicroscopy in this book provides compelling evidence that liquid dehydration followed by critical point drying should be discarded in favor of freeze-drying. Nevertheless, it is accepted that liquid dehydration in one of the primary, secondary, or polyhydric alcohols will still remain a method of convenience. This convenience must be weighed against the chemical extraction, distortion, and shrinkage which accompany these methods. For high-resolution SEM studies, and for investigations where one hopes to obtain some measure of the biological activity of the specimen, these techniques should be dispensed with and the water removed by freeze-drying.

The evidence against the use of critical point drying as a final step in the dehydration procedure is impressive. Following the first detailed study on this aspect of specimen preparation by Boyde *et al.* (1977), a number of papers have appeared which confirm the realization that critical point drying causes gross (up to 70%) and spatially unequal dimensional changes in most specimens.

These dimensional changes, which may be measured directly on the sample during drying by morphometric analysis using an image analyzer (Boyde *et al.,* 1977) or more simply by mapping the changes in relative position of externally applied fluorescent markers (Campbell and Roach, 1981), are found in plant, animal, and microbial tissues. It was originally thought that such changes were no more than a process of multidirectional miniaturization due to the pressure within the critical point bomb. There is no evidence to support this view as the dimensional changes vary within different parts of the same specimen and specimens frequently show a change in shape as well as dimension. Another explanation for the shrinkage is that it is due to solvent evaporation (Boyde and Maconnachie, 1979), a suggestion recently corroborated by Eskelinen and Saukko (1983).

In addition to the dimensional changes, there is evidence that critical point drying may also cause morphological changes. The use of lipid solvents as dehydrating and transition liquids can cause selective solubilization of cell components, and Boyde and Maconnachie (1979) observed that the plasma membrane was perforated in critical point-dried glutaraldehyde-fixed material. Boyde and Tamarin (1984) have developed an improved method of dehydration and critical point drying which leads to a marked reduction in morphological artifacts. The dehydration is via ethanol and the ethanol is replaced by Freon 113 by refluxing in a Soxhlet apparatus. Care was taken to prevent any air-drying, and the authors believe that the success of their method is based on rigorous exclusion of water and ethanol prior to critical point drying.

We have already discussed elsewhere the merits of freeze-drying (10–15% shrinkage) over critical point drying (60–70% shrinkage). In the absence of freeze-drying equipment, it is possible to diminish the deleterious effects of critical point drying by the inclusion of various additives to the stabilization and dehydrating fluids. Post-osmication and/or treatment with Ca^{2+} and Cu^{2+} ions (Boyde and Maconnachie, 1979); use of lithium and uranyl salts, and cetylpyridinium chloride (Boyde, 1980); successive treatment with glutaraldehyde, osmium, tannic acid, and uranyl salts (Wollweber *et al.*, 1981); and the use of tannic acid and guanidine hydrochloride to enhance osmium binding (Gamliel *et al.*, 1983) all reduce shrinkage, in some cases to as low as 5%. Figure 8.1 demonstrates the effectiveness of these methods during the preparation of animal cells. The selective tissue erosions and perturbation of surface morphology still remain a problem.

It would be wrong, however, to think that all critical point drying gives rise to a distorted sample. In a careful study on rat hepatocytes, Nordestgaard and Rostgaard (1985) found that both freeze-drying and critical point drying caused specimen shrinkage. At low magnification, i.e., up to 3000×, there was little to choose between freeze-drying and critical point drying, but at high resolution, critical point drying was superior to freeze-drying.

8.5. Exposing Internal Surfaces

One of the prime uses of a scanning microscope is to examine and analyze surfaces. Many of the surfaces we wish to examine are at the natural interface of an organism and its environment. Many more are hidden from view and we must seek ways of exposing them for examination.

One approach to exposing the internal contents is to make a replica of the object concerned as shown in Figure 8.2. Details of these procedures are given in our earlier book, and the recent papers by Ohtani *et al.* (1982) and Nowell (1983) provide an updated account of the methods

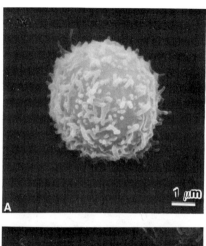

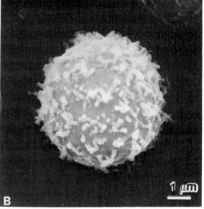

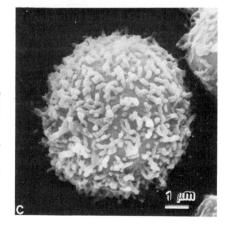

Figure 8.1. (A) Cells from a patient (A.Z.) with lymphoid leukemia, prepared for SEM by the conventional procedure of critical point drying after glutaraldehyde fixation. (B) Lymphoid cells from the same donor (A.Z.), critical point dried after glutaraldehyde and osmium tetroxide fixation. (C) Lymphoid cells from the same donor (A.Z.), critical point dried after GTGO treatment. (From Gamliel *et al.*, 1983.)

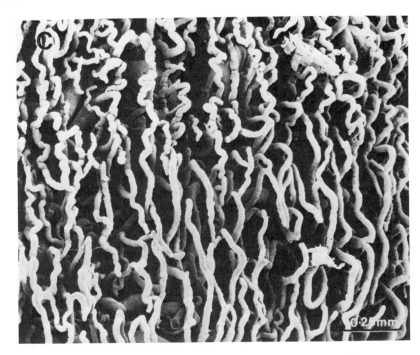

Figure 8.2. Serosal view of a microvascular cast of the uterine longitudinal muscle capillaries, showing their parallel arrangement along the longitudinal axis of the uterus. At the top of the micrograph, the capillaries are bunched and convoluted, indicating an area where the muscle was contracted at the time of casting. Below this area, the capillaries run straighter with few bends or kinks, showing an area where the longitudinal muscle fibers were relaxed. (From Rogers and Gannon, 1983.)

which may be used with biological tissue. A novel modification of the replica method is given by Grocki and Dermietzel (1984). These workers found that simultaneous perfusion of fibrinogen and thrombin formed fibrin inside cerebral blood vessels which could then be more easily excised from the brain tissue. Morrison and Buskirk (1984) have ingeniously combined sequential, *in situ,* microdissection in the SEM of methacrylate casts of the ciliary microvasculature of monkey eyes. A number of these methods—fracturing, sectioning, dissolution, and solubilization—are discussed in *SEMXM.* However, in the interim a number of new methods have been devised which are of particular interest for scanning microscopists. In most cases, it is usually necessary to embed the sample in resin or wax which, once polymerized or hardened, can be sectioned or fractured. These techniques are well established and need no further discussion. Westphal and Frösch (1985) have found that cells and tissues, when embedded in a hydrophilic melamine resin, are as hard as glass and can be easily fractured and used to give SEM pictures similar in quality to TEM images of freeze-fracture replicas. Bachhuber and Frösch (1983) have used this same resin to prepare thin sections which give images of exceptional fidelity when examined in the electron microscope. The newer low-temperature embedding methods are considered in Chapter 9 on cryomicroscopy, and are particularly useful when one wishes to maintain the chemical integrity of the specimen. Warner (1984) considers the metal gallium to be a useful alternative to plastic and paraffin embedding. Its low melting point (303 K), low toxicity, and high conductivity make it potentially very useful as an embedding medium for plastics and polymers. The gallium-embedded samples can be sectioned and fractured. Although gallium wets surfaces relatively easily, it does not penetrate samples and so cannot be used to infiltrate soft biological tissue.

Haggis *et al.* (1983) have extended their freeze-fracture-fix thaw technique to high-resolution SEM. Cryoprotected cells are rapidly frozen and fractured under liquid nitrogen. The fractured cells are thawed in a fixative solution which, with or without the aid of detergents, has the effect of removing a large proportion of the soluble material in the cell, exposing components of the cytoskeleton and the nuclear chromatin. These structures may be preserved and observed after critical point drying and rotary coating with platinum. Figure 8.3 shows an example of the use of these methods to reveal both microtubules and microfilaments in lym-

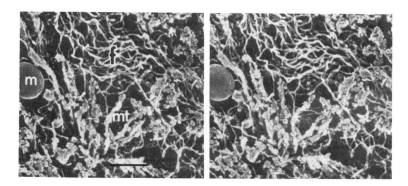

Figure 8.3. Ethanol fracture through a permeabilized concanavalin A-stimulated lymphocyte which appears to have responded maximally to stimulation, with cytoplasmic proliferation of a web of fine filaments. Below the web of filaments (f), microtubules (mt) are seen. The fine filaments seen here are probably, for the most part, intermediate filaments, since they have remained self-supporting after ethanol freezing and thawing, and after subsequent critical point drying. A mitochondrion (m) is seen at the left. Thin-section micrographs show swollen mitochondria in these permeabilized cells. Bar = 0.5 μm. Stereopair (0 and 10°). (From Haggis, 1983.)

phocytes. The results are quite impressive as the technique allows visualization of microtubules and intermediate filaments with the added advantage of seeing them dispersed within the three-dimensional space of the cell. The results obtained using high-resolution SEM are directly comparable with the information obtained by freeze-etch replicas. A more general approach to the use of freeze-fracture techniques for viewing internal cell structures by SEM is given in an earlier paper by Haggis (1982). The different methods for the selective removal of soluble cell components are discussed in more detail and include osmium digestion, glycerol extraction, delayed fixation, and treatment with detergents. A similar method has been devised by Inove (1983). Tissues are fixed with osmium tetroxide, rinsed with distilled water, and infiltrated with 5% DMSO before being quench-cooled. The tissue pieces are then cryofractured and the fractured pieces are rinsed in distilled water to remove cytoplasmic debris. Such methods allow three-dimensional visualization of mitochondria and endoplasmic reticulum in the SEM.

A different approach to the study of internal structures is given by Nagele *et al.* (1984) and Hawes and Horne (1985). The material is stabilized by conventional fixation and embedded in polyethylene glycol. The embedded tissue is sectioned to the desired region, immersed in solvent to remove the polyethylene glycol, critical point dried and examined in

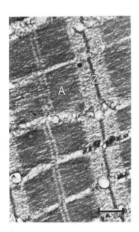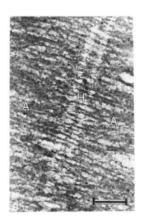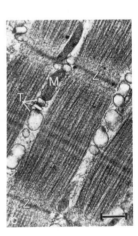

Figure 8.4. (A) A 150-nm-thick section of PEG-embedded mouse skeletal muscle. Z, Z-line; A, A-band. Bar = 0.5 μm. (B) Image of PEG-embedded mouse skeletal muscle. A, A-band; H, H-zone. Bar = 0.25 μm. (C) Image of a thin section showing the general appearance of mouse skeletal muscle after removal of the PEG embedment, subsequent embedding in Epon, and sectioning. M, mitochondria; T, triad of sarcoplasmic reticulum; Z, Z-lines. Bar = 0.25 μm. (From Nagele *et al.,* 1983.)

the SEM. As Nagele *et al.* have shown (Figure 8.4), this procedure allows clean fractures to be made through tissues with a minimum of distortion. Bauer and Butler (1983) achieved essentially the same result using polyvinyl alcohol (PVA). The tissues are gradually infiltrated with increasing concentrations of PVA, and the internal surfaces exposed by cryofracturing. The fracture faces may be etched with ethanol. The internal structures may also be exposed by fracturing paraffin wax-embedded tissues at room temperature (Shennawy *et al.*, 1983). Such samples can be used for light and scanning microscopy.

Jones (1981) has devised a method of ultraplaning to reveal the internal contents of tissues. Tissues are impregnated with osmium and uranyl acetate and embedded in a high-molecular-weight polymer of polyethylene glycol to give a hard block. The block face is then planed on an ultramicrotome to give a very smooth surface. The polyethylene glycol is removed from the block by repeated washes in water, and the tissue after staining with lead salts is taken through a dehydration–critical point drying regime before being examined in the SEM. A typical image is shown in Figure 8.5. An alternative procedure involves a celloidin–paraffin embedding, with the embedding medium being removed by xylene. The use of heavy metal impregnation lessens the need for coating. The advantage of the procedure is that it permits a controlled and accurately oriented plane of section to be made and allows one to view a large sur-

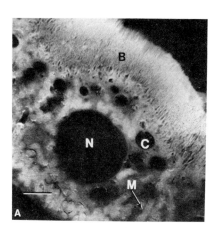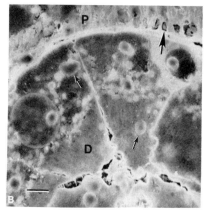

Figure 8.5. (A) Rat proximal convoluted tubule cell, revealing brush border (B), nucleus (N), mitochondria (M), and cytosome (C). Bar = 2 μm. (B) Experimental ischemic tubular injury in rat. Proximal (P) and distal tubule (D). Note the dilated basolateral spaces (large arrow) in the proximal tubule and presumed lipid droplets (small arrows) in a distal tubule. Bar = 2 μm. (From Jones, 1981.)

face area at low magnification. In addition, the quality of the preparation also allows high-resolution studies to be made on the same surface. This type of preparation would also permit the use of backscattered imaging.

Linton *et al.* (1984) have found that both ion-beam etching and radiofrequency etching are a useful way to selectively etch biological tissue and thus expose internal structures. The etching role for ion-beam sputtering appears to be related to the physical sputtering mechanism rather than the chemical activity of the incident ion. Heavy metal postfixation had no qualitative effect on the nature of the etching phenomena. Earlier work by Kuzurian and Leighton (1983) had shown that the oxygen plasma etching technique could be used on the entire block face of resin-embedded material. There was an increased visualization of tissue components when examined in the SEM. The authors have coupled the etcher with a small microtome and sputter coated inside the microscope chamber. This ingenious arrangement allows a continual process of cutting a smooth block face, etching the surface, and coating the etched surface, thus enabling a continuous three-dimensional analysis to be made of a piece of tissue.

8.6. Localizing Regions of Biological Activity and Chemical Specificity

One of the most important needs in all forms of microscopy is for high-resolution techniques to identify and localize specific macromolecules wherever they are present in cells. Whereas the identification and localization of elements is a more or less routine procedure by x-ray microanalysis, the same cannot be said of either molecules or macromolecules which form an important part of biological material. One approach is to couple x-ray microanalysis with well-tried cytochemical methods where the end product of the reaction is a heavy metal. The principles of this approach were discussed in *SEMXM,* and a recent paper by Sumner (1984) gives an updated summary of the advances made in this analytical procedure.

Various marker methods have been devised for use with the light and transmission electron microscope. These include: (1) enzyme cytochemistry where specific enzymes are detected; (2) the use of molecules that are specific ligands for proteins, i.e., hormones for receptors, myosin for actin, lectins for glycosylated lipids and proteins; (3) antibodies for antigenic sites; (4) autoradiography. In some cases, these molecules need to be labeled to identify the protein or substrate to which they bind. In other cases, the attaching molecule is sufficiently distinctive to be recognized on its own. Scanning microscopists have borrowed heavily from these methods and adapted them for their own use. In addition, they have devised new techniques which are quite specific for SEM. It is appropriate that we discuss some of these newer molecular localizing methods. For convenience, they will be discussed under three main headings: (1) immunocytochemical techniques, (2) radioactive labeling methods, (3) backscattered electron cytochemical methods.

8.6.1. Immunocytochemical Techniques

Immunohistochemical localization of antigens by SEM is a sophisticated and precise way of localizing and delimiting sites of specific biological activity in cells and tissues. It successfully combines the analytical and morphological advantages of the SEM and moves the microscope away from being solely involved with the descriptive anatomy of cells. It is difficult, in fact probably impossible, to identify antibody molecules by themselves and one requires a marker which can be linked to the antibody and is readily recognizable in the SEM. Such markers must be carefully chosen so as not to change the antibody's activity and specificity and they should have a net charge similar to the natural antibody to avoid any nonspecific ionic interactions. A good general review on scanning immuno-electron microscopy is provided by Gamliel and Polliack (1983).

There is neither space nor detailed expertise on our part to discuss the chemistry and structure of immunoglobulins and antibodies. The book by Nisonoff *et al.* (1975) provides a suitable introduction to the subject. Antibodies belong to the immunoglobulin G (IgG) class of proteins with a molecular weight of about 150,000 and are made up of four amino acid chains. Although the chemical basis for antibody specificity remains obscure, it is thought that certain amino acid residues within the N-terminal parts of the amino acid chains may form the basis of the antigen-combining site. Other regions of the four amino acid chains provide contact amino acids for bound ligands. It is these regions to which specific marker molecules may be attached. Immunoglobulins are a class of proteins made up of five types called IgG, IgA, IgM, IgD, and IgE, each with their own characteristic properties and molecular weight. The IgM immunoglobulins are of special interest as they have an increased combining power for most antigens and should prove useful for immunocytochemical studies. Although there are now many publications on immunocytochemical procedures generally (and somewhat less on SEM immunocytochemical methods), it is useful for readers to have a key reference to the subject. The most useful introduction and detailed exposition on methodology is the series by Bullock and Petrusz (1981, 1983).

There are several important prerequisites for a good cell surface marker for SEM. It must have distinctive properties of size and shape and be readily visualized against a cell surface background which itself may have a regular and/or complex surface topography. It must be small enough to allow good target-site localization and should form stable complexes with the particular antibody. Each type of marker will require its own method of attachment to the antibody and it will be necessary to consult the specialist literature dealing with this aspect of the procedure.

Four main types of markers are used in SEM immunochemistry: (1) viral, (2) emissive, (3) enzymatic, (4) particulate.

8.6.1.1. Viral

These were among the first type of markers considered and their usefulness lies in their distinctive and recognizable morphology. The long

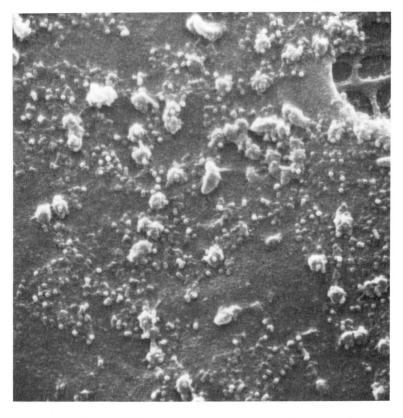

Figure 8.6. SEM of MMTV-infected Mm_5mt/c_1 murine cells labeled by the immuno-Hcy bridge. Both the cell surface and budding virions are labeled by a monoclonal anti-MMTV gp52 serum which is reactive with the envelope proteins of the virus. $\times 24{,}000$. (From Gonda *et al.*, 1981.)

helically constructed strands of tobacco mosaic virus, the tadpole shape of the bacteriophase T_4, and the near-spherical isodiametric shape of bushy stunt virus, all provide readily recognizable markers. The viral markers are now less popular in SEM work because newer, smaller markers have a greater affinity for the antibodies and give a better spatial resolution. Figure 8.6 shows an example of how these viral markers may be used to immunogenically localize sites of animal cells.

8.6.1.2. Emissive

This group includes fluorescent probes which were the type of marker suggested in the original work by Coons *et al.* (1941). The SEM counterpart of these fluorescent probes, which were designed for use with the light microscope, are chemical groupings which emit visible light when irradiated with an electron beam, i.e., cathodoluminescence. Cathodoluminescence is not a widely used method in biology due to problems of spatial resolution and poor signal-to-noise ratio. Although attempts have been made to obtain a cathodoluminescence signal from fluorescence-labeled antibody, the instability of this marker under the electron beam puts severe restraints on its usefulness. An alternative approach is to use a radioactive ligand as the marker (Cheng *et al.*, 1985). X-ray emission and backscattered electrons do, however, provide a useful signal for use in immunofluorescence studies. Hoyer *et al.* (1979) used x-ray microanalysis to visualize the simultaneous immunolabeling of ferritin and gold, and Hartman and Nakane (1981) made use of the backscattered signal for the intracellular localization of osmium–diaminobenzine–peroxidase-labeled antibodies.

8.6.1.3. Enzymatic

The use of an enzyme as a marker has considerable potential in immunocytochemical studies. It penetrates cells and tissues, forms stable immune reaction products, and has a high degree of sensitivity. One enzyme which has been used with some success is peroxidase, whose presence is detected using a diaminobenzidine–osmium complex which has a strong backscattered electron signal (Becker and DeBruyn, 1976). In a study on kidney tissue, Hartman and Nakane (1981) used this method on sections which had the added advantage that the osmium–diaminobenzidine deposits were seen as black granules in the light microscope, as electron-dense deposits in the TEM, and as a backscattered electron signal in the SEM. Figure 8.7 shows an example of this type of preparation and compares the backscattered electron (BSE) image with the secondary electron (SE) image.

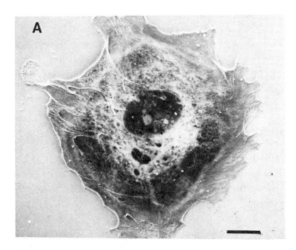

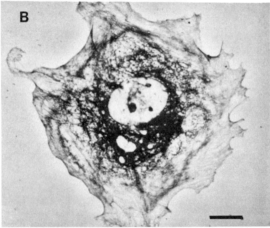

Figure 8.7. Scanning electron micrographs of a cell obtained from a primary culture of new-born mouse cardiac cells. Following trypsinization, cells were allowed to attach to a carbon-coated glass slide, fixed for 30 min with cold periodate–lysine–paraformaldehyde fixative, and stained by the indirect peroxidase-labeled antibody method using a rabbit antidesmin antiserum as the primary antibody. Following staining, the cells were dehydrated through a graded series of ethanols, critical point dried from liquid CO_2, and examined on a Philips 501 scanning electron microscope fitted with a GW Electronics solid-state backscattered electron detector. Photographs were taken on a Polaroid type 55 P/N film using an accelerating voltage of 30 kV, a spot size of 50 nm, and a line speed of 15 ms/line. (A) Secondary electron image; (B) backscattered electron image. Bars = 10 μm. (From Hartman and Nakane, 1981.)

8.6.1.4. Particulate

Particulate markers are probably the most useful marker for use in scanning electron immunocytochemistry. The type of particles which have been used fall into three main categories: (1) proteins such as hemocyanin and ferritin, (2) microspheres such as latex spheres and silica spheres, (3) metal deposits such as gold or silver.

8.6.1.4.1. Proteins. Hemocyanin is a stable monomeric conjugate approximately 35 × 50 nm in size. This large size may under some circumstances be a disadvantage as it limits the spatial resolution. The hemocyanin marker is recognized on the basis of its size and shape rather than its elemental composition. A study by Gonda *et al.* (1981) on cell surface antigens used hemocyanin linked to monoclonal antibodies as the marker. Ferritin is potentially a more useful marker because of its high electron density and smaller size. Ferritin is an iron-containing protein with a diameter of 10–12 nm, a molecular weight of 750,000, and 2000–3000 atoms of iron per molecule. There is wide experience with the immunoferritin methods in TEM where identification relies on its electron density. However, its small size limits its usefulness to high-resolution SEM studies and in spite of the high iron content, identification of the marker by x-ray microanalysis is difficult. Hsu (1981) reviews the use of this important marker molecule.

8.6.1.4.2. Microspheres. Monodispersed polystyrene latex spheres may be conjugated to specific antisera using glutaraldehyde. Provided the glutaraldehyde is later neutralized with glycine, this is a useful marker for fairly low-resolution scanning immunoelectron microscopy. The method has spatial limitations as the smallest latex spheres are approximately 100 nm. Alternatively, the larger-sized beads of Sepharose (40–200 μm), a bead-formed gel prepared from agarose, may be treated with the plant lectin concanavalin A, to provide binding sites for carbohydrate residues present in the biological sample. Millikin and Weiss (1984) show how this may be achieved for localizing glycosyl residues in algal flagella. The flagella are seen attached to the surface of the much larger Sepharose beads. Molday and Mayer (1980) have reviewed the application of very small microspheres to immunoelectronmicroscopy including a microsphere containing iron. These microspheres have a sufficiently high iron content to enable them to be detected using secondary electrons and x-ray microanalysis. Takahashi and Tavassoli (1983) give details of a simple method of processing polymeric beads to ensure they remain associated with the tissue.

8.6.1.4.3. Metal Deposits. Metal deposits, and in particular colloidal gold, are proving to be one of the most useful marker molecules for immunocytochemistry. Colloidal gold has been successfully applied in many TEM studies because it can be unambiguously detected in thin sections. It is more difficult to detect small (10–15 nm) particles using the SE signal because for high-resolution studies it is necessary to coat the sample, and this may obscure the SE signal from the very small particles. It is for the reason that a number of workers (e.g., see Walther *et al.,* 1984) have used the BSE signal which can readily detect individual gold particles in the range 10–15 nm. Colloidal gold sols range in color from orange to violet, have a strong secondary and backscattered electron coefficient, are electron dense, and have a distinctive x-ray signal. Figures 8.8 and 8.9 show that they are well suited for correlative microscopy. The gold particles range in size from 5 to 150 nm, are easily prepared, and have a very low nonspecific binding. Gold particles can be rapidly labeled with a variety of macromolecules including polysaccharides, glycoproteins, lectins (Takata and Hirano, 1984), and of course antibodies with little apparent change in biological activity.

It is possible to take advantage of the distinctive size range of the colloidal gold particles and devise a multiple marking technique. Thus, one antibody could be linked to a 10-nm colloidal gold particle while another antibody could be linked to a 100-nm particle. The size (~5 nm) of the smallest gold particle makes it particularly useful for studying binding sites and distribution of receptors or membranes where the density

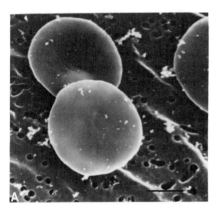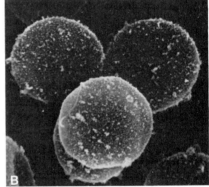

Figure 8.8. Secondary electron image of critical point-dried, platinum-coated human red blood cells (type O) fixed 1 h in 6% glutaraldehyde in 0.1 mol Sorensen's buffer pH 7.4, washed 3 × 30 min in 2 mol glycine (in PBS), either (A) neuraminidase-treated or (B) untreated, and labeled 1 h at 293 K with PNS-Au 35. ×4750. Bar = 2 μm. (From Goodman *et al.,* 1981.)

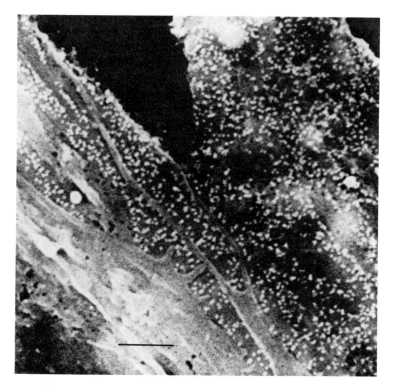

Figure 8.9. Scanning electron micrograph of Hell7 fibroblasts treated with anti-human fibronectin antibodies followed by gold (45 nm)-conjugated second antibody (immunogold procedure). The gold particles are located and aligned along the fibronectin strands and over occasional dense mats of fibronectin. Backscattered image. Bar = 1 μm. (From Trejdosiew-icz *et al.*, 1981.)

may result in separations as small as 5–10 nm apart. As discussed earlier, the only small disadvantage to the use of gold markers is that it is not possible to coat SEM samples with noble metals. The usual procedure in these situations is either to coat with carbon or use one of the bulk conductivity methods discussed elsewhere in this chapter. There are two comprehensive reviews on the colloidal gold marker system (Goodman *et al.*, 1980; Horisberg, 1983) which give full details of the use and application of this ubiquitous marker.

8.6.1.5. Fixation for Immunocytochemical Methods

Considerable care has to be taken over the specimen stabilization procedures in order to retain the biological activity and have good morpho-spatial resolution. Formaldehyde and glutaraldehyde very effectively immobilize and cross-link proteins. This can be a potential problem as the functionality and specificity of antibodies are dependent on their conformational features. Although some of the deleterious effects of the organic aldehyde may be alleviated by treatment with sucrose, washing (i.e., formaldehyde) or neutralizing with glycine (i.e., formaldehyde), it is probably best to avoid these fixatives if possible. Unfortunately, there is no good alternative. Bullock (1984) suggests using carbodiimides or parabenzoquinone which, although shown to be of use in light microscopy, have yet to be applied at the ultrastructural level. Alternative procedures suggested by Bullock include rapid fixation and dilute fixative (both of which would mitigate against good structural preservation). Bendayan and Zollinger (1983) find that treating glutaraldehyde- and osmium-fixed material with sodium metaperiodate enhanced the antigenic staining capacity.

The well-known protein-denaturing effects of dehydrating agents such as ethanol and methanol can to some extent be reversed by rehydration. But these too should be avoided as far as possible. This brings us back to some of the low-temperature methods discussed in Chapter 9, where tissues are mildly and rapidly fixed, dehydrated at low temperature with nonpolar liquids, and finally embedded in water-soluble resins. Under these conditions, most of the antigenicity is retained.

8.6.2. Radioactive Labeling Methods

Autoradiography is an analytical procedure in which specific radioactive molecules are incorporated into a known synthetic pathway either to reveal the spatial localization of the pathway in the tissue or to follow the synthesis, turnover, and movement of molecules in the cells. The presence of the radioactive label is revealed by the development of silver grains in a thin layer of photographic emulsion placed on the tissue in which the radioactive label has been incorporated. A one-to-one spatial juxtaposition is presumed to exist between the *site* of radioactivity in the tissue and its manifestation as a silver grain in the overlying emulsion.

Autoradiography has been used in light and transmission electron microscopy for a long time. It has only more recently been used in scanning microscopy. The principle of the method is the same, but there are important variations in the way the radioactive label is visualized in the SEM to warrant further discussion of the method. Whereas the silver grains appear black in light microscope images and electron dense in TEM images, they appear bright in SEM images due to the fourfold higher emissivity of the silver against the background biological matrix. The registration of the silver grains is further facilitated in the SEM because of the increased depth of focus. In addition, the presence of the silver grains can be confirmed using x-ray microanalysis (Sumner, 1982).

SEM autoradiography was, for a long time, a somewhat low-resolution analytical technique due to four main factors. SEM images are usually taken of rough surfaces, and the topographic contrast could frequently interfere with the signal from the silver grains. The detection of the radioactivity involves several wet–dry–wet sequences finishing with air-drying the samples. Such procedures severely distort the surface of the specimen. The presence of even a thin layer of gelatinous photographic emulsion on the specimen surface would mask fine morphological details. The usual coating procedures which involve noble metal would obscure the signals from silver grains. In the last couple of years, some new methods have been devised which alleviate some of these problems and make SEM autoradiography a more useful analytical technique.

The problem of autoradiography on rough surfaces cannot be easily resolved and better results will be obtained either from flat sections or ultraplaned surfaces (see earlier). The problem of alternating wet–dry–wet preparative sequences has been overcome by performing the autoradiography on samples maintained in the liquid state. Weiss (1980) took cells of a flagellate alga and incorporated the label during growth in aqueous culture. The labeled cells attached to polylysine-coated slides were briefly fixed and then passed sequentially through an ascending and descending ethanol–fluorocarbon water mixture. This dehydration and rehydration were found necessary to condition the cells. A thin ($\sim 20 \mu$m) layer of emulsion was applied directly to the wetted cells. Following a series of exposure times, the emulsion-coated samples were developed photographically, the excess emulsion removed, and and the samples finally critical point dried. Figure 8.10 shows that this procedure gives relatively undistorted cells in which silver grains may be easily identified. Weiss (1980) found that gentle washing with water and/or brief treatment with trypsin solutions remove most of the gelatin in the emulsion without excessive disturbance to the distribution of the silver grains. Satisfactory coating of autoradiographic samples can be achieved by using an extra-thick (i.e., 30–50 nm) layer of carbon.

Cheng *et al.* (1985) describe a method for SEM autoradiography whereby preservation of high-resolution cell surface details is retained together with a degelatination of the emulsion without gross loss or redistribution of silver grains. This technique provides a convenient medium-sized marker for topograhic studies of biosynthesized molecules and of cell surface receptors using radiolabeled ligands.

The modified procedures work reasonably well but it is still difficult to localize silver grains and read the autoradiographs from rounded cells. This can be made easier by examining samples at different focal planes

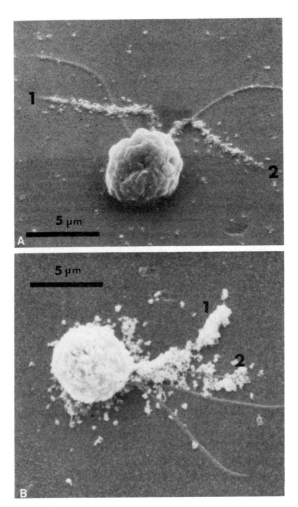

Figure 8.10. (A) Loop autoradiograph of quadriflagellate zygote. Two labeled flagella (1 and 2) with attached silver grains appear with two unlabeled flagella. The unlabeled cell body is convoluted from air-drying. Developed in D-19. (B) SEM autoradiograph of quadriflagellate zygote. Two heavily labeled flagella (1 and 2) appear with two unlabeled flagella. The cell body is round and heavily labeled with silver grains. Developed in D-19. (From Weiss, 1980.)

and using stereo pairs. It is important to combine the techniques of back-scattered imaging and the transmitted electron signal to localize the silver grains. A new procedure, autofluorography, described by Chang and Alexander (1981) makes SEM autoradiography even more attractive as an analytical tool. Specimen integrity is maintained by keeping the emulsion and biological material in a liquid phase until the final critical point drying. Autofluorography differs from autoradiography in that the energy from the decaying atomic nucleus excites a molecule of a scintillator which in turn emits a photon and exposes the emulsion. The exposure time is shorter than for autoradiography (hours rather than weeks), but the process may turn out to be less efficient than autoradiography. A variation of the autoradiographic technique has recently been described by Danscher (1984). In the method, which is referred to as autometallography, tissue sections are covered with a thin emulsion layer. During development, the chemical developer will penetrate the emulsion, pick up the silver ions, and the presence of reducing substances will penetrate the tissue. At this point, the developer has been turned into a physical developer, and any small traces of metals in the tissue, i.e., gold, silver, metal sulfides, and metal selenides, are amplified by being surrounded by shells of metallic silver. Probably less than ten catalytic atoms or molecules can be visualized by autometallography.

In all these radiographic techniques, special attention has to be paid to the tissue stabilization procedures to ensure that losses of radioactivity during processing are measured. There is also the problem of the fixation-induced losses of diffusible elements and small molecules.

8.6.3. Backscattered-Electron Cytochemical Methods

This is one of the analytical methods which is peculiar to SEM and has been developed to take advantage of one of the modes of signal acquisition.

Elastic scattering of the incident electrons occurs when they collide with the atomic nuclei of the specimen as screened by the orbital electrons. There is little loss of energy but there may be considerable change in trajectory. The production and nature of these so-called backscattered electrons are discussed in detail in *SEM XM*, because they form an important part of the imaging systems available on the SEM. The production of backscattered electrons increases roughly with mean atomic number such that ten times more of the incident electron beam is backscattered by gold than by carbon. It is these differences in backscattering coefficient which form the basis of the qualitative analytical procedure. A high-atomic-number inclusion in a low-atomic-number background will give a stronger backscattered signal which may be used to form contrast in an image to spatially localize the inclusion. Such inclusions could for example be a heavy metal dust particle inhaled into pulmonary tissue, a heavy metal ligand attached to the end product of an enzymatic reaction, or a heavy metal stain with a specificity for a given chemical grouping within a cell such as that achieved by Spicer *et al.* (1983) for carbohydrate moieties. The backscattered signal usually appears bright against a dark background. Biologists have frequently found it convenient to reverse this contrast so that regions of strong backscattering appear dark against a light background. As backscattered imaging is usually carried out on specimens also examined in the light microscope, the correlative microscopy is easier to interpret as the areas of interest appear dark in both caess.

DeHarven (1983) has proposed a number of conditions which should be met in order to make full and proper use of this analytical technique.

1. There should be maximal specific localization of high-atomic-number elements within the sample.
2. There should be minimal nonspecific distribution of high-atomic-number elements in and around the sample.
3. The cytochemical methods must result in an adequate level of preservation of cell structure.
4. The backscattered detector must have a high efficiency and should not interfere with the secondary mode of operation.
5. The accelerating voltages used should be selected to maximize the backscattered signal.

Before discussing details of the various cytochemical procedures which can result in the deposition of a heavy metal at a specific site in the tissue, it is useful to briefly discuss the types of detectors which can be used to measure these signals. A full discussion of these detectors can be found in *SEMXM*. The Everhart–Thornley detector (the original ET detector) can detect backscattered electrons, both in a very directional sense and in a diffuse sense by collection of remotely generated secondaries from the chamber walls. While the collecting efficiency could be increaesd by tilting the specimen toward the detector, this in turn gives rise to problems of spatial distortion of the image. The backscattered image is usually a mixture of specimen composition and surface topography and the ET collector is unable to distinguish these two signals, particularly on a rough sample. The newer annular detectors based on silicon surface barrier diodes can overcome some of these problems. The detectors, which are simple segmented disks with electrical leads, can be mounted just below the final lens concentric to the beam, looking down on the specimen. By electrically adding or subtracting the signals from one or more segments of the semiconductor disk, the backscattered signal may be separated into its compositional and topographic images to a first order. Adding the signals enhances the compositional image and gives reasonable atomic number contrast while subtracting them away produces good topographic contrast. In order to obtain maximum topographic contrast using secondary electrons with the conventional ET detectors, it is useful to be able to suppress the backscattered electron to secondary electron conversion above the specimen. This may be simply achieved using a device described by Volbert and Reimer (1980), and this can also be used to advantage in enhancing the backscattered image coming from the specimen. These annular detectors produce a higher resolution than the ET detectors and at much lower incident beam currents, thus reducing the problem of beam damage. There is more than adequate contrast available for most biological samples. In addition, depending on the beam energy, the method does allow us to look into the interior of biological specimens and obtain a backscattered electron signal from an inclusion 1–2 μm below the surface of the specimen. Detail on these and other detectors are given elsewhere in this book and in the paper by Becker and Sogard (1979).

A number of light-microscope cytochemical methods have been adapted for use in the SEM. This has the advantage that the techniques come from a well-tested pedigree and form a useful basis for correlative microscopy. We mention only a few examples here and readers should refer to standard histochemistry texts for further details and methods of application. Becker and Geoffrey (1981) provide an excellent review of the application of backscattered imaging to histochemical studies.

1. Silver methenamine staining, $Z = 47$: Aldehyde-fixed tissues are exposed to solutions of silver methenamine which is an effective, although not specific, stain for chromatin. Figure 8.11 shows how the stain works on human leukocytes.

2. Periodic acid–thiocarbohydrazide–osmium staining, $Z = 76$: This is a derivative of the periodic acid–Schiff technique used to reveal the presence of polysaccharides and mucopolysaccharides by oxidizing 1–2 glycol groups to aldehydes which react with the Schiff reagent. Thiocarbohydrazide is a multidentate ligand which is used as a bridging agent in cytochemical studies. As we shall see later in the section on methods for bulk conductivity, thiocarbohydrazide is also able to bind osmium to other metals, thus enhancing both their overall electron density and electrical conductivity.

3. Diaminobenzidine–osmium staining , $Z = 76$: Aldehyde-fixed tissues are treated with a solution of diaminobenzidine, thoroughly washed, and briefly exposed to aqueous osmium tetroxide. This method is widely used to demonstrate the presence of oxidases and peroxidases in both sectioned and bulk samples. The diaminobenzidine reaction can also be used in conjunction with nickel and cobalt salts.

4. Modified lead–Gomori method, $Z = 82$: Tissues are incubated in a phosphate-containing substrate, i.e., β-glycerophosphate, together with lead acetate at an adjusted pH. The acid and alkaline phosphatases split off the phosphate group which interacts with the lead ion to give an insoluble deposit of lead phosphate.

In addition to the active methods where a specific chemical reaction

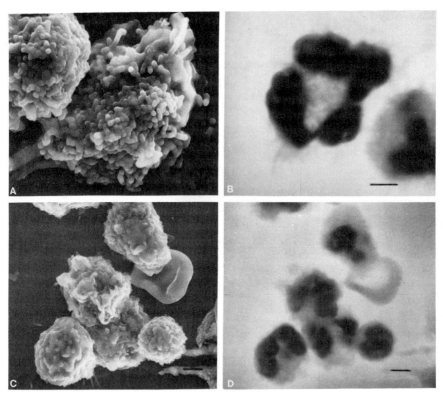

Figure 8.11. Normal human leukocytes after staining with silver methanamine. (A) Secondary electron image, 10 kV. (B) Backscattered electron image, 30 kV [same cell as in (A)]. (C) Secondary electron image, 10 kV. (D) Backscattered electron image, 30 kV [same cell as in (C)]. Bar = 2 μm. (From Soligo *et al.,* 1981.)

results in the localization of the heavy metal, it is also possible to exploit the situation where cells and tissues absorb or take up heavy metals. Three examples will suffice to illustrate this phenomenon.

5. Thorotrast method, $Z = 90$: Cells will take up colloidal thorium by a process of phagocytosis. The thorium will in turn be sequestered in particular cells of the tissue.

6. Iron carbonyl method, $Z = 26$: Soligo *et al.* (1981) have shown that iron carbonyl is a useful marker for phagocytic activity. Within 30 min of application, iron globules can be detected inside cells. Figure 8.12 shows the effectiveness of this method.

7. Uranium staining, $Z = 92$: Silyn-Roberts (1983) describes a simple method of estimating pore density and the ratio of blocked to unblocked pores in egg shells by staining with a dilute solution of uranyl

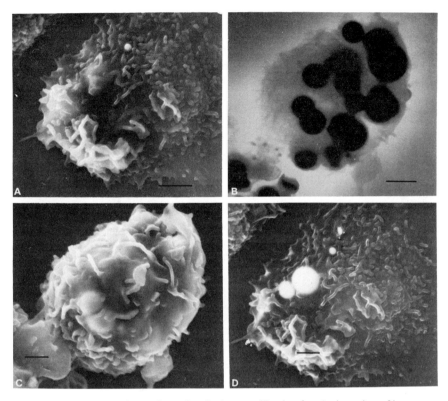

Figure 8.12. Human polymorphonuclear leukocytes 30 min after the ingestion of iron carbonyl. (A) Secondary electron image, 10 kV. (B) Backscattered electron image, 30 kV [same cell as the (A)]. (C) Secondary electron image, 10 kV. (D) Secondary electron image, 30 kV. Bar = 2 μm. (From Soligo *et al.*, 1981.)

acetate. Ulrich and McClung (1983) have used intense staining with uranyl acetate to produce a backscattered image of sufficient intensity to follow the movement of nuclei during cell fusion. These few examples should serve to illustrate the usefulness of this technique to analytical studies carried out on thick and thin sections and intact and fractured bulk material. Further details can be found in Soligo *et al.* (1983).

The rest of the specimen preparation is fairly straightforward with the usual attention being paid to the retention of the active constituent in the cells and tissue. Because one is looking for a heavy metal deposit in a low elemental matrix, the noble metals and their alloys are not the first choice of coating material. It is more usual to coat with carbon or possibly aluminum. The slight disadvantage of carbon is that heavier-than-usual (20–40 nm) coating layers are necessary which may obscure fine surface detail. Nevertheless, thin layers of noble metals have been used in situations where the heavy metal deposits are particularly well defined and strongly emissive. It is prudent to experiment with different accelerating voltages when examining the specimen. A compromise should be tried with a voltage high enough to elicit a strong backscattered electron signal, but low enough to minimize spread and penetration into the specimen.

The only problems which arise in the interpretation of the images are where the topographic contrast and composition contrast overlap. The best results have been obtained from sections and smooth surfaces. Problems can arise in interpreting the contrast differences from several granules in the same cell, especially if some granules protrude (strong signal) and others are embedded within the specimen matrix (weak signal).

8.7. Modifying Specimen Bulk Conductivity

The problem of charging and thermal instability in nonconductive specimens can be readily overcome by increasing the surface conductivity of the specimen by applying a thin film of a conductor, usually a metal. An alternative approach is to increase the bulk conductivity of the specimen by infiltrating it with either metal salts or deposits of metal.

The early attempts at these latter procedures were not very successful as they were based on extended fixation in heavy metal fixatives such as salts of osmium and manganese. While there was a marginal improvement, there were not enough natural binding sites in the specimens to obtain a sufficiently high loading of the heavy metals to make any substantial change in the conductivity. Similarly, staining during dehydration with sodium chloroaurate or uranyl nitrate also failed to make any significant change in the sample conductance.

By using reactive heavy metals such as osmium, lead, and uranyl ions together with mordants, some of which might be ligands, such as the thiocarbohydrazides, phenyleneidamines, and galloylglucoses, it was possible to make a substantial increase in metal loading on the samples and a significant improvement in conductivity. The process of mordanting is not new to microscopy; it has long been used for enhancing the staining ability of dyes. The mordant acts as a molecular bridge between the specimen and the dye (or heavy metal) and thus enhances the reactivity of the molecule of interest. Thiocarbohydrazide ($NH_2-NH-CS-NH-NH_2$) is a particularly useful mordant as it can form a bridge between osmium molecules. One terminal amine group reacts with the osmium previously applied to the tissue, and the other terminal amine group in turn binds to further osmium ions or, as Munger (1977) has shown, to uranyl or lead ions. The mordants phenylenediamine (Estable-Puig *et al.*, 1975) and tetramethyl ethylenediamine (Wilson *et al.*, 1979) are presumed to act in a similar fashion as a molecular bridge. In a detailed study on the galloylglucoses, usually referred to as tannins, Simionescu and Simionescu (1976) found that these substances act as a mordant between osmium and lead. At present, there is no satisfactory explanation of the chemical nature of the binding, but it is thought to involve carboxyl and hydroxyl groups. Of all the mordants and heavy metal ions which have been tried, osmium–thiocarbohydrazide and osmium–tannin are the most successful and examples of typical procedures are given below.

1. Osmium–thiocarbohydrazide–osmium method: Specimens are fixed in glutaraldehyde, washed, and postfixed in osmium tetroxide. The osmicated tissue is then thoroughly washed in buffer and incubated in the thiocarbohydrazide solution. After a second thorough wash to remove any unbound thiocarbohydrazide, the tissue is incubated for about 1 h in osmium tetroxide. Following a final thorough wash, the specimen is dehydrated and dried and is then ready for examination in the microscope. There are a number of variations to the method, the most important one being several alternating passes through thiocarbohydrazide and osmium.

2. Tannic acid-osmium method: Aldehyde-fixed tissues are soaked in a guanidine hydrochloride–tannic acid solution for several hours, thoroughly washed, and passed into osmium tetroxide for an equally long period. The samples are then washed, dehydrated, and dried.

3. Tannic acid–osmium–thiocarbohydrazide method: Aldehyde-fixed material is immersed in a glutaraldehyde–tannic acid mixture. After washing, the tissue is passed into an osmium solution, washed, and then placed in thiocarbohydrazide. After another wash, the tissue passes into a fresh osmium solution, and is subsequently washed, dehydrated, and dried. These alternating procedures can be repeated several times in order to increase intensification, as shown in Figure 8.13.

In addition to these three principal types of procedures, some success has been obtained with ammoniacal silver and with osmium vapor.

4. Silver nitrate method: Cells are fixed in a glutaraldehyde–DMSO solution, washed to remove excess aldehyde, and treated with ammoniacal silver nitrate. The tissue is then briefly immersed in photographic fixer, dehydrated, and dried.

5. Osmium–hydrazine vapor method: This method differs from the other methods in that the samples are exposed to the vapor of reactants rather than the solutions. Dried specimens are exposed to osmium tetroxide vapor followed by vaporized hydrazine hydrate which reduces the osmium salt to the metal. Although this method gives satisfactory results

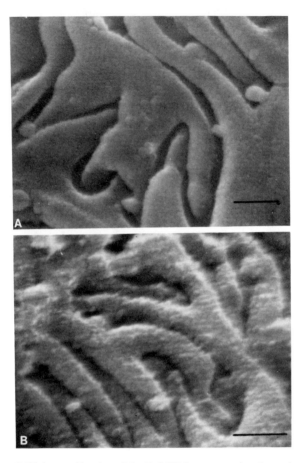

Figure 8.13. (A) High magnification of the TaOTO-impregnated and metal-evaporated surfaces showing granulations which are not seen in the nonevaporated surfaces. (B) High-magnification scanning electron micrograph of a tannin–osmium–thiocarbohydrazide–osmium–thiocarbohydrazide–osmium (TaOTOTO)-impregnated rat kidney. Note that the surfaces of the foot processes showed marked irregularities consisting of coarse granulations. Bar = 0.32 μm. (From Murakami and Jones, 1980.)

with plastics and polymers, it is not recommended for use with labile biological material due to the corrosive nature of the hydrazine vapor. It does, however, give good results with biological material when used in the liquid phases. Figure 8.14 shows an example of the application of the method to rat kidney tissue.

Full operational details of all these methods and the various variations which have been developed around a particular theme are given in the excellent review papers by Murphey (1978, 1980), Murakami and Jones (1980), Murakami *et al.* (1982, 1983), and Munger (1977).

The results of these bulk conductivity preparative techniques are impressive and high-resolution images have been obtained from completely uncoated samples. There are different degrees of success, the best images at magnifications of up to 150,000× being obtained from the tannic acid–osmium material at 20–25 kV and a 100-pA beam current.

The advantages of the bulk conductivity approach over the surface conductivity are as follows:

1. Metal-impregnated samples may be repeatedly dissected to reveal internal details without significant charging effects.
2. Very rough-textured or deeply indentated surfaces can be rendered conductive.
3. The surface conductivity is more even and there are less edge effects.
4. It makes it possible to obtain sufficient contrast from low-profile specimens.
5. Samples treated by these methods show considerably less shrinkage when critical point dried.
6. By substantially increasing the density of the sample by the inclusion of heavy metal ions, beam penetration is diminished and hence spatial resolution is increased.

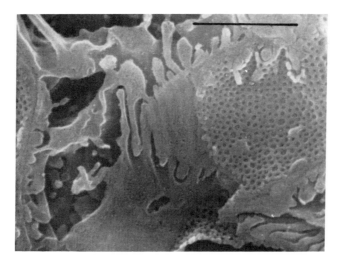

Figure 8.14. Scanning electron micrograph of a rat kidney block stained by the double liquid-phase osmium–hydrazine method (see text). Bar = 2 μm. (From Murakami *et al.*, 1982.)

Table 8.1. Thermal and Electrical Resistivity of Some Elements and Organic Materials

	Thermal conductivity (W/cm per K at 300 K)	Resistivity (Ohm-cm at 300 K)
Gold	3.17	2.40
Palladium	0.72	11.0
Platinum	0.72	10.0
Aluminum	2.37	2.83
Carbon	1.29	3500
Osmium	0.87	9.5
Lead	0.35	22.0
Uranium	0.28	30
Silver	4.29	1.60
Wood	0.05	10^{10}–10^{13}
Bone	0.05	10^8
Water	0.006	10^4–10^7

A simple comparison of the electrical and thermal properties of the metals (Table 8.1) which are used for these procedures shows that they compare favorably with the material used for thin films. The success of osmium is no doubt due to its optimal properties.

The main disadvantages are the increased length of time for specimen preparation, a signal with a somewhat lower S/N ratio, and in some cases a resolution lower than that from metal-coated samples. Some of the reagents, i.e., tannic acid, hydrazine, ammoniacal silver nitrate, can cause tissue damage, and prolonged exposure to osmium tetroxide would mitigate against high-resolution SEM at the molecular level. The presence of such high amounts of heavy metals precludes any attempts at analysis for elements of natural origin. In some instances, the conductive staining procedures are too successful and result in such a high backscattered electron coefficient that the topographic contrast is reduced. McCarthy *et al.* (1985) have modified the tannic acid procedure so that it may be used for specimens to be examined in both TEM and SEM.

It should be realized that the two methods for increasing specimen conductivity are not mutually exclusive. Some very useful images have been obtained from samples which have been impregnated with metal ions, critical point dried, and then lightly (i.e., 3–5 nm) coated with a thin metal coating. As Figure 8.15 shows, this method has the treble advantage if a substantial increase in bulk conductivity, diminished beam penetration, and high secondary electron emissivity from the metal layer.

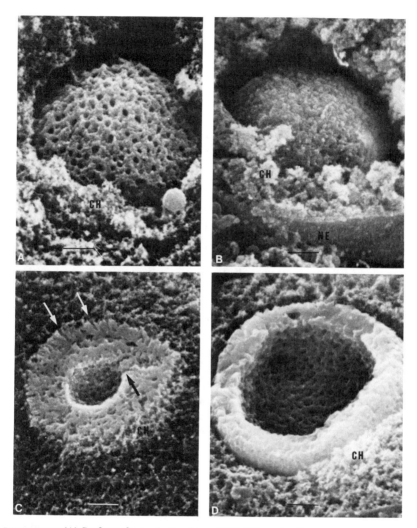

Figure 8.15. (A) Surface of a nucleolus. Pores 0.15–0.2 μm in diameter are surrounded by strands 0.15–0.2 μm in width. CH, chromatin. ×11,000. (B) Surface of a nucleolus. The nucleolus appears as a compact ball composed of anastomosing strands 0.1–0.15 μm in width. CH, chromatin; NE, nuclear envelope. ×11,000. (C) Fracture through a nucleolus. There is a deep depression in the center of the nucleolus, which may correspond to the zone called the nucleolar vacuole in light microscopy. The surface of the depression is porous, just as is the outer surface of the nucleolus. The pores on both surfaces of the organelle and the depression penetrate deeply into the main mass (arrows). CH, chromatin. ×11,000. (D) Fracture through a nucleolus containing a large, centrally located depression. Note many pores on the surface of the depression. CH, chromatin. ×11,000. (From Maruyama *et al.*, 1982.)

8.8. Specimen Mounting Procedures

Murphey (1982) in a monumental paper describes in great detail the procedures which one may use for mounting specimens. This is frequently a sadly neglected area of specimen preparation and one suspects that otherwise perfectly prepared specimens are spoiled by lack of attention to this final detail. Murphey, while agreeing that the materials and methods chosen for SEM sample mounting must necessarily be a compromise between the aims of the study, the characteristics of the sample, and the availability of instrumentation, provides practical details on how these procedures should be carried out.

The specimen stubs are usually made of a conductive material and care must be taken that the atomic number of the stub material does not interfere with backscattered and x-ray signals. For these two latter modes of operation, carbon, beryllium, and possibly aluminum are the material of choice. At least a dozen different stub types are available (e.g., flat, grooved, well) and they should all be cleaned before use and carefully checked that they fit into the microscope.

In some cases, it is more convenient to place the specimen on to a substrate which in turn is mounted on the stub. There are many different substrates, ranging from glass and plastic coverslips, metal and crystalline disks, plastics, waxes, and a whole range of membrane filters. Johansen *et al.* (1983) find that mica is a convenient support of biological samples, being more "charge" resistant than glass. Some progress has been made toward providing biologically active substrates. Tsuji and Karasek (1985) have found that cultured endothelial cells will reorganize on collagen disks, which can be easily processed for SEM. Kumon *et al.* (1983) found that gelatin-covered glass coverslips, impregnated with osmium vapor and coated with polylysine, eliminated charging artifacts. The choice of substrate will obviously be influenced by the specimen, and such factors as transparency to photons and electrons, solvent solubility, porosity, topography, composition, and conductivity must be considered.

It is frequently necessary to stick the specimen to the stub and/or the substrate to the stub. A bewildering number of adhesives are available for this purpose and the characteristics which must be considered include adhesive viscosity, stickiness, setting time, resistance to heat, solvent and beam damage, physical and chemical composition (many good glues have unaccpetably high vapor pressures which contaminate the electron microscope column), transparency and surface topography, and ease of application. Witcomb (1985) gives a comprehensive review of the glues which are available together with a list of their properties.

Thin adhesive layers are more easily produced using liquid glues, and one of the epoxy glues with or without a conductive additive is a useful starting material for dry samples.

8.9. High-Resolution Microscopy

To obtain the ultimate resolution from a SEM requires considerable attention to detail. No single preparative procedure, no single quirk of instrument design will guarantee high resolution; it is a combination of events. Leaving aside the instrumental route to high resolution, i.e., low-loss microscopy, STEM, field emission sources, minimum spot size, optimized working distance, and so on, all of which are discussed elsewhere in this book, it is instructive to see what may be done from the point of view of improvements to specimen preparation. Many of the methods which are used in high-resolution studies are no more than modifications of existing techniques discussed elsewhere in this chapter. An examination of the methods used in high-resolution SEM reveals a number of principles of specimen preparation. It is useful to briefly consider these principles which can be adapted to a specific experimental situation.

8.9.1. Isolation of Object of Interest

A cell is packed with structural features all bathed in a low-molecular-weight soup. Much of the effort toward optimizing preparative methods in electron microscopy has been centered on preserving everything *in situ*. This worked well for TEM which essentially provides a projected two-dimensional planar view of the object. Such procedures are usually satisfactory for routine SEM, but the presence of all the overlapping structures can limit the three-dimensional view which the SEM can provide. Figure 8.16 shows a high-resolution image of the surface of a spermatozoan and the internal details of a mitochondrion.

Thus, we must seek ways of isolating the object we wish to study, not by taking a reductionist approach and removing it from its natural environment, but by assuming a holistic approach and keeping it *in situ* and removing the obscuring structures. If we assume that no useful information can be obtained from the electron microscopy of small organic and inorganic molecules and water, it is permissible to remove these from the cell. One of the most successful ways of achieving this cytoplasmic catharsis is to use the freeze-fracture–thaw technique devised by Haggis and co-workers (for details see Haggis, 1982; Haggis *et al.*, 1983). This method removes much of the cytoplasmic matrix by thawing freeze-fractured tissue samples in dilute fixative. On the assumption that one wishes

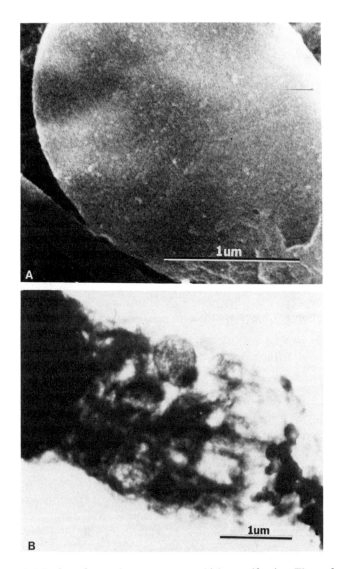

Figure 8.16. (A) Surface of normal spermatozoan at high magnification. The surface is even and finely granulated. OTO treatment, SEM, 20 kV. (B) Cytoplasmic body seen in STEM mode. The gray level is adjusted to show internal structures of spherical bodies. As a result, contour of axonemal filament complex is not well defined. Mitochondrial cristae are shown. OTO treatment, brightfield STEM, 100 kV. (From Okagaki *et al.,* 1980.)

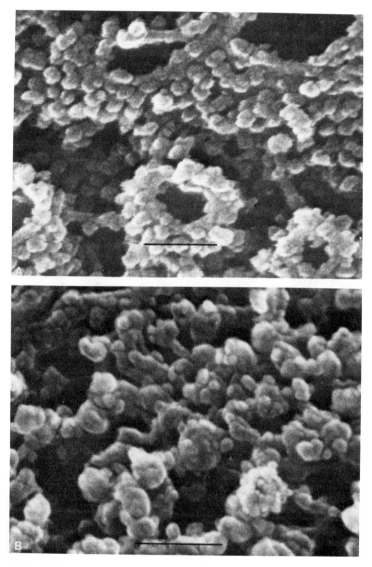

Figure 8.17. (A) A polysome observed on a rough endoplasmic reticulum A ribosome consists of two subunits. (B) Synaptic vesicles of a rat retina, which show various shapes such as spherical, cocoonlike and kidney shape. Bars = 100 nm. (From Tanaka, 1981.)

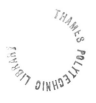

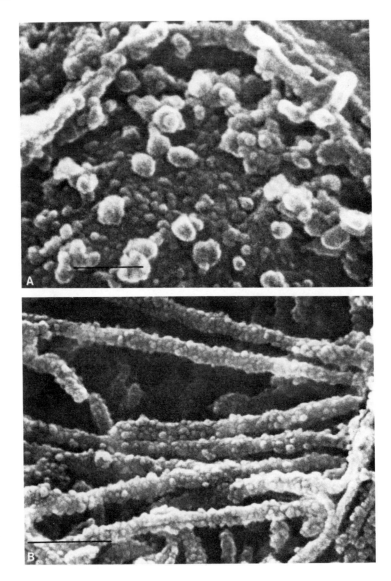

Figure 8.18. (A) Cytoplasmic surface of synaptic membrane in a rat retina. Many granules are seen on the synaptic membrane. (B) Highly magnified mitochondrial tubuli of hamster liver cell. On their surface, numerous particles are observed. Bars = 100 nm. (From Tanaka, 1981.)

to view the organelles and macromolecular components of the cytoskeleton, this method provides an excellent view of these structures.

A similar approach has been recommended by Yamada *et al.* (1983). Specimens were fixed in osmium tetroxide, conductively stained with uranyl acetate, dehydrated in ethanol, and then frozen and fractured. The critical point-dried material was rotary shadowed with a very thin ($\sim$ 2 nm) layer of platinum–carbon and showed the three-dimensional structure of *Cucurbita* prolamellar bodies.

8.9.2. Stabilization and Conductive Staining

Nearly all the high-resolution studies have employed some form of conductive staining method whereby the sample is infiltrated with heavy metal ions. These methods have been outlined elsewhere in this chapter. In addition, Tanaka and Mitsushima (1984) have devised a simple solubilization and conductive staining procedure involving successively treating the specimen with osmium and DMSO coupled with an osmium–tannic acid mordanting method. The DMSO facilitates removal of some of the soluble components, while the combination of osmium and tannic acid substantially increases the sample conductivity. Care must be taken not to allow any of the insoluble deposits which frequently form during conductive staining, to become deposited on the structures of interest. Figures 8.17 and 8.18 show the fine detail which can be seen in specimens prepared by these techniques.

8.9.3. Specimen Coating

A thin layer of a noble metal on a specimen whose electrical properties have been enhanced by conductive staining, improves the quality of the image. Full details of the coating procedures which could be used are given in Chapter 7, but they center around the application of thin layers either of low-atomic-number elements such as niobium or chromium, or very thin layers of noble metals. Peters *et al.* (1983) give examples of the type of images which can be obtained after coating with low-atomic-number elements. The success of this type of coating depends on minimizing backscattering in the beam–specimen interaction zone. It is important to only use the secondary electrons generated on the specimen surface by the incident electron beam. Tanaka and Mitsushima (1984) have obtained equally impressive results by ion-beam coating rotating specimens with a very thin layer of platinum.

Cryomicroscopy

9.1. Introduction

It is the purpose of this chapter to show how low temperatures may be used to advantage in the preparation, examination, and analysis of organic samples converting the liquid phases of the specimen to a solid. In this context, the temperature range which will be considered is that at which water is in a solid state, i.e., 0–273 K.

There appear to be four main advantages to using low temperatures in the study of organic material. (1) By lowering the temperature but still maintaining the liquid state, chemical reaction rates and transport processes such as viscosity and diffusion are slowed down. This slowdown makes such processes more amenable to study *in situ*. (2) In the solid state, water and many organic materials show an increase in mechanical strength as their temperature is lowered. This increase in mechanical strength allows these materials to be sectioned, fractured, or dissected to reveal subsurface details. (3) There is a diminution in the amount of damage to the specimen which is an inevitable consequence of using some of the imaging and analyzing systems. (4) There may be no need to use the deleterious chemical methods which are frequently required to stabilize and strengthen organic samples during specimen preparation for examination at ambient temperatures.

This is not to suggest that low-temperature microscopy may only be used to advantage in studying organic material. As Huebener and Seifert (1984) have shown, low-temperature SEM can provide new information on the properties of inhomogeneous samples by means of the two-dimensional voltage image and the phonon image. These techniques have an immediate application to thin-film superconducting structures, low-temperature solid-state physics, cryoelectronics, and electron beam testing. In addition, low-temperature electron microscopy can be used to study the interaction of electrons with condensed matter and enhances the cathodoluminescent spectra from semiconductors. However, unlike their organic counterparts, these types of specimen present little difficulty in sample preparation. It is these problems which will occupy most of our attention in this chapter.

It is probably misleading to think that low-temperature techniques involve purely physical processes. This would only be true if all the constituents of the specimen were in the same position relative to each other before and after the application of the low-temperature treatment. The phase transition from liquid to solid, while not changing the overall chemical composition, may well cause changes in local composition and variations in physicochemical properties. Nevertheless, the low-temperature approach offers the single most promising route to the study of organic and biological material at high spatial and analytic resolution. In addition, the low temperature approach also permits a study to be made of some of the biological processes which occur in the liquid state. Thus, the diffusion correlation time T_D (a measure of the movement of molecules) for ice is 10^{-5} s, whereas for pure water the figure is 10^{-11} s. Conversion of water to ice slows the process down by a factor of 10^6. Although these approaches would appear to be the panacea for studying organic and biological systems, they are not without serious theoretical and technical problems. Heide (1984) gives a detailed consideration of a number of these problems.

The conversion of liquid water to solid ice involves phase transformations and in some case phase segregations. The ideal goal at which all these techniques should be aimed is the vitrification of the liquid phase in which all the constitutent atoms, molecules, and ions remain in their relative position in the specimen before and after cooling. It is most unlikely that such a perfect state can ever be achieved in a heterogeneous, multiphase specimen and it is only rarely achieved in homogeneous single-phase samples. Leaving aside for the moment the vitrification of water which is a special case, many nonaqueous organic materials, liquids, elastomers, and plastics can be converted to a solid phase in which only the physical properties, i.e., density, heat capacity, viscosity, tensile strength, hardness, have been changed. Their chemical composition remains unaltered because of the low rates of transformation processes at low temperatures and the strength of the bonds between the atoms. Nearly all biological material and a surprising amount of nonbiological organic material contain a high proportion of water and it is the presence (and properties) of the water which give rise to most of the problems in cryomicroscopy. Pure water does not exist in nature. It is invariably bonded to hydrophilic materials and/or contains dissolved impurities. When liquid water, pure or "natural," is cooled, it undergoes a phase separation. The phase transformation from a disorganized liquid to a crystalline solid cannot be avoided, although the size of the individual crystallites can, if the cooling conditions are optimized, be reduced to very small dimensions. Because the ice crystallites are only formed from water, a phase segregation must occur when heterogeneous systems containing water are cooled below their freezing point. The extent of this segregation can to some extent be minimized. It would be quite naive to think we can avoid ice artifacts; it would be a dereliction of our scientific purpose not to seek ways of minimizing their effects. This chapter will not enter into a detailed discussion of the biophysics and biochemical properties of water and ice as this has been elegantly and concisely presented by Franks (1985). Neither will there be any discussion of the status of water in biological systems, a subject discussed recently by Beall (1983). It would seem more useful to consider some of the techniques that are being used to solidify liquid specimens, to discuss how such solid samples may be further processed for microscopy and analysis, and finally consider the problems of damage which may occur to specimens during the process of data acquisition. Much of what will be discussed will be centered on biological material for it is here that the problems associated with cryomicroscopy are most exacting. But the underlying principles will also apply to any system in which it is the intent to preserve and study the triphasic state of matter, e.g., soils, food products, emulsions, oil and brine mixtures, and so on.

9.2. Low-Temperature States of Water

At atmospheric pressure, water exists entirely as a vapor above 373 K, as a solid below 273 K, and as a liquid between these two extremes of temperature. It is this solid phase of water which we must now consider. Depending on temperature and pressure, the solid phase of water can exist in eight stable crystalline polymorphs, one metastable crystalline form, and one metastable amorphous form (Fletcher, 1970; Hobbs, 1974). Within this context, it is convenient to consider the three main forms of ice which cryomicroscopists might encounter: cubic, hexagonal, and amorphous or vitreous ice.

There has been some confusion about the terms *amorphous* and *vitreous ice*. In this chapter, the terms will be used synonymously even though the two forms of ice may be different. *Amorphous ice* forms when water vapor condenses on a cold surface held at below the glass-transition point ($\sim$ 143 K). It is a form of ice in which no long-range order is present and where no crystalline order can be detected. *Vitreous ice* is believed to form when thin layers consisting of a few nanometers of liquid water are rapidly cooled below the glass-transition point. Vitreous ice is, as the name suggests, a glasslike, noncrystalline form of ice in which no crystallites have been detected.

The basis of the current misunderstanding is as follows:

1. There are serious doubts [see Rasmussen (1982) for detailed discussion] whether vitreous ice can be formed by cooling liquid water.
2. Angell (1982) considers that vitreous ice and amorphous ice have different physical properties.
3. Dubochet *et al.* (1983a) have compared the electron diffraction patterns and recrystallization temperature of amorphous and vitreous ice. They found that, as far as these two properties are concerned, the two forms of ice are identical.
4. X-ray diffraction studies by Narlen *et al.* (1976) show that two forms of amorphous ice exist: a low-density form ($\delta = 0.94$ g) and a high-density form ($\delta = 1.1$ g). The low-density form is similar to hexagonal ice (I_H), whereas the high-density form is closer to liquid water. At temperatures below 70 K, the low-density form can be transformed to the high-density form by electron exposure. By increasing the temperature to 60–80 K, the high-density form spontaneously changes to the low-density form.
5. Indiscriminate use of the term *vitreous ice* has occurred for a form of ice in which no crystallites could be observed but where the observations and measurements have been carried out at a resolution lower than that of individual ice crystallites, i.e., ice crystals could be present but were not observed or measured. The hypothesis such that because no ice crystals can be detected, no ice artifacts exist, is false.

The actual form of ice to be found in a given specimen will depend on a large number of factors including the water-binding capacity of the system, its temperature and thermal history, and the volume of the sample being cooled.

The liquid-to-solid transformation is initiated by nucleation events of which there are two types. *Homogeneous nucleation* occurs when the random movement and clustering of water molecules produces a cluster of the right proportions onto which more water molecules can condense. There is a specified temperature range at which this probability event occurs—the homogeneous nucleation temperature—and it is possible to subcool water to this temperature (~ 233 K) at which point the water clusters are considered to be sufficiently icelike that they act as nuclei for spontaneous crystal growth. Thus, if one can carefully subcool water, the crystallization process results in many small ice crystals. As Franks *et al.*

(1983) and Mathias *et al.* (1984) have shown, it is more common for water, particularly in biological systems, to undergo *heterogeneous nucleation* where a foreign particle within the aqueous matrix acts as the catalyst on which ice nuclei growth is initiated. It is assumed that living cells would abound with structures of the correct dimensions ($\sim$ 10 nm) and correct physical state to provide nucleation sites. The transition of liquid water to ice is a first-order phase change and the ice crystal grows by accreting pure water at its surface. This is the process by which hexagonal ice crystals are formed.

There are four important consequences of ice crystal formation in living cells and tissues. *First,* the process of crystallization is accompanied by a release of the latent heat of crystallization (334 J/g at 273 K). Unless this heat is quickly removed from the system, undesirable melting and recrystallization may occur, resulting in fewer, larger ice crystals. *Second,* as the water is removed from the liquid phase, the concentration of any soluble species will increase. As the crystallization proceeds, the liquid phase contains an increasing concentration of ions which are also eventually converted to a solid phase consisting of hexagonal ice crystals and hydrated salts. The temperature at which a salt solution may no longer exist in liquid form is known as the eutectic point. Although the eutectic point of many salts in water is known, it would be impossible to calculate the eutectic point of cell and tissue fluids because of the large number of different dissolved salts involved and the complex interactions of such salts with organic macromolecules in the cell matrix. It is generally accepted that phase separation in biological systems proceeds to about 253 K after which complete solidification occurs. However, because one rarely deals with equilibrium systems, eutectic crystallization probably does not arise in practice. This freeze concentration can lead to undesirable pH and osmotic effects, polymer denaturation, and enzyme inactivation. *Third,* the various forms of hexagonal ice crystals (e.g., dendritic, spherulitic) may grow to such a size that they can cause a gross disorganization of the cell contents and in some cases rupture the limiting confines of the cell. *Fourth,* unless the frozen specimen is kept below the recrystallization point of ice ($\sim$143 K), the ice crystals will continue to grow by long-range migration of water molecules even though the specimen is in a solid frozen phase. All four undesirable consequences of ice crystal growth are exacerbated by slow cooling and may be minimized by rapidly cooling the specimen and maintaining the frozen specimen at low temperatures.

Amorphous ice is formed when water vapor condenses at temperatures below the glass-transition point of ice (143 K). Falls *et al.* (1983) point out that because there is always a partial pressure of water in an electron microscope, a uniform layer of water will invariably be deposited on substrates maintained at below 143 K. This fact emphasizes the importance of having adequate anticontamination traps in the vicinity of frozen specimens. It is also a warning that claims for vitrification (see later) must have rigorously excluded the deposition of amorphous ice on specimens examined at temperatures below 143 K. When amorphous ice is warmed above the glass-transition point, the water molecules undergo relaxation and reorientation and an irreversible process of crystallization occurs. In this instance, the transition is a devitrification and the amorphous ice changes to cubic ice. The temperature range in which water vapor condenses as cubic ice (I_C) varies between 130 and 150 K at the lower limit and between 175 and 195 K for the upper limit (Heide, 1984). As the temperature is increased, further recrystallization occurs which includes the resumption of growth of preexisting nuclei or crystallites, the formation of new crystals from amorphous solids, and the growth of larger crystals at the expense of smaller crystals. The actual kinetics of these processes are unclear, but they are certainly temperature dependent. A further transformation occurs at temperatures above 163 K and the cubic ice is slowly but irreversibly changed to hexagonal ice. At 273 K, this hexagonal ice melts to form liquid water. These crystalline forms of ice can, like any crystalline material, contain matrix defects such as grain boundaries, dislocations, bend contours, and stacking faults as shown in Figure 9.1 (Falls *et al.,* 1982). Such defects may affect the properties of ice during manipulations such as fracturing and sectioning. An interest-

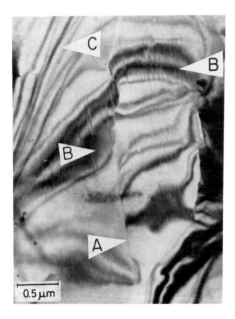

Figure 9.1. A frozen specimen of distilled water about 1.2 μm thick between two polyimide films, each about 30 nm thick. In the ice we see a grain boundary (A), stacking faults (B), and bend contours (C). The picture was taken in a JEOL JEM-100CX microscope at 100 kV, 93 K, with a JEOL EM-SCH cooling holder. (From Falls *et al.,* 1982.)

ing exception to this $I_A \rightarrow I_C \rightarrow I_H$ transformation is given by Lepault *et al.* (1983). These workers were able to reverse the process, i.e., transform crystalline ice I_H and I_C into amoprhous ice by cooling to 70 K and irradiating thin layers with 100–500 e^-/nm^2. The mechanism for this transformation is not clear. Heide (1984) reports a closely analogous situation where I_C irradiated with electrons at below 70 K is transformed into the high-density form of amorphous ice.

Although water can be vitrified in the presence of high concentrations of nonionic solutes and hydrophilic polymers (Franks, 1980), the claims (Brügeller and Mayer, 1980; Dubochet and McDowell, 1981; Mayer and Brügeller, 1982) that water can be vitrified from the liquid state are ambiguous. Figure 9.2 shows images and electron diffractograms of the three forms of ice. Rasmussen (1982) provides a powerful physicochemical argument which shows that it is impossible to obtain the vitreous phase of water by rapidly cooling liquid water. For even in thin (10 nm) layers and small (1 μm) droplets, the nucleation of ice cannot be avoided by rapid cooling. The hope that the thermal energy of a liquid can be extracted fast enough to prevent the clustering of water molecules with the resultant formation of a rigid glassy solid in which the distribution of the nonaqueous phase remains unaltered is unlikely to be realized. At best, all we can hope to do is to form microcrystalline ice, but even for high-resolution cryomicroscopy this may be good enough.

The cryo-pragmatist may argue that this distinction between microcrystalline and amorphous or vitreous ice, is a question of semantics. This is not so, for accepting that microcrystalline ice is a practical possibility and that bulk vitrified water is a theoretical dream, will allow us to better understand what is happening when water in biological systems is cooled. It is hoped that the foregoing discussion explains some of the problems associated with cryomicroscopy and can provide us with a better understanding of how to minimize the inevitable ice crystals.

9.3. Conversion of the Liquid to the Solid State

This initial phase of specimen preparation can be considered under two general headings: (1) specimen treatment before cooling, and (2) methods of rapid cooling.

9.3.1. Specimen Pretreatment

9.3.1.1. Chemical Fixation

On the assumption that chemical fixatives cross-link and stabilize macromolecules, some forms of mild, nonoxidizing fixatives have been

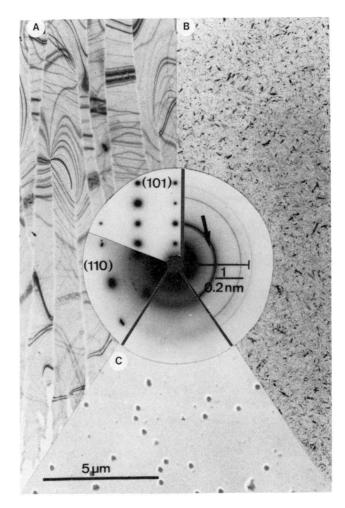

Figure 9.2. Typical images and electron diffractograms of the three forms of ice. The direct images are all at the same magnification (×10,000). (A) I_H obtained by rapid freezing of a thin water layer spread on a carbon film. The thickness of the layer shown in the micrograph is 50–80 nm. The diffractograms which are taken from other specimens show the (110) and (101) planes. (B) I_C obtained by warming a layer of I_V. The small contribution of the (100) form of I_H has been marked on the diffractogram (arrow). The I_C layer is approximately 70 nm thick. (C) I_V obtained by deposition of water in the electron microscope on a film supporting polystyrene spheres. The layer is approximately 70 nm thick. The shadowing effect seen in this preparation demonstrates that the flux of water molecules hitting the specimen in the microscope was anisotropic. (From Dubochet *et al.,* 1982a.)

used at ambient temperatures in the preparation of specimens for morphological studies. Such studies fall into two main categories, freeze-etching and low-temperature embedding procedures and cryoultramicrotomy. Much of the earlier work on freeze etching made use of mild fixatives such as some of the organic aldehydes which stabilized and strengthened the cell structure and caused sufficient changes in membrane permeability to permit the easier access of cryoprotecting agents. These fixatives play no part in minimizing ice crystal formation and growth, but because they strengthen organic material, they may help to minimize ice crystal damage. More recent work dispenses with such pretreatment as it has been shown that these chemicals are responsible for creating their own artifacts (Sleytr and Robards, 1982). Brief and mild chemical fixation is still employed in connection with the low-temperature embedding methods, details of which will be discussed later in this chapter. As will be shown, these methods appear to preserve ultrastructural integrity with high fidelity. There is, however, a nagging uncertainty that such images may not truly represent what is present in living tissue. For morphological studies, chemical fixatives are best avoided until such times as we know exactly what these materials are doing to macromolecules. In analytical studies where one is concerned with measuring and localizing diffusible substances in cells and tissues, the answer is quite unambiguous. No chemical fixatives should be used. There is an overwhelming body of evidence to show that even the mildest chemical fixation can cause dramatic changes in cell permeability so that many of the soluble constituents are either relocated in, or irretrievably lost from the tissue. These changes are not, however, universal for *all* elements in *all* tissues. Insoluble crystalline deposits and covalently bonded elements are much less mobile than soluble ions so some prudent compromise might be possible.

9.3.1.2. Artificial Nucleators

As discussed earlier, one important factor determining the size of ice crystals is the rate of formation of water clusters of a critical size to initiate the nucleating event. The higher the nucleation rate, the smaller are the ice crystals. As it is not possible to vitrify specimens of a size convenient and practical for most cryomicroscopy, it would be appropriate to settle for the next best thing in which the water had been converted to a large number of very small ice crystals. To this end, a number of artificial nucleators have been proposed; the idea being that the introduction of such compounds into cells and tissues would promote nucleation, in the same way that silver iodide crystals are used to seed a rain-cloud to form rain. Unfortunately, the likely candidates for biological artificial nucleators are either toxic, e.g., chloroform, or difficult to use, e.g., liquid CO_2. In any case, it is doubtful whether artificial nucleators would be of much use in the cytoplasm of cells, because there is already a large number of hydrophilic macromolecules and inclusions of the appropriate size and dimension in the cytoplasm which would act as heterogeneous nucleators. At the present time, artificial nucleators in biological and heterogeneous organic systems appear to be a lost cause. It would, however, seem useful to further explore the use of artificial nucleators to accelerate ice crystallization in the large, highly aqueous vacuoles and intercellular spaces in mature plant tissues and the cell-free spaces and collecting ducts which exist in many animal tissues. This method of seeded nucleation appears to be a strategy employed by some cold-tolerant plants (Krog *et al.*, 1979) and although the chemical concerned has not been positively identified, it is thought to be a high-molecular-weight polysaccharide. Certain polar fish (Knight *et al.* 1984) have glycopeptides and peptides in their blood which prevent the formation of ice crystals in water at temperatures down to 272 K. These organic compounds appear to be incorporated into growing ice and not separated like normal solutes. Although the mechanisms of freeze inhibition are not clearly understood, these and related natural compounds warrant further study as potential antifreeze agents in experimental systems.

9.3.1.3. Cryoprotection

Two terms have been used to describe these chemicals which minimize the disruptive action of ice crystals. The term *cryoprotectant* is used for chemicals which are used in studies where maintenance of vitality is of prime importance. The term *cryofixative* is reserved for chemicals which are used to help achieve and maintain the solid state of water with a minimum of distortion and crystal damage for microscopical and analytical studies. It is for this reason that I shall use the latter term in this chapter. However, in many instances the same chemical can be effective both as a cryoprotectant and as a cryofixative, i.e, glycerol. A further term, *cryofixation*, is used to indicate a low-temperature physical fixation where no chemicals are employed.

It has been known for some time that certain chemicals can protect cells and tissues from the disruptive action of freezing and thawing. To be effective, a cryofixative must lower the nucleation temperature, i.e., the temperature at which there is measurable nucleation, slow down the rate at which water molecules diffuse to the growing crystal, and reduce the release of latent heat which occurs as water crystallizes. The cryofixatives used in cryomicroscopy may be divided into those which penetrate cells and tissues and those which do not.

9.3.1.3.1. Penetrating Cryofixatives. Most penetrating cryofixatives (methanol, ethanol, DMSO, glycerol, ethylene glycol, and some sugars) alter the permeability of the cell membrane which invariably results in a redistribution of ions. Although penetrating cryofixatives should not be used in studies involving the analysis of diffusible ions, they have been used to great effect in freeze-fracture morphological studies. The most widely used penetrating cryofixative is glycerol. It penetrates most animal and some plant tissues quite readily, effectively lowers the freezing point of the cell contents, and retards ice crystallization. It is also toxic to many cells and produces a series of artifacts, many of which are recognizable in freeze-fracture images (Sleytr and Robards, 1982; Skaer, 1982). It is also difficult to freeze-dry or deep-etch (i.e., remove a surface layer of ice by sublimation) tissues which have been infiltrated with glycerol, for although initially the water component of a glycerol–water mixture can be removed by sublimation, a limit is set by the low vapor pressure of glycerol which is unetchable to any appreciable extent except at very high vacuum. In spite of the various problems associated with the use of glycerol, it is an effective and popular cryofixative for morphological studies.

9.3.1.3.2. Nonpenetrating Cryofixatives. Most nonpenetrating cryofixatives [serum albumin, dextran, polyethylene glycol, and more effectively polyvinylpyrrolidone (PVP) and hydroxyethyl starch (HES)] do not appear to penetrate cells to any appreciable extent [see Barnard and Hall (1984) as a possible exception], and exert their effect from outside the cell. Studies by Franks and Skaer (1976) showed that buffered solutions of PVP effectively diminished ice crystal damage in insect tissue. A similar effect was seen by Barnard and Hall (1984) who used dextran as the cryoprotectant. Figures 9.3 and 9.4 show plant and animal cells which have been treated with PVP. These studies were extended to a wide range of plant and animal tissues (Franks *et al.*, 1977; Echlin *et al.*, 1977; Skaer *et al.*, 1977) where it was shown that solutions of PVP and HES gave acceptable preservation as demonstrated in frozen sections, freeze fracture images, and microanalytical studies. Because these polymers do not penetrate the tissues, they allow ice to be sublimed from the interior of cells. This is particularly useful for examining the fracture faces of bulk frozen material for although it is possible to see the cell outlines in unetched specimens, removal of a surface layer of ice facilitates visualization of cellular detail. This is not to suggest that these polymers are ideal for all investigations as there are indications that even after brief exposure, some of these molecules can affect the natural physiological processes of some tissues. The polymers may also exert a noncolligative osmotic pressure resulting in shrinkage, and adequate cryofixation has not been achieved in all tissues. In the case of plant cells, Wilson and Robards

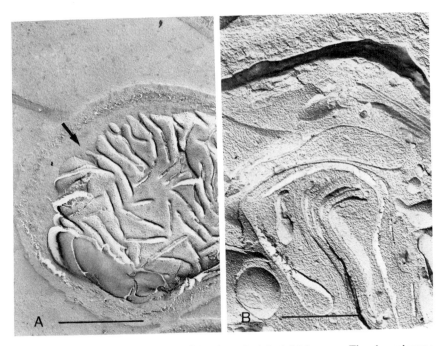

Figure 9.3. (A) A yeast cell showing slight plasmolysis in 1.5 *M* sucrose. The plasmalemma has pulled away from the cell wall (arrow) as a result of the osmotic pressure exerted by the external sucrose solution. ×28,000. (B) Cultured soya cells cryoprotected in 25% polyvinylpyrrolidone without chemical fixation. The cell wall, plasmalemma, and internal membranes are clear and the degree of ice crystal growth is low. ×25,000. (From Skaer, 1982.)

(1982) have calculated that PVP is likely only to coat the outermost cell layer of a given tissue as the polymer molecule is unable to penetrate the cellulose cell walls. Skaer (1982) has shown that there is a substantial increase in ice crystal damage in tissues where the highly aqueous phases are inaccessible to the incubating polymer. It is important that the period of incubation is long enough to ensure the polymer mixes at the tissue surface, without causing cell shrinkage. Unlike the use of glycerol in association with morphological studies, there is no ideal nonpenetrating cryofixative and it is necessary to establish the optimum conditions for each polymer with each tissue examined.

The mode of action of cryofixatives is not clearly understood. They are all very soluble in water and their presence will perturb solutions to the extent that they can no longer be considered in an ideal state. The ability of penetrating cryofixatives such as glycerol to minimize ice crystal damage is believed to lie in their increasing the viscosity of solutions,

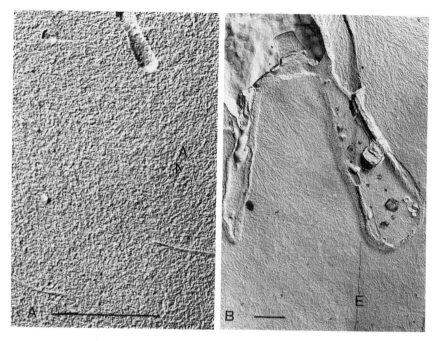

Figure 9.4. (A) Higher magnification of polyvinylpyrrolidone-protected tissue from the nervous system of the cockroach, showing the very low level of ice crystal growth. ×35,000. (B) A cultured soya bean cell in 25% polyvinylpyrrolidone exhibiting an unusual form of plasmolysis, where the cell wall appears to have acted as the semipermeable membrane (presumably as a result of the very high molecular weight of the solute). As a result, the cell collapses rather than plasmolyzing as in Figure 9.3. ×9000. Bars = 1 μm. (From Skaer, 1982.)

thus slowing down the movement of water molecules to growing ice crystals and in their ability to act as a solvent, thereby keeping potentially harmful salts in solution as they undergo freeze concentration. The presence of ¬enetrating cryofixatives inside cells will also lower the nucleation temperature and thus diminish the size of ice crystals.

The nonpenetrating cryofixatives probably act in the same way as their penetrating counterparts. They too have high solution viscosities which effectively retards crystallization. Our studies have shown that the polymer solutions in which the tissues are embedded must be vitrified during the cooling process to ensure effective cryoprotection of the cells. This suggests that prevention of freezing *outside* the cells delays nucleation inside, so that ice crystal formation is only initiated at the nucleation temperature of the cell cytoplasm (Skaer *et al.*, 1977, 1978). A more detailed discussion of chemical cryofixatives and cryoprotectants including a summary of the use of these chemicals on a wide range of biological tissues is given by Skaer (1982) and Barnard and Hall (1984).

9.3.1.4. Embedding Agents

It has long been known that it is useful to embed pieces of tissue in 10–20% gelatin prior to freezing. The gelatin provides additional support to frozen samples and allows them to be more easily sectioned or fractured. Following these earlier studies, serum albumin, methylcellulose, polyethylene glycol, and dextran have also been used for the same purpose and effective encapsulation has also been achieved using polymeric cryofixatives such as PVP and HES. The use of PVP and HES has the added advantage in that solutions of these materials vitrify when frozen. Such vitrified solids are more readily sectioned and fractured than crystalline materials. Experience has shown that plant tissues invariably require encapsulation in order that they may more easily be sectioned and fractured in the frozen state. The presence of large watery vacuoles and a cellulosic cell wall makes frozen plant tissue very brittle and more difficult to cryosection and fracture smoothly. The external embedding agent appears to facilitate initiation of the sectioning process and helps to confine a fracture to more or less the same plane.

9.3.2. Nonchemical Pretreatment

The preparative procedures outlined in the preceding sections all suffer from the disadvantage that they involve the addition of foreign substances to the cells and tissues. It is, however, possible to carry out some manipulations which are compatible with life processes in biological systems. One of the greatest problems in freezing tissues is the extraction of heat from the sample. From this, it follows that the size and shape of specimens is an important parameter when it comes to optimizing cryofixation, and one should maximize the surface to volume ratio (A/V) of the sample. It is no accident that the best cryopreservation has been obtained in individual cells spray-frozen in microdroplets or in thin films of liquid suspensions placed between metal foils of high thermal conductivity. In many instances, we have no opportunity of dictating the size and shape of the specimen, but we should always seek to use specimens as small as is compatible with the physiological and morphological aims of the experiment. The simple expedient of cooling specimens to a few degrees above the freezing point of water, will lessen the temperature range through which the sample must pass to arrive below the recrystallization point of ice (143 K). Such prefreezing cooling must of course not affect the normal vitality of the specimen. Rebhun (1971) described a series of experiments in which different specimens were coated with a variety of organic insulating substances or finely powdered nucleating materials before freezing. He found that these surface modifications substantially increased cooling rates by promoting nucleate boiling of the cryogen. There is unfortunately very little we can do to biological tissue without affecting its physiology. One thing is certain—ice crystal damage is reduced by rapidly cooling the sample, and we will now discuss the ways this important part of the preparative procedure is currently being carried out.

9.4. Methods of Rapid Cooling

In the absence of any chemical pretreatment, specimens for ultrastructural and analytical studies should be cooled as rapidly as possible. The reasons for this should now be self-evident, but they include minimizing phase separation and redistribution of solubilized materials, and a rapid cessation of the dynamic processes which take place in the aqueous phase.

As Bachmann and Talmon (1984) point out, quench cooling a sample in a liquid cryogen is a relatively complicated heat transfer problem. The rate of heat removal Q is given by

$$Q = Ah(T_c - T_s) = mC_p \frac{dT}{dt}$$

where A = surface area, h = heat transfer coefficient, T_c = temperature of the coolant, T_s = surface temperature, C_p = specific heat of the sample, and m = mass. More succinctly, Bachmann and Talmon consider that in order to maximize cooling rates, A/V should be large, h should be optimized, and T_c should be as low as possible.

The rate of cooling at the center of a specimen is dependent on the shape and size of the sample, the temperature difference between the sample and the cooling medium, as well as the density, specific heat, and thermal conductivity of both sample and cooling medium. The greatest problem in cooling samples which contain a substantial amount of water is the removal of latent heat, because the ice which is formed has a low thermal conductivity. This means that even with very rapid cooling, although the surface layers of the sample may have acceptably small ice crystals, about 10 nm, there will be a progressive increase in crystallite size the further one progresses into the sample. Hence, the necessity exists of removing the heat as rapidly as possible.

Fletcher (1971) has calculated that a cooling rate of 10^{10} K/s would be necessary to vitrify pure bulk water. A rate of between 10^5 and 10^6 K/s would be needed to vitrify the water in the superficial layers of a reasonably sized biological sample (Brügeller and Mayer, 1980). Jones (1984) has described a mathematical model to estimate the freezing times and cooling rates in the first 10 μm of a specimen. A simple analysis of heat transfer during rapid freezing of biological samples shows that cooling rates in excess of 40,000 K/s are associated with freezing times of less than 0.5 ms. These cooling rates may be achieved either by rapid immersion in cryogen liquid or by freezing on a metal block. These are the rates, i.e., something of the order of a temperature drop of a million degrees per second, we should aim for in order to obtain *vitrification*; as will be shown, we are at present somewhat short of the goal.

A number of ingenious methods have been devised to facilitate rapid cooling, and Plattner and Bachmann (1982) discuss these in detail. These and other methods will be discussed in turn and a value given for the optimal cooling rate which has been achieved with each technique. These values are probably all underestimates, and it is doubtful whether they are strictly comparable because no one group of experiments has compared all techniques. All the individual experiments have been evaluated using different-sized thermocouples and samples and with the temperature drop measured at different points on the cooling curve. Nevertheless, a general trend does emerge.

9.4.1. Plunge Cooling

As the name suggests, the sample is plunged, mechanically or manually, into a liquid cryogen. A number of cryogens have been used including propane, fluorocarbons, liquid nitrogen, and liquid nitrogen slush. There is still some controversy over which is the best cryogen for rapid cooling. Liquid nitrogen has for a long time been considered inadequate because the closeness of its melting and boiling temperatures causes a vapor phase to form around the specimen which slows down the cooling rate. Bald (1984), in a theoretical paper on the relative efficiency of cryogenic liquids, has come to the surprising conclusion that subcooled liquid nitrogen, because of its fast cooling capacity, high liquid density, and low viscosity, is potentially the *best* cryogenic fluid for ultrastructural preservation. However, this potential will only be realized if the minimum plunge depth and velocity criteria are such to prevent any vapor formation around the sample. A new derivative of liquid nitrogen cooling is that suggested by Sybers *et al.* (1983) who found that a container of slush made from liquid nitrogen and powdered graphite kept cool by an outer chamber containing liquid nitrogen, gave a 10- to 20-μm ice-free zone in heart tissue. Elder *et al.* (1982) have summarized the different ways plunge cooling may be achieved and the precautions it is necessary to take to achieve the optimal rate of cooling. The method has the advantage of being simple and inexpensive and avoids the disadvantage of mechanical damage associated with metal block cooling. These workers found that propane at its equilibrium freezing point gave a rate of about 20,000 K/s. Elder *et al.* emphasize the need for small sample size with a high entry velocity. The sample should be placed at the leading edge of the plunging device, and the cryogen should be vigorously stirred and fill a 30-mm-deep container. Although faster cooling rates (27,000 K/s) have been measured using small (25 μm) bare thermocouples (Pscheid *et al.*, 1981), the work of Elder *et al.* appears to be most applicable to small (0.5–0.3 mm) biological samples. The best estimate of the rate at the *center* of a 100-μm sample is of the order of 2000 K/s. Marchese-Ragona (1984) has obtained good tissue preservation in freeze-substituted protozoans which had been mechanically propelled into ethanol super cooled to 143 K. This cryogen is much safer than propane.

9.4.2. Spray Cooling

This is a rather specialized method in which specimen suspensions (cells, organelles, macromolecules) are sprayed as ∼20-μm droplets, with a spray gun into a liquid cryogen (Bachmann and Schmitt, 1971). The cells show good preservation but it is unclear whether this is due to the small size of the specimen or fast contact with the cryogen. A recent modification of the spray-freezing method has been devised by Mayer and Brügeller (1982). These workers projected a 10-μm jet of water at 400 atm pressure into a liquid cryogen. Using this technique, they claim to have vitrified pure water. It is difficult to give a cooling rate for spray freezing but an extrapolated rate would be approximately 100,000 K/s.

9.4.3. Jet Cooling

In this procedure, a jet of cryogen at several atmospheres pressure is sprayed onto a specimen from one or both sides simultaneously. This ensures a rapid renewal of the cryogen during cooling and presumably a rapid removal of heat from the sample. Knoll *et al.* (1982) demonstrate how this method is carried out. The sample is sandwiched between a thin copper sheet and an insulated layer, and melting propane used as the cryogen. The method is simple to use and avoids the hazard of passing through the cold gas phase which is a feature of plunge cooling, and the mechanical damage associated with metal block cooling. Rates of cooling appear to be marginally better than can be achieved with plunge cooling, i.e., ∼30,000 K/s.

Espevik and Elasgeler (1984) claim that liquid propane jet freezing is a simple inexpensive alternative to liquid helium block freezing. Using the jet-freezing method, these workers have obtained images of cytoskeletal structures comparable to those obtained by impact freezing.

9.4.4. Metal Block Cooling

Specimens are rapidly pressed against a highly polished metal surface maintained at or near the temperature of liquid helium (4 K). The main advantage of this method is that although metals such as copper or silver have a thermal capacity about the same as organic liquids, they have a much higher thermal conductivity and consequently the same amount of heat is transferred 10,000 times faster through copper than an organic cryogen such as propane. The method, which was originally devised by Van Harreveld and Crowell (1964), has been improved by Heuser *et al.* (1979) and Escaig (1982). It involves rapidly propelling the specimen against a polished block of high-purity copper held at 4 K; and calculated rates of cooling are in the region of 100,000 K/s. The metal surface must be scrupulously clean as contaminants such as amorphous ice can substantially lower the surface conductivity. The purity of the copper is also important, because only ultrapure copper (99.999%) has the high thermal conductivity to ensure maximum cooling rates. White and Woods (1955) showed that copper containing 0.056% iron had a thermal conductivity of 13% of the high-purity metal. Heath (1984) discusses the implications of metal impurities versus cooling rates in his paper describing a simple liquid helium-cooled slam freezer.

Any impact cooling device should ensure that there is immediate and continued contact between the specimen and cold metal surface. Phillips and Boyne (1984) have addressed this particular problem and have constructed a simple but highly effective bounce suppression device to ensure the specimen does not oscillate at the cold metal interface. Their results are impressive and they have been able to demonstrate ice-artifact-free zones as deep as 25 μm in postfreezing chemically substituted tissue. Although the method gives very high cooling rates, the rapid contact of the initially soft sample with the metal surface can cause superficial mechanical damage. A recent study by Bald (1983) has shown, using finite element numerical techniques, that pure silver blocks at 15 K can give a cooling rate twice that which can be obtained at 4 K. This is because at 15 K, silver has a substantially higher ability to remove heat from the sample than at the *lower* temperature. Bald also postulates that a composite material made of copper containing minute gold rods arranged parallel to the direction of heat flow would cool specimens faster than a pure silver block. Bald calculates that such a composite block held at 15 K should give an average cooling, at 10 μm below the surface, of

3×10^6 K/s. Although these are theoretical calculations, they are exciting because they provide a practical way forward to achieve the ultrarapid cooling necessary to vitrify the water in the superficial layers of a specimen.

9.4.5. High-Pressure Cooling

An examination of the phase diagram of water will show that vitreous water should form when liquid water is cooled under high pressure. The freezing point of water at 1.1 kbar is reduced to 251 K. Diminishing the temperature range over which crystallization can occur, increases the chance of vitrificaiton or, at the very best, microcrystalline ice. Moor and his colleagues [see Hunziker et al. (1984) for the latest developments] have exploited this phenomenon and have built a high-pressure cooling device. Specimens are subjected to pressures of 2-0 kbar by applying a jet of liquid propanol on each side of the specimen a few milliseconds before it is cooled by a jet of liquid nitrogen also applied on both sides of the specimen. It is estimated that the tissue water was frozen within 40 ms of the initiation of the pressure buildup. This simple idea has been difficult to achieve in practice and it has only recently become commercially available. The results are impressive and with cooling rates in the region of 10^4 K/s, it has been shown that some organisms can survive the high pressure and that good structural preservation is maintained with vitrification in tissue samples up to 600 μm thick.

One of the difficulties in assessing the relative usefulness of the different methods of cooling is to obtain some comparative measurement of cooling rates. These rates may be calculated from theory (Bald, 1983; Jones, 1984) deduced from variations in certain electrical coefficients during cooling (Heuser et al., 1979) or directly measured using thermocouples. Although thermocouples give consistent results when used to measure the *mean* cooling rate of a given cryogen, it is very difficult to use them to measure a cooling rate in the middle of an organic sample. Thermocouple measurements also have an inherent disadvantage that they probably underestimate the cooling rate at the surface of the specimen, and at best probably only give an average value at the center. This point is discussed in some detail by Jones (1984) who considers that many of the published *mean cooling rates* are difficult to interpret as they ignore two fundamental measures of freezing: (1) the times at which the various regions are frozen; (2) the cooling rate at which freezing occurs. The cooling rates given in Table 9.1 are an average value for a thin (100–200 μm) sample and should only be used as to compare the different values. The values given are an underestimate of the cooling rate at the surface and a gross overestimate of the value at the center of the sample. A

Table 9.1. Comparison of Cooling Rates

Method	Best rate (K × 10³/s)	Artifact-freeze zone (μm)	Cryogen (temp.)
Plunge	20–30	5–10	Propane (83 K)
Spray	100	20	Propane (83 K)
Jet	30–40	10	Propane (83 K)
Block	50–60	15–20	Helium (4 K)
Pressure	100	600	Nitrogen (77 K)

more detailed analysis of the cooling rates obtained by the different methods is given by Plattner and Bachmann (1982) and Jones (1984).

If one is only concerned with the surface of the sample, then there is little to choose among the five methods. If one is concerned with obtaining the smallest ice crystals in a reasonably sized sample (∼ 1 mm³) with relative ease and a minimum cost, then plunge and jet cooling using propane as cryogen would give the best result. If very small (i.e., less than 10 nm) ice crystals or vitrification is the goal, then metal block cooling at 15 K would appear to be the best approach.

Having successfully cooled the specimen, it is important to keep it below the recrystallization point of water (143 K). A storage dewar of liquid nitrogen is a convenient and inexpensive way of storing specimens. Rigler and Patton (1984) and Williamson (1984) give details of some simple inexpensive storage devices. It has always been assumed that specimens stored in liquid nitrogen would be safe for an indefinite period of time. Rebiai *et al.* (1983) suggest that this may not be the case. These workers found an unexpectedly high solubility of water in cryogenic liquids and suggested that this could lead to desiccation of biological specimens stored for long periods of time in direct contact with liquid nitrogen. However, the draconian predictions are probably unfounded as most storage dewars contain liquid nitrogen saturated with water due to repeated exposure to the atmosphere. Nevertheless, it would probably be unwise to expose thin sections to pure liquid nitrogen.

9.5. Sample Handling after Rapid Cooling

There are a number of options open to the experimenter regarding the further treatment of the sample after it has been rapidly cooled. These options include (1) sectioning, (2) fracturing, (3) etching and replication, (4) chemical substitution, and (5) freeze-drying. Before deciding which of these options will be used, it is important to decide whether the specimen is to be examined in the frozen-dried or the frozen-hydrated state and whether the external surface or the internal contents are the subject of the investigation. A frozen-dried specimen is one in which the solid water has been removed by sublimation under vacuum. This is a thermodynamic process and therefore requires thermal movement of molecules. This same mobility can also lead to recrystallization and the consequent formation of artifacts. By comparison, a frozen-hydrated sample is one in which the solid water is retained *in situ* throughout preparation, examination, and analysis. Some workers (Gupta and Hall, 1981) prefer to work in the partially hydrated state. This approach is subject to grave uncertainty about how much water is actually present in the sample at a given stage of the experiment. The process of dehydration is a dynamic process and although the *average* value of hydration of a sample may indicate a value between 0 and 100%, the actual value at a given point would be either 0 *or* 100%. There are *a priori* reasons why a specimen should be anything but fully hydrated or fully dried. This uncertainty about the degree of hydration in a partially dried sample is exacerbated in studies where an accurate measure of the specimen mass is important.

Irrespective of what happens to the specimen after it is quench cooled, the sample must be held in some sort of clamping device. Placing the sample in the clamping device *before* quench cooling is an easy answer to this problem, provided the size of the clamping device does not affect the cooling rate. This problem may be overcome either by using small holders which fit into a larger holder [see Echlin *et al.* (1982b) for a practical solution to this problem], or by attaching rapidly cooled specimens to the sample holder. This latter procedure calls for some sort of low-temperature glue or embedding medium and the use of *n*-heptane by Steinbrecht and Zierold (1984) gives a satisfactory answer to the problem. Its low melting point (182 K), high vapor pressure, and chemical inertia at low temperatures, make it ideally suited for either embedding small samples prior to sectioning, or attaching larger specimens to the cryomicrotome specimen holder. Toluene (Karp *et al.*, 1982) and *n*-butylbenzene (Saubermann and Echlin, 1975) have similar properties. These procedures may be used to assemble small frozen droplets which had previously been quench cooled by spray freezing into a more manageable size for subsequent sectioning or fracturing.

9.5.1. Sectioning

A convenient way of exposing the internal features of a solid sample is to section it into slices thin enough to be examined by some form of transmitted illumination. In a homogeneous sample such as a polymer or a frozen salt solution, only a few sections will be necessary as it is presumed that a single section is representative of the solid specimen. In a heterogeneous sample, there is a greater uncertainty and it may be necessary to take a series of sections through the whole specimen. Although there is still a great deal of controversy about the physics of the process of cryosectioning, it is convenient to consider thin (50–100 nm) and thick (0.2–2.0 μm) sections separately.

9.5.1.1. Thin Sections

The nature and success of cryoultramicrotomy is very dependent on the way the specimens have been prepared. Specimens which are prepared with a minimum phase separation of the aqueous and nonaqueous components either by infiltration with cryoprotectants or by rapid cooling, can be sectioned more thinly, more easily, and at lower temperatures. Figure 9.5 shows a frozen-dried cryosection of skeletal muscle from a frog. In other words, the larger the ice crystals, the thicker the section and the warmer the sectioning temperature has to be in order to obtain smooth sections. The reverse is also true. This fact can be demonstrated by cutting sections of a rapidly cooled aqueous solution of 25% PVP. Such a solution will truly vitrify on cooling and it is as easy to cut thin sections of this material at between 115 and 193 K as it is to cut resin sections at ambient temperatures. The only difference is that much slower sectioning speeds (0.1–1.0 mm/s) are used in cutting cryosections. Another important variable in the sectioning process is of course the nature of the specimen. The lower the amount of free or unbound water in the sample, the better the freezing and the easier it is to section. Thus, while an elastomer such as rubber or a well-glycerinated piece of biological material is easily sectioned at 143 K, it is virtually impossible to consistently obtain smooth sections of an untreated mature vacuolate plant cell. Extending this to heterogeneous specimens, Wendt-Gallitelli and Woeburg (1981) were able to cut thin sections at 143 K on muscle tissue cooled by the metal block process at 4 K. It was not possible to obtain thin sections from material in which ice crystals larger than 50 nm were visible. Zierold (1982b) has cut thin (100 nm) sections at 173 K of yeast suspensions cooled by using the propane jet method, and McDowall *et al.* (1983) have cut thin, crystallite-free sections from what they claim to be vitrified samples maintained below the recrystallization temperature (147 K). Figure 9.6 shows images of sections of vitreous ice and of vitrified rat liver. These and numerous other studies demonstrate that thin cryosections can be cut at between 173 and 143 K from a variety of frozen solutions, tissues, and polymers by using glass or diamond knives. Space will not permit a detailed explanation of the procedure for cutting thin sections, for although the basic procedures are the same, important dif-

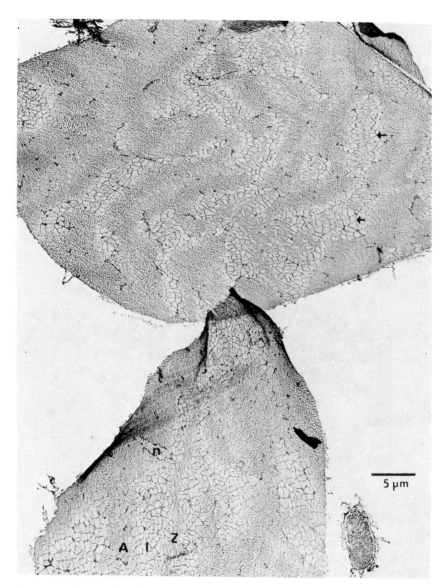

Figure 9.5. Cryosection of skeletal muscle (frog semitendinosus) fibers oriented transversely using toluene as a low-temperature cement. Individual fibrils surrounded by reticulum (arrows) are clearly seen in the light regions corresponding to the I-band (I) and can also be resolved at higher magnification in the darker A-band (A) regions. The darker areas (Z) within the I-band of the lower fiber correspond to the Z-band. n, nucleus. (From Karp *et al.*, 1982.)

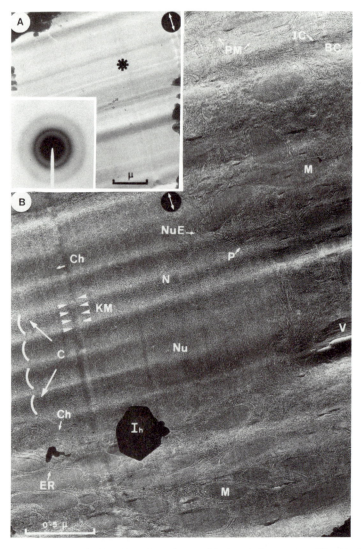

Figure 9.6. (A) Frozen-hydrated section from a block of vitreous ice. The block was obtained by condensation of water vapor at 10^{-1} Pa for 2 h on a specimen holder kept at boiling nitrogen temperature. Sectioning temperature 100 K. The thickness at the point marked by the asterisk is 118 nm. $\times 12,600$. The corresponding electron diffractogram is shown in the inset. The first ring corresponds to 0.37 nm. (B) Frozen-hydrated section from an untreated rat liver sample vitrified by the metal mirror freezing method. Sectioning temperature 120 K; thickness 180 nm. $\times$ 52,000. N, nucleus; Nu, nucleolus; NuE, nuclear envelope; P, nuclear pore; JC, junctional complex; BC, bile canaliculus; PM, plasma membrane; Ch, chromatin; M, mitochondria; ER, endoplasmic reticulum with ribosomes; V, vacuole with ice in hexagonal form; I_h, contaminating hexagonal ice crystals; KM, knife marks; C, chatter. (From McDowall *et al.,* 1983.)

ferences exist for the various cryomicrotome types and whether the section remains in the hydrated state or whether it is subsequently dried. A good general introduction to the subject can be found in Sitte (1982), Frederik (1982), Frederik *et al.* (1982), and Barnard (1982). The recent article by Parsons *et al.* (1984) emphasizes the practical aspects of routine cryoultramicrotomy.

9.5.1.2. Thick Sections

Cryosectioning of thick (i.e., 10–20 μm) sections is a standard procedure in many pathology laboratories. However, although such sections are suitable for light microscopy, they are too thick to be examined and analyzed using electron beam instruments. In addition, the relatively warm sectioning temperature ($\sim$250 K) introduces too many recrystallization artifacts to make such sections useful for ultrastructural studies. In the past few years, there has been a move to carrying out microanalysis on thick sections (0.2–2.0 μm) using the SEM. The sectioning procedure is basically the same as for thin sections, except that warmer temperatures (193–233 K) appear to give better results, i.e., smooth sections. The thicker sections are cut using glass, diamond, steel, and tungsten carbide knives (Saubermann, personal communication) and it is interesting to note that the use of metal knives permits warmer sectioning temperatures to be employed. Saubermann *et al.* (1981b), Biddlecombe *et al.* (1982), and Zierold (1982c) review the current procedures used in cutting these thicker cryosections.

Irrespective of the method of cryosectioning, it is important that the section does not melt during the process of cutting. Earlier studies indicated that this may indeed have been a problem, particularly with thin sections. More recent work based on careful measurement of the energy input into the specimen (Saubermann *et al.*, 1977), sectioning material of known melting point (Karp *et al.*, 1982), and microscopic examination of freeze-dried and embedded cryosections (Frederik and Busing, 1981) all indicate that there is neither through-section melting nor growth of ice crystals at sectioning temperatures between 143 and 243 K. Although it is unlikely that section melting occurs, there is some evidence that phase transitions may result as a consequence of the cutting process. Chang *et al.* (1983) observed a series of bands in cryosections cut at below 143 K in material they considered had been vitrified during cooling. Chang *et al.* interpret this periodicity as representing cutting-induced devitrification. Frederik and Busing (1980) do not consider that migratory recrystallization makes a significant contribution to the ice crystal damage seen in most frozen sections. The ice crystal damage occurs during the initial cooling process. A closely related problem associated with cryosectioning is that the thin section does not dry out during temporary residence in the microtome, transient passage in a transfer device, and semipermanent residence on the cold stage of the microscope. Freeze-drying (see later) is all too easy with a thin section in the high vacuum of an electron microscope. The only way to ensure that sections remain in a fully hydrated state during transfer to, and examination in the microscope, is to keep the *sample* below the ice recrystallization point. The sublimation rate of ice from sections in the cryomicrotome has until recently been an unknown quantity. Zingsheim (1984) has shown that the sublimation rate of ice in a nitrogen-filled cryochamber of an ultramicrotome is four to five times smaller than sublimation *in vacuo* at the same temperature. This finding is reassuring because it means that the danger of even partial dehydration of semithick sections (0.5–1.0 μm) is less serious than previously assumed. The situation is less certain with ultrathin (30–50 nm) sections.

9.5.1.3. The Sectioning Process

In spite of the advances in cryomicrotomy, the nature of the cutting process is not fully understood. There appears to be general agreement that in samples which show significant phase separation as a result of slow cooling, it is progressively more difficult to section as the temperature of the block is decreased, i.e., the larger the ice crystals, the more difficult it is to section. It is also clear that cryosectioning is influenced by both temperature and speed of sectioning. Leunissen *et al.* (1984) have shown that fractures appear on specimen blocks (and hence it is believed on the derived sections) cut at 90 mm/s and below 200 K, whereas at slow speeds (0.1 mm/s) fractures were only seen at below 150 K. The near-complementary ripples on the sections are considered to originate from plastic deformation of the section near the knife edge. Saubermann *et al.* (1977) were able to show that with thick sections at temperatures of about 193 K, the sectioning process was a discontinuous fracture process producing small rough chips of material and that smooth sections were only produced at 233 K. This does not appear to occur with thin sections, although a peculiar structure with a periodicity of 10–30 nm has been observed in hydrated thin sections cut at low temperatures. It is not clear whether this is another manifestation of the continuous fracturing process observed in thick sections, a phase transformation, or whether it represents plastic deformation. Frederik *et al.* (1984) considers sectioning as a flow process with the inherent characteristics of fracture, compression, and deformation. He considers that a "slip and stick" type of fracture occurs between the section and knife which causes the shear plane to oscillate. With increased friction, the shear plane moves toward the block face resulting in a thicker section, and as the friction decreases the sections become thinner. Frederik *et al.* (1984) confirms Chang *et al.* (1983) who considered that the heat input at the knife edge may result in phase changes in the ice. Frederik also revives the earlier notion that a very thin layer of water may be responsible for diminishing friction at the knife edge. This might explain why relatively smooth sections can be obtained at higher cutting temperatures. It is important to distinguish *fracturing* which is a brittle fracture of the crystallite components and *cutting* which is a flow process and probably involves plastic deformation of the crystallites. In fracturing, the crack propagates some distance from the knife edge or from where the force is exerted. In cutting, the separation occurs at the knife edge. Little attention has been paid to the amount of plastic flow of ice which increases as the temperature is raised.

The question remains whether the smooth, thick sections produced at 233 K are the result of transient melting or represent true sectioning of the material. All the evidence would point to the latter. The use of metal knives with a thermal conductivity 40 times that of glass would more quickly dissipate any heat generated at the cutting edge. The absence of smearing in gradients of frozen mixtures of salts, the slow cutting speeds, and the increased ductility (and hence plastic flow) of ice at warmer temperatures would all indicate that no significant melting had occurred.

Although the success of cutting is a reflection of the quality of cooling, a firm theoretical and practical base for understanding cryomicrotomy has yet to be established. It will be necessary to cut thick and thin sections at a variety of different temperatures from a standard sample cooled at different rates. Only then can we begin to understand what is happening during cryomicrotomy and in turn interpret the features seen and analyzed in the sections.

9.5.2. Fracturing

An alternative way of exposing the internal surfaces of a hydrated or frozen-dried sample is to fracture the sample at low temperature and examine and analyze either the frozen-dried or the frozen-hydrated surface. The fracturing procedure is a relatively straightforward process. Specimens are rapidly cooled and transferred under liquid nitrogen to the precooled stage of the fracturing device. Although a number of simple devices have been constructed, more success has been obtained with equipment which ensures that the fracturing is carried out below the recrystallization point of ice and under high vacuum. Such a device has been constructed by Pawley and Norton (1978) and consists of a chamber attached to the side of a microscope column which permits samples to be fractured, etched, and coated at low temperatures (100 K) and in a clean, high vacuum (50 μPa). The fracturing is by means of a fixed angle cold metal knife, the height of which is controlled by a microtome. The ability to control the level of the fracture plane means that it is possible to obtain relatively smooth fracture faces which may be used for x-ray microanalysis. The facility of being able to surface etch the specimens means that

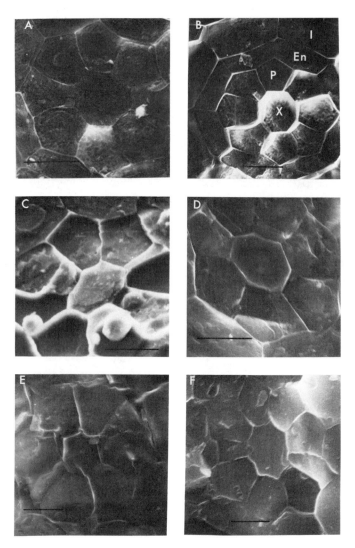

Figure 9.7. Frozen-hydrated bulk samples fractured to reveal internal contents. Sample is root tip of *Lemna* minor. All samples fully hydrated, samples (A) and (B) lightly etched. Carbon coated. 15 kV, 100 K. X, xylem; P, phloem; En, endodermis; I, inner cortex. Bar = 10 μm.

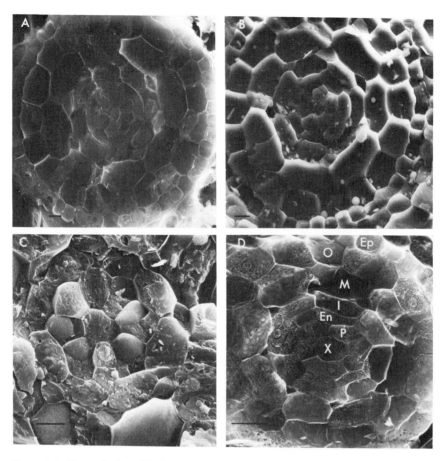

Figure 9.8. Frozen-hydrated bulk samples fractured to show internal contents. Sample is root tip of *Lemna* minor. Samples (A)–(C) fully hydrated with no etching. Sample (D) fully hydrated, surface etched. Carbon coated. 15 kV, 100 K. X, xylem; P, phloem; En, endodermis; I, inner cortex; M, middle cortex; O, outer cortex; Ep, epidermis. Bar = 10 μm.

a thin (0.1–1.0 μm) surface layer of water may be sublimed from the fracture face to enhance specimen morphology while the bulk of the specimen remains in a fully frozen-hydrated state. Figures 9.7 and 9.8 are typical fracture faces of plant material maintained at approximately 100 K.

Recent papers by Marshall (1982a) and Echlin *et al.* (1986) show how the fracture technique is used in conjunction with x-ray microanalysis of biological material. The studies by Beckett *et al.* (1982, 1984) on plant material, Carr *et al.* (1983) on animal material, Kalab (1981) and Schmidt and van Hooydonk (1980) on foodstuffs, and Pesheck *et al.* (1981) on porous oil-bearing rock samples, serve to illustrate how this technique can be used to expose the internal surface morphology of specimens (Figure 9.9).

Haggis *et al.* (1983) provide further refinement of their freeze-fracture thaw technique for examining the morphology of specimens at high resolution in the SEM. Cryoprotected cells and tissues are rapidly frozen and fractured at low temperature. The fractured pieces of tissues are then thawed in fixative, dehydrated in ethanol, critical point dried, and rotary coated. The method gives good details of both microtubules and intermediate filaments with considerable depth of structure. Alternatively, Maruyama and Okuda (1985) found that pieces of tissue may be quench frozen in the *absence* of a cryoprotective, fractured, and thawed in an aldehyde fixative containing DMSO. The presence of a cryoprotectant in

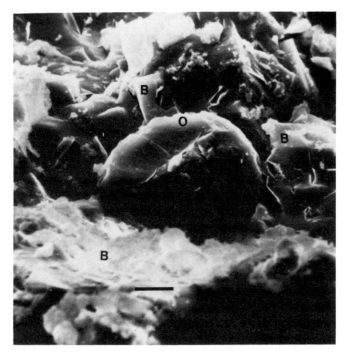

Figure 9.9. The fracture face of a ⅛-inch-diameter cylinder of berea sandstone which was filled with oil phase (consisting of 90% eldorado crude oil and 10% *n*-iodohexadecane to facilitate oil phase identification by x-ray microanalysis) and then flooded with an aqueous solution of 1% NaCl and 0.5% sodium dodecylbenzene sulfonate. The rock was then mounted, frozen in melting nitrogen, broken, surface flushed, coated, and examined. The magnification is ×1060, and the bar is 10 μm long. Features labeled "B" are brine (Na and Cl x-rays) and "O" is oil since it gave a very strong iodine signal. (From Pesheck *et al.*, 1981.)

the thawing solution contributed to good preservation of cell structure. When the tissue was pretreated with cryoprotectant before quench cooling, there was evidence of both shrinkage and structural damage. A similar phenomenon was seen by Blackmore *et al.* (1984) in cryofractured faces of *Aucuba japonica* leaves where the cytoskeletal components were only visible in unfixed and uncryoprotected leaves.

An alternative approach to fracturing hydrated samples is to chemically fix the material and infiltrate it with an organic solvent prior to cooling and fracturing (Dahlen *et al.*, 1983). Fracture faces of frozen ethanol and of frozen epoxy resin-infiltrated materials reveal a wealth of morphological detail, but the use of chemicals during specimen preparation precludes the use of this technique in connection with analytical studies.

9.5.3. Etching and Replication

Freeze-fracturing and freeze-etching are now a standard primary preparative technique for ultrastructural investigation at the molecular level. A variety of different instruments and methods has been described since the technique was introduced 25 years ago by Russell Steere, but the basic procedure remains the same. Rapidly frozen specimens are fractured at low temperatures in a high vacuum and a heavy metal/carbon replica made either of the fracture face or of the etched fracture face from which a surface layer of water has been removed by sublimation. Refinements to this basic method have included fracturing at much lower temperatures and at ultrahigh vacuum in order to reduce the level of recognizable contamination (Niedermeyer, 1982); and deep etching combined with rotary shadowing with refractory materials to improve the fidelity of the replicas (Heuser *et al.*, 1979). Fisher (1982) has used monolayer freeze-fracture with electron microscope autoradiography, thus combining a high-resolution ultrastructural technique with a method which gives cytochemical information. A diagrammatic outline of the procedure is shown in Figure 9.10.

It should be stressed that the conventional freeze-fracturing technique only provides replicas of fractured surfaces and while they give a great deal of highly significant structural information at the molecular and macromolecular level (i.e., membranes), such replicas are generally devoid of any chemical information about the specimen. Some recent studies have shown however, that the freeze-fracture procedure may be combined with cytochemical studies. By labeling tissues with the polyene antibiotic filipin, it is possible to detect filipin–β-hydroxysterols in soybean (Herman *et al.*, 1984) and filipin–cholesterol in red blood cells (Behnke *et al.*, 1984). Pinto de Silva and Kan (1984) have developed a

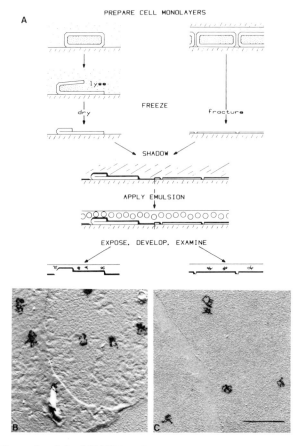

Figure 9.10. Synopsis of the MONOFARG method. (A) Sequence for preparing intact membranes (left) and fractured "half" membranes (right). (B, C) TEM autoradiographs of a radioisotopically labeled, freeze-dried RBC ghost (B), and its paired freeze-fractured RBC counterpart (C). Areas of the autoradiographs (B, C) selected to approximately correspond to the diagrammatic representation (A). (A) Cells are labeled with radioisotope, column-purified, and applied to a planar cationic surface, PL-glass, either after dilution (left) or as a thick slurry (right). Intact membranes of double thickness [E surface (ES) exposed] and single thickness [cytoplasmic surface (PS) exposed] are prepared by lysing and freeze-drying bound cells (left). Split membranes [E fracture face (EF) exposed] are prepared by mono-layer freeze-fracture (right). Intact and split samples are processed together for heavy metal shadowing and autoradiography. After exposure and photographic processing, emulsion-coated replicas are stripped from the glass and examined by TEM. (B, C) Electron micro-graphs of portions of a freeze-dried, Pt-C-shadowed (shadowed direction: bottom to top) human RBC ghost (B) and freeze-fractured RBC (C) coated with Ilford L4 autoradiographic emulsion, exposed at 278 K for 63 days and developed in D-19 for 2 min at 293 K. Silver grains overlie double-membrane extracellular surfaces (ES) and single-membrane cyto-plasmic surfaces (PS) or split-membrane E fracture faces (EF) on PL-glass (PL). ×20,000. Bar = 1 μm. (From Fisher, 1982.)

"label fracture" procedure which allows the observation of the distribution of a cytochemical label such as colloidal gold on a cell surface. Freeze-etching has its own set of artifacts which must be recognized in newly examined material (Rash and Hudson, 1979). Some of these artifacts are shown in Figure 9.11.

9.5.4. Chemical Substitution

The rapidly cooled sample may be dehydrated by a process of low-temperature chemical substitution using organic liquids. The dehydrated sample is then infiltrated at low temperature with a liquid resin which is polymerized to a solid from which thin sections may be cut. Although the main force of the investigations has been directed toward preserving the morphological integrity of the specimen, there is now sufficient evidence to suggest that freeze substitution might also be a useful preparative tech-

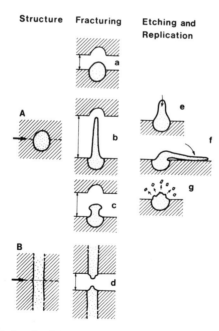

Figure 9.11. Schematic drawing illustrating the events during fracturing of a two-phase system (polymer in an ice matrix). The globular polymer (A) may either separate "cleanly" from the surrounding matrix (a) or may undergo complete (b) or partial (c) deformation. Fibrillar polymer structures (B) generally deform in a symmetric fashion (d). Exposed deformed structures can be affected during etching and/or replication. Structural changes such as elastic recontraction (healing) (e), collapse (f), or total disintegration (g) may occur. (From Sleytr and Robards, 1982.)

nique for microanalysis. The review by Harvey (1982) discusses the wide range of methods which have been applied to biological tissue. Figure 9.12 shows the detailed structures which may be seen using freeze substitution combined with chemical fixation.

The whole procedure of substitution, resin infiltration, polymerization, and sectioning must be carried out under strictly anhydrous conditions and in the initial phases, at low temperatures. Such requirements can create technical problems as atmospheric water vapor is very rapidly absorbed by desiccants at low temperatures. For this reason, the changes and transfers are either carried out in a glove box maintained at a slight positive pressure with dry nitrogen, or in sealed containers fitted with exit and entry ports. To be effective, freeze substitution must be carried out below the ice-recrystallization temperature, which for pure water is 148/K and for most biological tissues is between 163 and 193 K.

A number of different organic liquids have been used as substitution fluids. No strict times can be given and it is necessary to vary the proce-

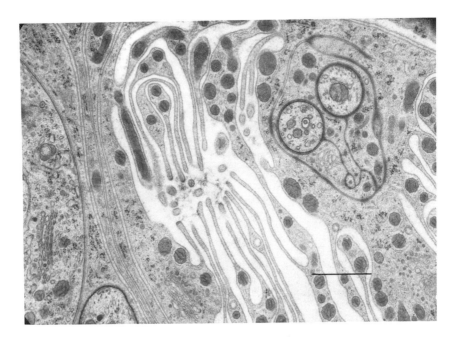

Figure 9.12. *Bombyx mori* antenna quickly frozen and freeze substituted according to routine procedure. The profiles of receptor dendrites are round in cross section, membranes and junctions follow a smooth course, microvilli and microfolds bordering the receptor-lymph space are straight and regular; such features are not observed after chemical fixation. The picture was taken close to the antennal surface; ice-crystal ghosts are not discernible. Bar = 1 μm. (From Steinbrecht, 1982.)

dure for different samples. Large samples substituted at low temperatures will take longer to complete the process. Thus, substitution of plant cytoplasm in an acetone–acrolein mixture at 193 K is completed within 10 days (McCully, 1985), whereas dimethylether at 160 K requires at least 4 weeks. To aid structural preservation, a fixative such as OsO_4 or uranyl acetate can be added to the substituting fluid, but the presence of a heavy metal can seriously compromise the analytical quantitation. Thus, Nagele et al. (1985) were able to show that a double fixation protocol of freeze substitution in glutaraldehyde/ethanol at 183 K followed by OsO_4/ acetone at 183 K gave good structural preservation but with little retention of tissue immunogenicity. Substitution in glutaraldehyde/ethanol alone allowed the tissue to be processed for immunocytochemical analysis.

A typical substitution procedure would be as follows. Small pieces of tissue in an open-mesh wire basket are rapidly cooled in liquid propane at 83 K. The frozen samples are transferred to anhydrous acetone at 193 K and the cold acetone changed every day for 3–4 days. The most convenient drying agent for the substitution fluid is pellets of Linde Molecular Sieve or anhydrous silica gel, but care must be taken not to get pieces of the desiccant in the specimen as it makes it difficult to section properly. A recent study of Ross et al. (1983) showed that molecular sieves release varying amounts of sodium, potassium, and calcium which would compromise any analytical studies. Silica gel was found to be an excellent solvent desiccant lacking these problems. Following substitution at 193 K, the samples are slowly allowed to warm to 233 K and then gradually infiltrated with increasing concentrations of liquid resin in acetone. The anhydrous conditions must be retained during this 3-day infiltration and the temperature of the specimen slowly allowed to rise to 293 K. The resin is polymerized at 333 K. Alternative methods rely on low-temperature polymerization of the resin using UV light. Humbel et al. (1983) have combined freeze substitution with low-temperature embedding to ensure the specimen never gets warmer than 243 K. Such an approach gives good structural preservation as well as retaining tissue immunogenicity. Sections are cut from the polymerized resin block either using a dry knife, or a trough liquid which will not dissolve the soluble contents of the specimen.

The promising results obtained by a number of workers should not be taken as an indication that freeze substitution is an ideal method of preservation. There is considerable variation in the solubility (and hence extraction) of electrolytes in the substitution fluids. Thus, Weibull et al. (1984) found that acetone extracted approximately 5% of the lipid from bacterial cells, methanol 15–45%, and resin negligible amounts. Elemental displacement and relocation can occur during the substitution process.

In spite of these shortcomings, freeze substitution is a useful technique for specimens with a dense matrix.

9.5.5. Low-Temperature Embedding

Although not strictly a low-temperature technique, in as much that the samples are not initially rapidly cooled, low-temperature embedding procedures are assuming greater importance in the preservation of ultrastructure while at the same time retaining enzymatic activity and immunogenicity. Conventional (ambient temperature–wet chemical) preparative techniques impose limitations on the information which may be seen using electron beam instruments. Such techniques disrupt molecular complexes and invariably result in structural deformation of proteins. This is due to organic solvent denaturation during dehydration, and heat denaturation during the polymerization of the embedding resins. High-resolution details are further obscured by the deposits of heavy metals used as fixatives and stains. There is now sufficient knowledge about the chemistry of cell components to show that in order to preserve the true ultrastructure of living tissue, it is necessary to optimize the dielectric constant, polarity, and pH of the solvent used during preparation. The macromolecular order will only be preserved if complete dehydration is avoided, mild inter- and intra-molecular cross-linking of proteins is achieved, and a polar environment is maintained during preparation. Inaddition, low temperatures favor these processes. Figures 9.13 and 9.14 show some of the results which may be obtained using the low-temperature embedding procedures. There have been a number of different approaches to this problem, and the papers by Sjostrand (1982), Arbruster *et al.* (1982), and Carlemalm *et al.* (1982a) should be consulted for detailed application of these procedures.

The basic procedure involves brief (in some cases only a few minutes) fixation in a dilute aldehyde which stabilizes the proteins without causing extensive cross-linking and denaturation. Dehydration is carried out using ethylene glycol, which is a weak denaturing solvent, or avoided entirely by infiltrating the sample with a water-soluble resin. The dehydration and/or infiltration is carried out at low temperature, i.e., 238 K, but care is taken not to allow the aqueous phases to crystallize by the simple expedient of raising the concentration of the organic solvent stepwise as the temperature is decreased. New resins have been developed (Carlemalm *et al.*, 1982a; Arbruster *et al.*, 1982) which can be polymerized using UV light at low temperatures, i.e., 238–245 K.

Although these methods are relatively new, the results are quite impressive. Embedded crystals of aspartate aminotransferase maintain

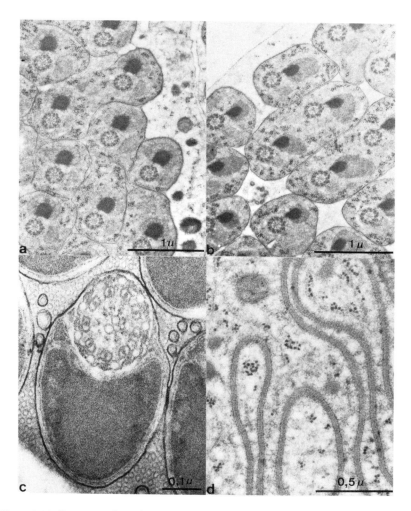

Figure 9.13. Representative micrographs of biological specimens embedded in HM20. The micrographs are from testes of *D. melanogaster* that were glutaraldehyde fixed, dehydrated at low temperature (223 K), and embedded in HM20. (a, b) Regions of spermatid bundles containing nonindividualized syncytial spermatids surrounded by an interstitial (or cyst) cell. The microtubules of the axoneme are quite distinct and the delicate cyst cell membranes are intact. The stage of development of these two bundles is clearly evident by the extent of differentiation in the mitochondrial derivative. (c) An individualized spermatid embedded in a matrix of minute tubules. The axoneme substructure appears quite well preserved. (d) Part of the septate junction girdle created by the two interstitial cells which surround a spermatid bundle. (a–c) Aqueous uranyl acetate stain; (d) uranyl acetate and lead citrate stain. (From Carlemalm *et al.,* 1982a.)

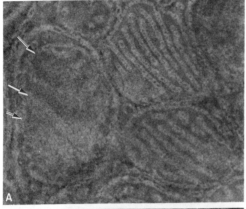

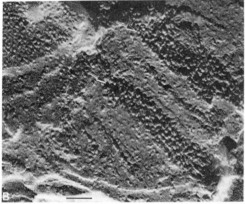

Figure 9.14. (A) Three mitochondria in a proximal tubule cell of a rat kidney. The tissue was embedded according to the paper by Sjostrand (1982). The cristae are oriented at different angles relative to the direction of the electron beam in the three mitochondria. The orientation is parallel to the beam in the mitochondrion located in the lower left quadrant of the picture, somewhat obliquely in the mitochondrion in the upper left quadrant, and almost perpendicular to the beam in the mitochondrion in the right half of the picture. In the latter mitochondrion, several cristae are viewed (arrows). With increasing obliqueness of their orientation, the cristae show more clearly a particulate structure. The appearance of the mitochondria is basically the same in frozen-dried low-temperature-embedded material. Bar = 100 nm. (B) The same type of mitochondrion as shown in (A) after freeze-fracturing. When the fracture plane passes through the cristae (arrows), the exposed face shows a coarse particulate structure. This appearance is consistent with that of the cristae in low-denaturation embedded material if we assume that the particles observed in the freeze-fractured specimen correspond to the less intensely stained areas in these specimens. This assumption is reasonable on the basis of the anomalous staining, which means that the mass density is high in spite of the low opacity of the staining. Bar = 100 nm. (From Sjostrand, 1982.)

molecular order down to the 0.6 nm level; catalase to 0.8 nm (Carlemalm *et al.* 1982a). The peptidoglycan layer of *E. coli* cell envelopes has been preserved for the first time (Arbruster *et al.*, 1982) and new information obtained about mitochondrial membranes (Sjostrand, 1982). Weibull *et al.* (1980) have used these low-temperature procedures to preserve chloroplast ultrastructure, and were able to retain some of the photosynthetic enzymatic activity, i.e., photosystem I remained intact. In addition to the impressive retention of ultrastructure, these low-temperature resins are also being used to prepare material for immunocytochemical studies (see

Chapter 8). Rey (1984) demonstates how this method may be used to localize plant pathogen antigens in Lowicryl-embedded tissue.

It would appear that as far as molecular integrity is concerned, the low-temperature embedding methods are a useful compromise between the problems of phase separation invariably associated with standard cry-ofixation, and the disruptive procedures associated with conventional wet chemical fixation. These low-temperature embedding methods have recently been shown to be applicable to some forms of elemental analysis. Wroblewski and Wroblewski (1984) have shown the retention of ions to be better in freeze-dried or freeze-substituted tissue which were embed-ded in Lowicryl-HM20 than in conventional epoxy resins, although the mass loss in the electron beam was greater in the Lowicryl samples.

9.5.6. Freeze-Drying

Freeze-drying is a process of ice sublimation under vacuum and may be used to remove or etch water from frozen specimens. It is by no means the ideal technique and it is necessary to balance the problems associated with the inevitable formation and growth of ice crystals with the advan-tage of being able to avoid the tissue coming into contact with any chem-icals during the preparative process. Optimal preservation has usually only been obtained from specimens in which there is a matrix remaining after the freeze-drying is complete. It would not be a good preparation method for regions normally filled with an aqueous phase alone. Another advantage of freeze-drying is that the amount of tissue shinkage is gen-erally less than by other drying methods, i.e. critical point drying [Nordestgaard an Rsotgaard (1985) provide an interesting exception]. It is difficult to give a precise figure because of the biological variability, but the typical range is 5–15%.

Freeze-drying for microscopy and analysis is a somewhat empirical process and it is impossible to set out a protocol which will work for all specimens. The procedures are probably best designated after considering some of the physicochemical aspects of freeze-drying. Much has been written about freeze-drying (it is an important process in the industrial preparation of drugs and foodstuffs) and the papers by MacKenzie (1977) and Franks (1980) provide a good theoretical basis of the method. A deep-frozen aqueous sample consists of a mixture of pure water (ice) and the matrix, the so-called frozen eutectic mixture. The ice phase consists of the "unbound water" which is an important component of most bio-logical systems. The matrix consists largely of heteropolymers and elec-trolytes together with a variable amount of "bound" water. Freeze-drying can readily remove the ice but it is much more difficult to remove all the bound water which inevitably forms an integral part of the biological polymers. Wildhaber *et al.* (1982) have followed the course of freeze-drying under high vacuum conditions where the sample water is exchanged with heavy water (D_2O) (which could be detected using a mass spectromeoter). The thin (10–20 nm) membrane samples were dried at 193 K. By measuring the D_2O, it was found that the unbound water around the membranes sublimed in about 2 h at a pressure of 100 μPa. The maximum sublimation rate of the bound water occurred at between 233 and 238 K, and prolonged drying at 238 K revealed no further loss of water.

Sublimation of water vapor from the pure ice crystals in the eutectic mixture occurs when the partial pressure of the water vapor of the frozen surface is greater than that of the atmosphere adjacent to it. The rate of sublimation for an ice crystal is a function of the temperature of the specimen which governs the escape of water molecules, and the partial vapor pressure of water in the immediate vicinity of the specimen which governs the return of water molecules. This relationship can be expressed as

$$Q_n = 0.25(P_T - P_A)T^{-1/2}$$

where Q_n is the amount of water lost in g/cm^2 per s, P_A is the ambient vapor pressure (Pa) of water, and P_T is the saturated vapor pressure (Pa) of water at the specimen temperature (T, K). Provided the vacuum pressure is sufficiently low or a sufficiently dry atmosphere surrounds the specimen, then the specimen temperature will determine the sublimation rate. Thus, at 273 K, the maximum evaporation of ice is 8.3×10^{-2} g/cm^2, whereas at 173 K the rate is 100,000 times slower (5.0×10^{-7} g/cm^2). It should be remembered that because of withdrawal of latent heat of evaporation, the sample will cool during freeze-drying with a concomitant decrease in the ice sublimation rate. However, there is usually sufficient radiative and conductive heat from the equipment and the environment to balance the cooling effects of water sublimation. There are a number of different freeze dryers available but the basic features are as follows.

1. The drying chamber should contain a cold stage which should cool low enough (173–193 K) to avoid excessive recrystallization and growth of ice crystals. Facilities should be available to backfill the chamber with dry nitrogen.

2. A vacuum system capable of maintaining a pressure of between 10 and 100 μPa in the drying chamber. At high vacuum the mean free path of the subliming water molecules increases and the heat conduction between the sample and the condensing surface is minimized. The vacuum is usually achieved with a diffusion pump and a rotary pump,

although when freeze-drying is carried out at warmer temperatures the diffusion pump may not be necessary. The vacuum line should contain a chemical or low-temperature water-vapor trap.

3. A system to maintain a steep water vapor gradient at the solid phase boundary. This is best achieved by placing a liquid nitrogen-cooled metal plate close to the sample. A chemical desiccant such as phosphorus pentoxide or one of the zeolites is nearly as effective. The cold trap should be at least 20° cooler than the specimen. In order to effectively retain the water vapor subliming from the sample, the distance between the sample and the cold trap should be less than the mean free path of the water vapor molecule, which at 10–100mPa is between 50 and 500 mm.

The drying rate depends on a number of factors including specimen temperature, size and shape, the relative amounts of bound and free water in the sample, and, to some extent, the vacuum pressure of the drying chamber. The greatest impediment to fast drying is the object itself and in particular the resistance of the drying shell. Specimens dry from the outside inwards and water molecules subliming inside the specimen must pass through the dried areas once occupied by ice crystals in order to be removed by the vacuum system. This dry organic shell increases in thickness as the freeze-drying proceeds through the specimen and offers progressively more resistance to the water molecules which may undergo many collisions before reaching the surface. The drying rates for crystalline ice are slower than those measured in the metastable vitreous and amorphous ice. Dubochet *et al.* (1981) consider that recrystallization precedes freeze-drying when vitrified or amorphous ice is the starting material. Smaller ice crystals dry more rapidly than large ones. The drying rates for crystalline ice embedded in an organic matrix are even slower. Umrath (1983) has calculated the times required for freeze-drying at different temperatures. Although the computed sublimation rate is based on pure water, it does provide a guide to the drying rate of biological material. Thus, at 223 K and a pressure of 4 Pa, a millimeter of pure water is sublimed in about 4 min; at 193 K and 50 MPa, the time is increased to about 4 h; and at 173 K and 1 MPa, the time is about 6 days. At 113 K and 10 MPa, the time is 2 million years. Umrath considers that the drying times for biological material of equivalent thickness are anywhere between 10 and 10,000 times longer than for pure water. There is also considerable variation in the drying rate of different tissues.

The temperature at which drying should take place is a question of much debate. It is a compromise between structural preservation and sublimation at low specimen temperatures and a reasonable drying time. At low temperatures, recrystallization and growth are minimized but the drying time is inordinately long. Small (10–100 μm) samples and thin cryosections (50–500 μm) have been successfully dried at 173 K. Drying at warmer temperatures increases the risk of ice crystal growth but allows a faster removal of water. The warmer temperatures also increase the risk of collapse of the solute matrix with a concomitant loss of the structural integrity of the sample. Draenert and Draenert (1982) give details of some of the ice crystal damage which can occur during freeze-drying.

Most freeze-drying is carried out at between 213 and 203 K, at which a 100-μm monolayer is dried in a few hours whereas a sample several millimeters thick may take several days.

Samples should be as small as practicable, and as much as possible of the surface water should be removed. Prefixation with mild fixatives may only be used in connection with morphological studies. Penetrating cryofixatives should not be used, but nonpenetrating ones can be used as they more readily give up their water during freeze-drying.

Samples are cooled by one of the several methods mentioned earlier and should then be transferred under liquid cryogen as rapidly as possible to the precooled platform of the freeze dryer. Transferring the sample under liquid cryogen minimizes the formation of amorphous ice on the surface, which at warmer temperatures will crystallize and possibly distort the specimen surface.

Although no hard and fast procedure can be set for drying times and temperatures, the following general procedure appears to work for many specimens. The initial drying is started at 190 K and a pressure of 1–2 mPa. The temperature is slowly allowed to rise to ambient over a period of 24–48 h. The condenser is kept at 77 K. Once the specimen has reached ambient temperature, the sample should be swung away from the condenser and the latter allowed to warm up. Depending on the nature of the sample, it is prudent to warm the specimen to 303 K while maintaining the high vacuum to remove the last traces of water. Once drying is complete, the apparatus should be backfilled with a dry inert gas and the sample quickly placed in a desiccator as a properly frozen-dried sample is extremely hygroscopic. Alternatively, instead of removing the dried specimen, it may be infiltrated *in situ* under vacuum, with resin or wax, and thin sections subsequently cut for examination and analysis.

Boyde (1980) has suggested an alternative freeze-drying procedure for specimens whose surfaces are to be examined in the SEM and where the ice crystal dimensions inside the specimen are of no consequence. On the basis of continuous measurements on the area of a sample during freeze-drying, Boyde found that most specimens only shrank 6% at 223 K, and that there was a further 1–2% shrinkage when the samples were warmed to 238 K. The total shrinkage appeared to be unaffected by the rapidity of drying, which means that the whole drying process could be made faster. Boyde recommends using a pressure in the range 100 mPa to 10 Pa, and keeping the previously frozen specimen at 223 K for 30 min to remove the surface layers of ice. This is followed by 20 min at 265 K after which the specimen is allowed to rise to ambient temperature. There is a further small shrinkage at this higher temperature as the "bound" water is removed. The total drying would be on the order of 1–2 h, which is shorter than the times for critical point drying.

Thick and thin frozen-hydrated sections may be frozen-dried by exposing the material to a slow stream of dry cold nitrogen gas at atmospheric pressure and at a temperature between 200 and 170 K. Drying is completed within a few hours. Freeze-drying can give rise to a number of artifacts and it is important that these are recognized. If the drying is carried out at too high a temperature, the internal ice will melt and quickly evaporate with sufficient force to distort the sample. A certain amount of shrinkage occurs during freeze-drying, but this is considerably less than has been observed using other dehydrating methods.

An alternative freeze-drying procedure involving cryosorption has been described by Edelman (1979). A cooled specimen support loaded with frozen specimens is sealed in a closed vessel containing a molecular sieve. The sealed container is plunged into liquid nitrogen and the subsequent freeze-drying carried out at 203 K for 3 days and 213 K for 6 days. No vacuum is needed and the system works because of the high trapping capacity of the molecular sieve which at 77 K can produce a vacuum equivalent to 6.5 nPa.

9.6. Microscopy and Analysis

Up to the present point, we have considered only the preparation of specimens using low-temperature techniques. It is now necessary to consider some of the problems associated with the transfer and examination of the specimens by different forms of microscopy.

9.6.1. Specimen Transfer

This is an important part of the procedure, and unless due care is taken, a well-prepared specimen can all too easily be ruined during the transfer to the microscope. The exact procedures which must be followed are dictated by the exigencies of the instrumentation, but the following general principles apply in all cases. Frozen-dried specimens must be kept dry once the water has been removed by sublimation. This can be conveniently acheived by enclosing sections between two thin carbon films. Bulk specimens are more of a problem and it is usually convenient to transfer the samples in containers with a small amount of desiccant. Frozen-hydrated specimens have the added problem of being kept dry and cold in order to prevent contamination, melting and recrystallization. If frozen-hydrated samples are to be kept before being examined and analyzed, they should be maintained below 143 K, which is the recrystallization point of pure ice. This is considerably lower than the recrystallization point of active cells, i.e., 190–200 K. These constraints require special transfer devices, examples of which can be seen in the papers by Saubermann *et al.* (1981a,b), Hax and Lichtenegger (1982), Sitte (1982), and Perlov *et al.* (1983). Speed is of the essence in the transfer of frozen-hydrated specimens.

9.6.2. Specimen Stages

. Frozen-dried specimens can be examined in most forms of electron beam and visible photon beam microscopes without modification of the specimen stage. Frozen-hydrated specimens can only be examined at low temperatures and this requires specially designed cold stages. These come in a variety of forms, depending on the complexity of movements required in the specimens and the space available in the area around the point of interaction of the focused beam with the sample. The simplest form of cold stage is where a precooled specimen is held by an insulated sample holder. Studies are made while the sample warms up to the recrystallization point. Such stages have a limited usefulness. Alternatively, stages can be kept cool continuously either by conduction through a flexible conducting braid or rod connected to a reservoir of coolant, or by having the coolant circulating around the immediate area where the specimen is located. The use of a flexible braid helps to damp out the random movement of the cryogen in the reservoir and gives the stage more controlled movements and will, if properly constructed, maintain the specimen below 143 K. Lower temperatures can be achieved by circulating the coolant around the specimen holder but this can cause vibration, particularly if liquid coolants are used. Liquid nitrogen is the most common stage coolant, but stages have also been constructed which use liquid helium and cold helium or nitrogen gas. The sample temperature may be varied by the use of a small electrical heater attached to the stage. This allows initially frozen-hydrated samples to be frozen-dried at a controlled temperature in the high vacuum of an electron beam instrument. It also allows a sample to be warmed to the different phase transitions of ice.

One of the most versatile cold stages is that manufactured by AMRAY Corporation (Pawley and Norton, 1978). This is based on a Joule–Thompson refrigerator which takes advantage of the fact that a fine jet of high-pressure gas (usually nitrogen) will cool when allowed to expand into a large volume maintained at ambient pressure. Such refrigerators can be an integral part of the microscope cold stage and the only connections which are needed are a flexible high-pressure (1500–3000 psi) dry gas inlet line and a flexible outlet line. This puts little constraint on the sample which may be moved around with a much greater degree of freedom and without the problems of vibration.

Heidi (1982a), Gibson and McDonald (1984), Perlov *et al.* (1983), and Taylor *et al.* (1984) review the recent advances in the design of cold stages for TEMs; Robards and Crosby (1979), Saubermann and Echlin (1975), and Taylor and Burgess (1977) give details of cold stages for SEMs; and Diller (1982), Wharlon and Rowland (1984), and Kourosh and Diller (1984) comprehensively review cold stages for use with light microscopes.

9.6.3. Specimen Visualization

This section will consider the problems of imaging, contrast, and interpretation which are peculiar to frozen specimens examined by different types of microscopes. Frozen specimens abound with artifacts and even when these are appreciated and recognized, the appearance of the specimen is frequently very different from that seen in samples prepared by more conventional means. It is only in the last two or three years that microscopists have begun to recognize the morphology of frozen specimens and as a consequence the catalog of accepted "reference" images is far from complete.

9.6.3.1. Light Microscopy

The images obtained by this form of instrumentation are usually evaluated qualitatively by observing and recording changes in morphology and texture together with differences in the phases of the liquid and solid components and the various manifestations of ice crystal formation and cell injury. Light microscopy allows us to study the dynamic phases of these processes, and can give a real-time assessment of variations in cooling rates, shrinkage, volume, and crystallization. Image contrast is usually not a problem and considerable advances have been made in linking video recording systems to cryomicroscopes followed by digital computer processing of the images. The gross effects of ice crystal damage are readily observed, but the recognition, interpretation, and categorization of many of the consequences of sample freezing are difficult and inaccurate. The real strength of the cryomicroscope lies in its ability to visualize dynamic processes with a minimum of instrument-induced artifact as shown in Figure 9.15. Excellent reviews of the subject are found in Diller (1982) and Scheiwe and Korber (1982).

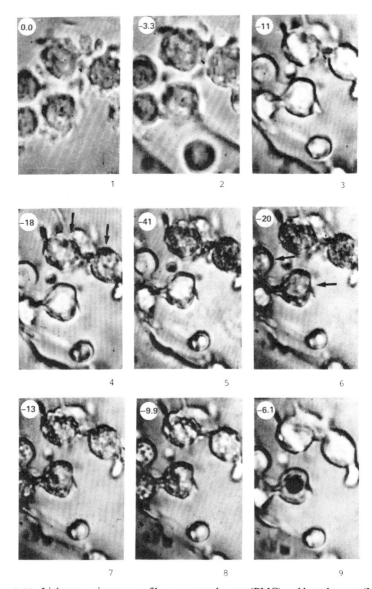

Figure 9.15. Light cryomicroscopy of human granulocytes (PMC) and lymphocytes (MNC). Cooling rate: 100°C/min; starting temperature = 303 K; lowest temperature: 213 K; warming rate: 100°C/min. Pictures were taken during cooling at (1) 273 K, (2) 269.7 K, (3) 262 K, (4) 255 K, (5) 232 K, during warming at (6) 253 K, (7) 260 K, (8) 263.1 K, (9) 266.9 K. ×1200; Leitz Orthoplan Microscope, brightfield illumination. At −18°C, two PMC crystallize internally; at 253 K upon rewarming, two additional PMC recrystallize/devitrify internally. At 260 K upon rewarming, an MNC recrystallizes/devitrifies internally. A gas bubble builds up in one PMC at 266.9 K. (From Scheiwe and Korber, 1982.)

9.6.3.2. Transmission Electron Microscopy

The main problem with visualizing frozen sections in the TEM is the inherent lack of specimen contrast. This problem can be fairly easily resolved by introducing high-atomic-number elements into the sample— so-called "staining." This may be achieved in the liquid or vapor phase and may result in positive or negative contrast. Alternatively, the image contrast of unstained sections can be increased by using darkfield microscopy as shown in Figure 9.16 and the so-called Z contrast available in STEM instruments as discussed by Carlemalm and Kellenberger (1982). In another paper (Carlemalm *et al.*, 1982b) where they explore the use of negative contrast resins, these workers suggest the possibility of incorporating low amounts of heavy metal into the ice matrix surrounding unstained biological samples. This is an interesting suggestion but would require careful selection of a salt which would remain within the ice matrix. R. Freeman (EMBL, Heidelberg) has suggested that Metrizamide, an iodinated substituted glucose, would make a suitable contrast embedding medium for frozen specimens. It should also be possible to use solutions of gold–thioglucose for the same purpose. Chiu *et al.* (1983) have found that it is more difficult to recognize protein crystals embedded in ice than in glucose, particularly when the ice is thick.

With a few exceptions, the image quality of frozen-dried sections is less clearly delineated than that of conventionally prepared material

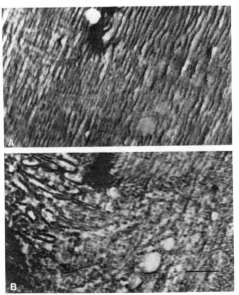

Figure 9.16. (A) Fully hydrated cryosection of rat kidney. Conspicuous section marks such as knife marks and a peculiar form of chatter can be observed. Recording temperature 93 K; STEM-DF mode. ×6800. (B) Fully dehydrated cryosection of rat kidney [same areas as (A)]. Subcellular structures can be recognized. Recording temperature 173 K; STEM-DF mode. ×6800. Bar = 2 μm. (From Frederik *et al.*, 1982.)

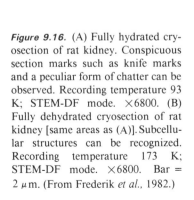

which relies on deposits of heavy metals to give contrast. Microscopists have become so conditioned to accepting chemically fixed samples as a true respresentation of the sample morphology that there is now an inherent resistance to accepting the poorer morphological details of frozen-dried sections. Paradoxically, these sections probably more closely represent the true state of the organic sample and it behooves microscopists to re-educate themselves to the new morphology.

Frozen-dried sections are not without other problems, for unless the drying is carried out slowly and at a low temperature, there will be sufficient ice crystal growth to severely distort molecular structures, as well as causing 25–30% shrinkage of the sections (Chang et al., 1983). Indeed, McDowall et al. (1984) consider that devitrification occurs at a temperature below the sublimation point for ice in a conventional electron microscope. This would mean that some ice crystal damage is an inevitable consequence of freeze-drying previously vitrified specimens. The problem of contrast is even more complicated in unfixed, frozen-hydrated sections where the presence of ice in the specimen gives rise to multiple electron scattering with a consequent degradation of image quality. The same effect is seen in images of frozen cell suspensions maintained in a microcrystalline ice matrix. Bachmann and Talmon (1984) consider that is is important to distinguish between *mass thickness contrast* which is the dominant contrast mechanism in vitrified specimens and *diffraction contrast* which is seen in the hexagonal ice matrix. The low contrast in "vitrified" frozen-hydrated specimens is of course due to the small mass differences between the aqueous and nonaqueous phases. However small this contrast difference may be, it is sufficient to obtain electron micrographs, particularly when recorded well under focus (Lepault and Pitt, 1984). Stewart and Lepault (1985) have used this technique to obtain micrographs of unstained tropomyosin magnesium crystals suspended in thin films of vitreous ice. There is only a marginal improvement to image contrast if the STEM mode is used. Jones and Leonard (1978) found an increase in contrast when images were mixed, and Zierold (1982a) found a similar contrast enhancement by dividing the brightfield image from the central detector by the darkfield image from an annular detector in a STEM instrument as shown in Figure 9.17. A more recent study by Zierold (1984) reverses this earlier finding and it now appears that frozen-hydrated sections have more contrast in CTEM than in STEM, although it is uncertain whether the ice matrix is amorphous or crystalline. There is considerable improvement in contrast when a frozen-hydrated specimen is frozen-dried and the low contrast of frozen-hydrated sections is now accepted as being a good indicator that the samples contain ice. The preparative methods for producing cryosections has now reached the point where, in the hands of some workers—

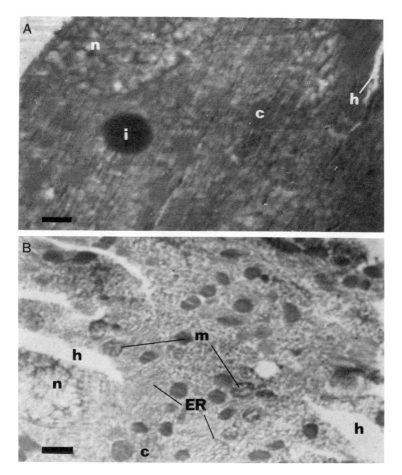

Figure 9.17. (A) A 100-nm-thick frozen-hydrated cryosection of rat liver tissue. STEM brightfield signal divided by darkfield signal. c, cytoplasm; n, nucleus; i, contaminated ice crystal; arrow indicates a crack in the section; h indicates a hole in the section. Bar = 1μm. (B) A 100-nm-thick freeze-dried cryosection of rat liver tissue. STEM brightfield image. c, Cytoplasm; ER, endoplasmic reticulum; m, mitochondria; n, nucleus; arrows indicate cracks in the section; h indicates a hole in the section. Bar = 1 μm. (From Zierold, 1982b.)

Dubochet *et al.* (1983a), Lepault *et al.* (1983a), and McDowall *et al.* (1984)—it can be more or less routinely used to obtain new biological information. Thus, Dubochet *et al.* (1983a), on the basis of comparing the images obtained from frozen-hydrated sections of bacteria with those obtained by more conventional means, consider that one of the long-accepted "organelles" of bacteria, the mesosome, is after all an artifact of wet chemical preparative methods.

The contrast problem is less exacting in thin sections and thin films of organic material within an ice matrix. The thin films are of particular interest as this is the method which appears to provide the most complete and accurate morphological description of the organic macromolecules which have been examined. Thin aqueous films are prepared within a strongly hydrophilic double carbon film sandwich. Any excess liquid is blotted away, resulting in regions of the aqueous film which are thin enough to be "vitrified" by quench cooling. A detailed description of the preparation technique is given in Milligan *et al.* (1984), which also contains high-resolution images of ribosomes, bladder membranes, and gap junctions. A similar process has been devised by Jaffe and Glaeser (1984); with the thinning process being achieved by evaporation rather than blotting. Glaeser *et al.* (1979) have shown good contrast in frozen-hydrated protein crystals suspended in an ice matrix. In this case, it was shown that the protein had a density 30–50% higher than the density of ice which was presumably enough to give a contrast difference. These workers showed that such specimens should not be contaminated as even a small amount of ice above and/or below the specimen will reduce contrast. Lepault *et al.* (1983b) have demonstrated a significant contrast difference between phage embedded in a 100-nm layer of amorphous ice and catalase crystals embedded in a 300-nm layer of hexagonal ice as shown in Figure 9.18. These workers make a clear distinction between bound water which they believe will vitrify and unbound water which they consider will crystallize and degrade the quality of the image of a frozen-hydrated specimen. It is difficult to remove the bulk water and still preserve the specimen in a hydrated state. It appears that good structural preservation can only be obtained for specimens completely embedded in ice which in turn results in low usable contrast. In a later paper (Lepault, 1984), it was found that the rate of freezing had an indirect effect on contrast. If the cooling rate is slow, large ice crystals form and suspended objects such as phage or protein crystals are expelled from these crystals. The expelled objects concentrate on the surface of the frozen layer where dehydration may take place, with a concomitant increase in contrast.

Talmon (1982a) has shown good contrast between lecithin vesicles suspended in an ice matrix and considers that because there is such a small mass difference between the two materials, the contrast is due to diffraction contrast. Eusemann *et al.* (1982) have made a detailed study of electron scattering in ice and organic materials and provide data for the interpretation of the scattering absorption contrast in brightfield CTEM and darkfield STEM images of amorphous organic material. Using these data, they have been able to determine the "angular mass thickness" of the principal organic components of biological material and

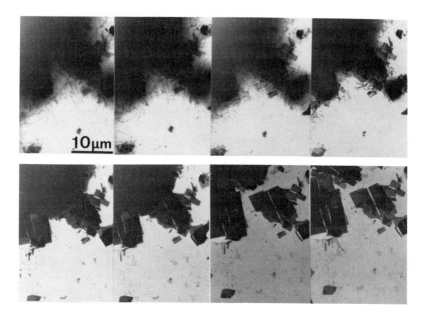

Figure 9.18. Images of catalase crystals recorded during freeze-drying by increasing the temperature of the specimen holder from 100 K to 200 K in about 20 min. Images 3–7 were taken within 5 min. ×1400. (From Lepault *et al.*, 1983b.)

have shown that significant differences exist between the mass per unit area of a thin layer of ice and a thin layer of carbon which can be used to provide contrast in unstained preparations. Lepault (1984) and Adrian *et al.* (1984) provide excellent examples of the high quality of information which may be obtained from thin vitrified layers of unfixed, unstained, and unsupported suspensions. The same general approach has been used to study specimens by electron diffraction. Downing (1984) has obtained electron diffraction patterns from thin frozen-hydrated platelet crystals of DNA which extend to 0.35 nm and with lattice images of 0.65 nm.

In all these examples of thin frozen sections or suspensions, image contrast is improved if the specimens are frozen-dried.

As far as contrast in frozen-hydrated sections is concerned, the following interpretations are beginning to emerge. In thin (i.e., <250 nm) samples where the unbound water has been converted to a microcrystalline–vitreous state, the contrast difference between the organic material and the aqueous phase is sufficient to obtain an image. The contrast and image quality is improved by using different imaging modes and by drying. In thick sections, or in thin sections contaminated with ice, the image contrast is poor, and can be only marginally improved by using different modes of microscope operation. The quality of these poor images is enhanced by drying. At the time of writing, the best image contrast and quality in unfixed, unstained, and uncryoprotected frozen-hydrated sections has been obtained from thin sections cut at slow speeds and maintained below 148 K in which the unbound water is microcrystalline or vitreous. Examples of such sections are seen in the studies by McDowell *et. al.* (1983) and Chang *et al.* (1983).

9.6.3.3. Scanning Electron Microscopy

Fracture faces of frozen-hydrated bulk material are readily examined in the SEM (Echlin, 1978). The image quality is improved if a surface layer of water is removed by sublimation, but this is now not considered to be absolutely necessary. Echlin *et al.* (1979) have shown that good secondary electron images may be obtained from frozen-hydrated fracture faces which have been coated with noble metals. Acceptable images can also be obtained from carbon-coated frozen-hydrated fracture faces (Echlin *et al.*, 1980b, 1981, 1982b). When examining new material, it is probably useful to slightly etch the frozen-hydrated fracture face in order to increase the quality of the image. However, with experience, it is possible to recognize the main features of cells in unetched samples. Contrast enhancement can be achieved by mixing the secondary and backscattered signals. Marshall (1981) has successfully used a backscattered signal to obtain good contrast from unetched samples of animal material. Figure 9.19 shows an SEM image of a frozen-hydrated insect Malpighian tubule.

As a general principle, it is advisable to use the lowest accelerating voltage and beam current conducive to the optimal resolution and information that are required of the specimen because there is an increase in signal current at low kilovolts. The production efficiency of secondary electrons is better and specimen penetration is reduced. Charging is reduced because the average number of secondary electrons emitted from the sample for each incident primary electron is greater than unity at low accelerating voltages.

Although most frozen fracture faces are coated with either a noble metal for morphological studies or carbon, chromium, or beryllium for analytical studies, there has been some success in examining uncoated samples. There is some discussion whether there is more or less charging of uncoated samples when they are surface dried. In a series of studies on insect tissue and gels containing known amounts of electrolytes, Marshall (1974) showed that there was diminished charging in frozen-hydrated bulk specimens that had been surface etched. Fully frozen-hydrated specimens charged even at low beam energy. Marshall considers that the charging is due to a decrease in charge carrier mobility at low tempera-

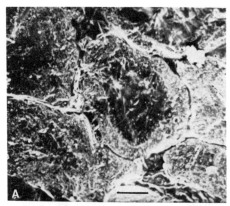

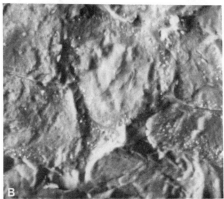

Figure 9.19. (A) Secondary electron image of fractured frozen-hydrated insect Malpighian tubule. Beryllium coated. 5 kV, 100 K. (B) Backscattered electron image of the same specimen using a solid-state detector mounted on the collimator of an energy-dispersive detector set at 40° takeoff angle. Beryllium coated. 15 kV, 100 K. Bar = 25 μm. (From Marshall, 1982b. © 1982 Pergamon Press, Ltd.)

tures. Ice is a good insulator and it is well known that ice crystals on fracture faces will rapidly charge. Work with plant material (Echlin, 1978) showed that fully hydrated frozen-fracture faces charged *less* than the surface-dried and frozen-dried samples provided low beam currents were used. The observed differences are really only one of degree and probably revolve around the number of available charge carriers in the frozen sample, the extent of electrical conductivity between sample and specimen holder, and differences in instrumental operating parameters.

It is much easier to obtain images of frozen samples using the SEM in one or more of its reflective modes of operation. In contrast to sections, fracture faces are much rougher and it is usually necessary to take stereopair photographs to interpret the surface properly. Many of the artifacts associated with sectioning are not seen on fractured faces of frozen samples. Provided the fracture is a real fracture and the knife is not allowed to scrape across the surface, knife marks are not apparent. It is thus of prime importance to have a large free-knife angle when fracturing. The fracturing can give rise to frozen fragments, some of which may land on the freshly exposed fracture face, but these are quickly recognized because of the characteristic charging patterns. Fracture faces exposed to a poor vacuum quickly become contaminated with ice crystals and it is important to use equipment like the AMRAY Biochamber which can give consistently high-quality frozen-fracture faces for both morphological and analytical studies. It is important to recognize the presence of artifacts in fracture faces which have been frozen-dried. Figure 9.20 shows such a fracture face in which the cell vacuole appears filled with beaded filaments. These structures are of no biological significance but are a result of differential sublimation rates of pure ice and the salts–water eutectic. On the basis of the small number of morphological studies which have been carried out on frozen-fracture faces, there is less shrinkage compared with frozen-dried and critical point-dried material. Beckett *et al.* (1984) compared the dimensions of fungal spores prepared by different methods. Although there was considerable variation, there was a progressive decrease in spore size in the order: "wet" untreated < frozen-

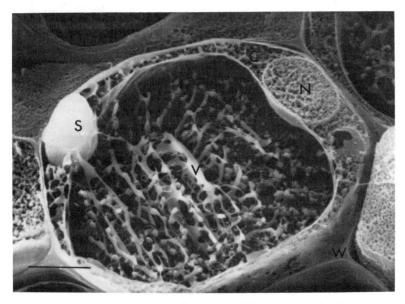

Figure 9.20. Frozen-dried fracture face of a cortical cell from the root tip of *Lemna minor*. The root has been quench frozen, fractured at 100 K in a clean vacuum, and frozen dried. The beaded-filamentous appearance of the vacuole is an artifact of drying, as such structures are not seen in a fully hydrated sample. C, cytoplasm; N, nucleus; S, starch grain; V, vacuole; W, cell wall. Coated with gold. 20 kV, 170 K. Bar = 5 μm. (From Marshall, 1982. © 1982 Pergamon Press, Ltd.)

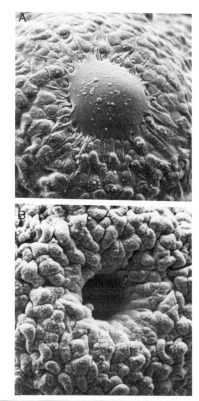

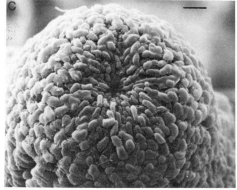

Figure 9.21. (A) *Sordaria humana.* Mucilaginous "perithecial sap" plugging the ostiole. Frozen-hydrated specimen. (B) *S. humana.* Open ostiole with thin coating of mucilage over the cells of the periphyses lining the opening. Frozen-hydrated specimen. (C) *S. humana.* Ostiole occluded by the shrunken and recurved tips of the periphyses. Note almost complete absence of mucilage and the exaggerated separation of cells. Critical point-dried specimen. Bar = 8 μm. (From Beckett *et al.,* 1982.)

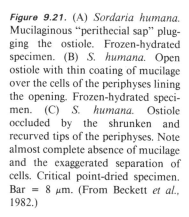

hydrated < frozen-dried < critical point dried. Similar findings on other material have been reported by Eveling and McCall (1983), Sargent (1983), and Beckett *et al.* (1982). Figure 9.21 shows the tip of a fungal perithecium prepared by the three methods of freeze-dyring, critical point drying, and frozen-hydrated sampling.

9.6.3.4. High-Voltage Electron Microscopy

Fotino and Giddings (1983) and Fotino (personal communication) have developed a cryostage for a high-voltage electron microscope. The increased voltage allows both whole cells and thick sections to be examined and although their work is at an early stage of development, they have obtained images of both frozen-dried and what appear to be partially hydrated cells and organelles. The operating problems, maintenance of low temperatures and transfer of fully hydrated specimens are no less exacting than with other forms of microscopy. It remains to be seen whether a combination of high acceleration voltage and decreased specimen temperature brings about any substantial decrease in specimen damage.

9.6.4. Artifacts of Microscopy

In addition to the problems associated with contrast in frozen-hydrated sections, there are a number of image perturbations which are recognized as artifacts associated with specimen preparation. Frederik (1982) and Frederik *et al.* (1984) review a number of the artifacts associated with thin sections. These artifacts, together with those associated with thick sections, will be discussed here.

9.6.4.1. Ice Crystal Damage

This is very difficult to observe in fully frozen-hydrated sections but appears as a series of voids in the frozen-dried section. These voids increase in size the farther the initial freezing point is away from the specimen surface and sectioning becomes increasingly more difficult with an increase in crystal size. Frederik and Busing (1980) have shown that the ice crystal damage is a result of the initial act of fast cooling and not a consequence of subsequent ice crystal growth in the frozen section. They also showed that ice crystal damage which could be observed in fully frozen-dried sections, disappeared when the sections were rehydrated. The rehydration also caused a number of deleterious structural changes as shown in Figure 9.22. McDowall *et al.* (1984) argue that only when the specimen is vitrified can one be sure there is no ice crystal damage.

Saubermann and Echlin (1975) showed that thick sections invariably contained a series of continuous deep fractures. In a later paper, Saubermann *et al.* (1981b) showed that these deep fractures were less evident at warmer cutting temperatures. An interesting series of artifacts have been observed in specimens which have been quickly cooled, freeze-dried, and

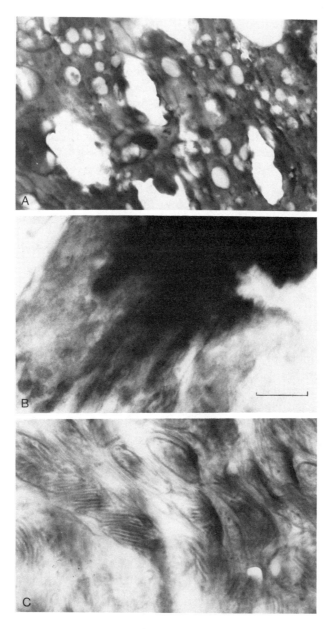

Figure 9.22. Transmission images from frozen thin sections obtained at 168 K. (A) Section heated for 1 s to about 293 K. Circular profiles may be seen overlaying the section, indicating melting artifacts. (B) Section heated for 60 s at 293 K. The ultrastructure is disrupted by melting. (C) Control section not heated. Bar = 1 μm. (From Frederik *et al.*, 1982.)

then replicated by rotary shadowing methods. Miller *et al.* (1983) found that virtually any buffer or salt solution formed structures remarkably like the microfilaments component of the cytoskeleton. It is suggested that when an aqueous solution is rapidly cooled, the resultant frozen solid is in a state in which pure ice crystals are separated by a network of eutectic regions. When such a solid is freeze-dried, the pure ice sublimates rapidly, leaving behind the less volatile eutectic which produces the filamentous artifacts. A similar appearance is seen in some scanning micrographs of frozen-dried fracture faces as shown earler in Figure 9.20.

9.6.4.2. Crevasses

More recently, Chang *et al.* (1983) have reported a series of lines in thin sections running parallel to the knife edge. It is thought that they represent fractures going deep into the section. They are found in nearly all sections. The crevasses only appear on the block side of the section and are absent from the block face.

9.6.4.3. Graininess

Sections can sometimes have a grainy appearance of 50- to 100-nm particles uniformly distributed across the sample. This effect has been seen in both cryofixed (Leunissen *et al.*, 1982) and unfixed (Chang *et al.*, 1983) samples and appears to be associated with higher cutting speeds, and higher cutting temperatures. The artifact is considered to represent transient melting during cutting followed by recrystallization. During the transient melting, salts dissolve and form small concentrates which appear as electron-dense deposits. Figure 9.23 shows images of these artifacts.

9.6.4.4. Chatter

This appears as a series of variations of section thickness along the cutting direction. These variations which can have a periodicity of 100 nm to 5 μm can be regular or irregular and are thought to be due either to mechanical vibration of the microtome or repeated stress and relaxation of the specimen. Frederik and Busing (1981) demonstrated a 0.5-μm chatter artifact in both the sections and on the frozen block face from which the sections were cut. They consider that the relative amounts of vitrification versus crystallization in the specimen influenced the amount of chatter. At high cutting temperatures, the chatter has a sawtooth appearance; at low cutting temperatures, it was in the form of a sine wave.

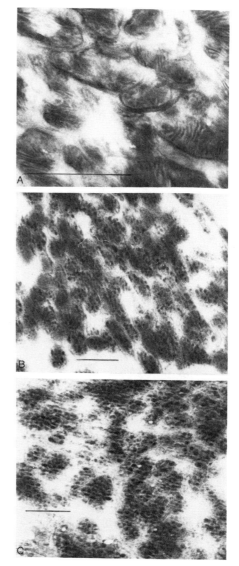

Figure 9.23. Rehydration of frozen thin sections. Sections (cutting temperature 193 K) were collected "dry" and pressed onto Formvar-coated copper grids (LKB-cryotools). (A) Control preparation. Section lyophilized and fixed in OsO_4 vapor. Membranes are clearly visible. Mitochondria have few (and small) granules. Bar = 1 μm. (B) Short rehydration. Section lyophilized and transferred to a petri dish with a wetted filter paper on the bottom. During exposure to a moist atmosphere, granules are formed in the mitochondria. Bar = 1 μm. (C) Prolonged rehydration. Section lyophilized and exposed to a moist atmosphere for prolonged period. Mitochondrial membranes are almost buried under granules. Bar = 1 μm. (From Frederik and Busing, 1980.)

9.6.4.5. Compression

As in resin sections, the solid matrix of the frozen sample can be deformed during sectioning. Chang *et al.* (1983) show that compression is more evident in thin sections but appears to be independent of sectioning speed and temperature. McDowall *et al.* (1983) show that 30–60%

compression can occur along the cutting direction even at temperatures as low as 123 K with minimal changes in the perpendicular direction.

9.6.4.6. Block and Section Noncomplementarity

A number of workers (Chang *et al.*, 1983; Leunissen *et al.*, 1984) have made carbon–metal replicas of both the frozen specimen block and the most recently cut frozen section. At high cutting speeds and temperatures below 200 K, the block face was made up of a series of fractures. Such features were absent in the corresponding frozen sections, although a gently rippled appearance was seen on both sides of most sections independent of temperature. There is no complementarity between block face and section and it is obvious that some changes are being brought about in the section due to the cutting process. These changes are probably related to plastic deformation and multiple slippage (Saubermann *et al.*, 1981b; Falls *et al.*, 1983).

9.6.4.7. Knife Marks

This is a characteristic feature of nearly all frozen sections particularly when a glass or metal knife is used in preference to a diamond knife. Knife marks which run at right angles to the direction of cutting are usually only found on one side of the section and also appear on the block face.

9.6.4.8. Ripples

A number of workers (Chang *et al.*, 1983; Leunissen *et al.*, 1984; Karp *et al.*, 1982; Frederik *et al.*, 1982; Zierold, 1984) have observed a series of fine bands running parallel to the knife edge in frozen sections. They have a much finer periodicity than chatter marks and range from 10 to 300 nm. Frederik *et al.* (1982, 1984) found that the fine distortions occurred at sectioning temperatures between 123 and 193 K, although they were less evident in thinner sections. Chang *et al.* (1983) consider this is a cutting-induced devitrification artifact. In a later paper, Frederik *et al.* (1984) were able to show that cryosections cut below 143 K were usually smooth except for a few knife marks. Occasionally, shear forces at the specimen–knife interface would give rise to ripples whose frequency could be related to cutting speed. Ripples tended to be absent in thinner sections. Frederik *et al.* consider plastic deformation to be an important component of cryosectioning.

9.6.4.9. Melting

The early literature on cryosectioning contained frequent references to section melting. It was thought that the sectioning process would either involve transient melting or that there would be sufficient energy released at the point of impact of knife and block to cause melting. With the possible exception of the very thin (a few molecules thick?) layer of water, which would be too thin to detect, but which would help explain the cutting process, there is no evidence to suggest that melting occurs during sectioning. To the contrary, Frederik and Busing (1981) and Frederik *et al.* (1982) have examined cross sections through frozen-dried and embedded sections and could find no melting artifacts. One surface of the cryosection is smooth whereas the other side is rough. These same workers have found that brief fixation with osmium vapor gave freeze-dried sections protection against structural alteration induced by rehydration. Provided there is minimal energy input into the sectioning process, i.e., low cutting speeds; good heat conduction at the knife–specimen interface, i.e., metal knives; and small ice crystals in the sample, section melting, either transient or complete, is not an artifact of cryosections. The presence of the very thin liquid water layer postulated earlier would not affect the microanalysis of thin sections as even the thinnest sections would be thick in comparison to the water layer. There is now sufficient morphological and analytical work on frozen-hydrated sections to show that such sections can be produced from many different samples using a variety of equipment. In addition to these artifacts, frozen sections can all too easily be contaminated with ice crystals during transfer and examination of the sample. It is important to appreciate the nature and extent of these artifacts and to realize that although an artifact observed in the frozen-hydrated state may disappear when the sample is dried, the damage caused by this artifact may still be present. Images of cryosections are difficult to interpret, particularly if they come from pieces of tissue and correlative microscopy may be the only answer.

9.7. Analysis

Most of the analytical studies which have been carried out on a frozen specimen have made use of x-ray microanalysis. The advantages and limitations of this technique are discussed elsewhere and the processes and problems of specimen preparation are identical to those associated with morphological studies. If anything, one has to be even more precise in the choice of the preparative protocol and avoid the use of any chemical fixatives. In addition to the problems of specimen visualization which have already been discussed, the analysis of frozen specimens presents its own catalog of problems.

At the outset, it should be made clear that the basis of the analytical procedure, i.e., the production of x-ray photons by high-energy electrons, is the same at 100 K as at 300 K. The analysis may be carried out on frozen sections or frozen-fractured bulk material. There are advantages and disadvantages to both approaches and both methods can be complementary; neither is mutually exclusive.

9.7.1. Thin Sections

The inherent difficulties of the thin section method center on the problems of tissue preparation and subsequent cell identification in the fully hydrated state, the ease by which the specimens can rapidly become dehydrated, and the relatively low mass of elements in the thin sections which are used. These disadvantages are, in many instances, outweighed by the improved spatial resolution (50–100 nm) compared to that which may be obtained from bulk specimens and the much simpler quantitative interpretation of the x-ray spectra. Hall and Gupta (1982), Saubermann *et al.* (1981b), Bulger *et al.* (1981), Nagy (1983), and Zierold (1982a,b,c, 1983) cover the recent advances in the analysis of thin sections.

9.7.2. Bulk Samples

The main advantages of using bulk frozen material are: (1) samples are much easier to prepare and maintain in a frozen hydrated state and (2) within the limits imposed by the reduced spatial resolution (2–5 μm), the morphological identification of tissue components is comparatively easy. Marshall (1981, 1982a) and Echlin *et al.* (1982b) give details of the progress that has been made with the analysis of bulk frozen samples.

The problems associated with image interpretation of a fully frozen-hydrated section continue to present a real challenge. Zierold (1984) considers the answer lies in using the combined dark- and brightfield image of a STEM system on thin sections. Saubermann *et al.* (1981b) propose a combination of x-ray mapping of selected elements and image storage with STEM images of the specimen in the hydrated and dry state. Gupta and Hall (1981) believe that selective partial drying of the sample produces sufficient contrast for tissue identification.

One of the many advantages of analyzing frozen-hydrated samples is that it does allow quantitative measurement to be made of the water content of the sample. This requires some modification to be made to the quantitative procedures which have been developed for microanalysis and an absolute assurance that the specimen remains fully hydrated throughout analysis. Hall and Gupta (1982) and Bulger *et al.* (1981) give details of modifications which can be applied to frozen sections. The quantitation of x-ray microanalysis of frozen bulk samples is less accurate, and Marshall (1981, 1982a), Roomans (1981), Lai and Hayes (1980), Echlin *et al.* (1982b) and Echlin and Taylor (1986) provide a review of the advances which have been made.

9.8. Specimen Damage

An unfortunate consequence of irradiating an organic sample with a beam of high-energy electrons is that the process of information transfer damages the specimen. This fact has been known for some time, but it has only been realized in the last few years that frozen specimens or specimens maintained at low temperature appear to suffer less damage than specimens maintained at ambient temperature. This apparent amelioration of the effect of beam damage should not, however, be taken as a signal that one can disregard these effects when working at low temperature. It is convenient to consider specimen damage under two headings, thermal damage and ionizing radiation damage.

9.8.1. Thermal Damage

Much of the energy transferred by the beam to the samples will eventually end up as heat. A temperature rise of 50–60 K could signal the onset of volatilization of organic material, phase transformation of crystallites, and a redistribution of solutes in the sample. Although the thermal conductivity of ice (5–7 W/m per K) is low compared with most metals (400–500 W/m per K), it is significantly higher than most organic materials (0.1 W/m per K). Talmon (1982a) calculated the thermal conductivity of frozen-hydrated tissue (70% water, 30% organic matter) to be 2.4 W/m per K. All the evidence would suggest that in the TEM, STEM, and SEM, the thermal conductivity of the frozen specimens would limit temperature rises to between 15 and 20 K. Thus, a *sample* maintained at 100 K would still remain below the recrystallization point of ice when irradiated by an electron beam provided it was in good thermal contact with the specimen support. In a seminal study of the subject, Talman (1982b) shows that even at a probe current of 10 nA, the temperature rise in a bulk sample is within the range 15–20 K. Talmon also shows that beam heating is an even smaller problem in thick sections and bulk samples because of the larger area available for heat dissipation. Heide (1984) confirms these findings which in practical terms means that polycrystalline continuous ice layers which have good contact with either the supporting film or the grid do not heat up significantly. The situation with amorphous ice is less clear, but even there it is not expected to show extensive thermal excursions at current densities of 1000 e^-/nm^2 per s.

These encouraging results are, however, no cause for complacency and it is important to optimize the following factors to avoid any danger of beam heating. The cold stage should be made of high-thermal-conductivity material, with the individual components in very close mechanical contact. It should be run at its lowest possible temperature; the specimen should be in good thermal contact with the specimen support; the sample should if possible be coated with a conducting film layer; low beam currents should be used whenever possible. Beam heating can be a problem with frozen-dried and organic samples because of their significantly lower thermal conductivity. In experiments where frozen-hydrated and frozen-dried samples are examined and analyzed, both sets of observations should be made at low temperatures.

Finally, it is very difficult to measure the actual temperature of the specimen, and the best one can do is to use a thin-film thermocouple which can also act as a specimen support (Clark *et al.*, 1976). In this way, one may achieve a reasonable value for the support temperature, and to be on the safe side one should assume the specimen temperature is about 10 K warmer.

9.8.2. Ionizing Radiation

The primary interactions of an electron beam with a specimen are excitation, ionization, and displacement of the constituent atoms. Because organic material is generally made up of light elements, the displacement of atoms is a relatively rare event, especially as most studies are carried out in the range, 15–100 keV. The excitation and ionization of atoms give rise to some of the signals we use in imaging and analysis, i.e., x-rays, cathodoluminescence, and also to secondary effects which can damage the specimen. Such secondary effects include heating, charging, phase transformation, bond rupture, cross-linking, and mass loss of both organic and inorganic constituents. Radiation damage to organic crystals at ambient temperature can be reduced by sandwiching the specimens between continuous carbon films and by the addition of an inorganic halide to the specimen (Fryer *et al.*, 1984). By working at low temperatures, in some cases as low as 4 K, many of these deleterious effects are lessened even further. The extent to which these effects are ameliorated is a subject of intense experimentation, discussion, and speculation. There is little disagreement that mass loss is greatly reduced, even at temperatures only as low as 100 K. Thus, a careful study by Egerton (1982) has shown that the mass loss from purely organic samples is reduced by two orders of magnitude when the temperature is reduced from 300 to 100 K. The situation with regard to the other effects remains confused. Knapek and Dubochet (1980) reported that L-valine could tolerate a one to two order of magnitude greater electron dose at 4.2 K than at room temperature as measured by the disappearance of the diffraction pattern. A similar figure was also found for other organic molecules (Knapek, 1982). More recent work by Lamvik *et al.* (1983) has been unable to confirm these findings and considers the improvement to be an order of magnitude less, i.e., only 4–6 times. Downing (1983) found a 10- to 15-fold increase in resistance to damage in hydrocarbon monolayers held at 6 K as compared to 300 K. Lepault (1984) found little difference in the amount of beam damage on ice-embedded catalase crystals between 160 and 4 K. It thus appears that the hoped-for increase in resistance at 4.2 K, due to the increased stability of chemical bonds at this temperature, has yet to be realized.

The presence of water in or near the specimen complicates the effects ionizing radiation may have on organic specimens. Taub and Eiben (1968) have shown that ice will undergo radiolysis by high-energy electrons to form free radicals and reactive molecules, which at temperatures warmer than 80 K will react with organic material. Even pure ice will undergo considerable mass loss at quite moderate electron doses. This problem is particularly acute in organic samples held at low temperatures, for unless extraordinary precautions are taken to remove all residual water molecules, the cold sample will quickly become covered in a layer of ice. If the ice deposition occurs in an irradiated region, Heide (1984) has shown that each arriving water molecule will remove one carbon atom. At 50 K, 240 electrons are needed to remove one molecule of water. As the temperature decreased, there was a corresponding decrease in the etching rate. Dubochet *et al.* (1982b) found that at 25 K, only 60 electrons were needed to remove a molecule of water. In specimens containing ice, the radiation damage is manifest as bubbling, holes, migration of solutes, and observable movement of the irradiated area. Figure 9.24 shows an example of bubbling in vitrified water. Glaeser and Taylor (1979) and Talmon (1982b) have shown that most of the visible damage to frozen-hydrated specimens occurs in the vicinity of organic material. Using polymer latex spheres embedded in ice, Talmon (1984) was able to show rapid etching occurs at the ice–organic material interface. No such damage was seen in an aqueous suspension of silica particles, which suggested that free radical reactions involving chemical species from the ice and the organic material were responsible for the damage. Vitreous

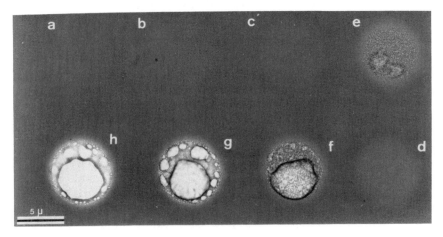

Figure 9.24. Bubbling in vitrified water. A specimen of 0.160 g/m² vitreous water obtained by condensation of low-pressure vapor on a cold carbon-coated Formvar film was irradiated at 100 K in areas a–h by electron doses of 5, 20, 40, 80, 120, 240, 340, and 450 ke⁻/nm², respectively, applied at the rate of 2 ke⁻/nm² per s with 80-kV electrons. Original magnification ×3400. (From Dubochet *et al.,* 1982b.)

ice was more susceptible than crystalline ice. The exposures are two to three orders of magnitude greater than those used in low-dose microscopy.

 Dubochet *et al.* (1982b) come to the same conclusion in the study of the effect of electron radiation on frozen water and aqueous solutions. However, they consider that it is the organic material which is the culprit because water is more easily damaged in the presence of organic material. These effects are reduced by using low electron doses and working at a low magnification. Figure 9.25 shows examples of the images which may be obtained using these techniques. Some success has been achieved by associating the sample with so-called "scavenger" molecules which react with the damaging free radicals produced by specimen irradiance. Henglein (1984) describes the various types of reactions of the primary radicals formed in liquid water. Although radical scavengers can exert a protective effect on the radiolysis of the organic substrate, this effect may be less pronounced at low temperatures as the rate constant of the reactions are expected to converge at the diffusion-limited value. The free radicals remain quite mobile above 90 K. Alternatively, so-called "protector molecules" could donate hydrogen atoms to damaged molecules (Zeitler, 1982). These are practical solutions for many morphological studies, but a problem still remains with x-ray microanalysis where higher beam currents are necessary. Talmon and Thomas (1978) have calculated that most of the water is lost in a 1-μm-thick frozen-hydrated section irradi-

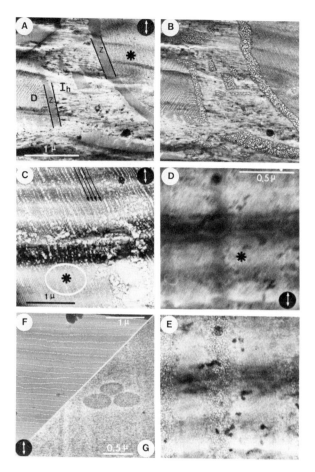

Figure 9.25. Electron beam damage on poorly frozen catalase crystal. I_h denotes a region of crystalline interstitial water. Z indicates the zone of dehydrated protein surrounding the crystal. D is a region with freezing-induced regularly spaced domains. The cutting direction is marked by the circled arrow. The thickness of the section at the site marked by the asterisk is 150 nm. ×24,500. (A) Image recorded with an accumulated dose of ~2000 e^-/nm². (B) Same region as in (a) after an accumulated dose of ~20 e^-/nm². (C) Freezing-induced damage in catalase crystals exposed to an irradiation of 8000 e^-/nm². The striation in the circled region has a period of 40 nm. Bubbling taking place in dense domains is indicated by arrows. Sectioning temperature 130 K; thickness 120 nm; ×22,400. (D) Freezing-induced band pattern in catalase crystals. The same area is shown recorded after a total electron dose of 1200 e^-/nm² and 8000 e^-/nm². (E) A severe drift blurs the low-dose image. Note that bubbling and mass loss take place only on the originally dense bands. The structure of the catalase crystal is visible only on the originally more transparent bands. Freezing in boiling nitrogen. Sectioning temperature 130 K; thickness 140 nm; ×54,000. (F) Band pattern from beam-induced damage. Bubbling in 35% gelatin solution. Sectioning temperature 100 K; sectioning speed 0.2 mm/s; thickness 100 nm; electron dose ~ 10 e^-/nm²; ×18,000. (G) Striation in 20% gelatin solution containing polystyrene latex particles. The section was rewarmed for 10 min at 150 K in the electron microscope. Sectioning temperature 110 K; sectioning speed 0.2 mm/s; thickness 220 nm; electron dose ~ 10 e^-/nm²; ×2700. (From Chang *et al.*, 1983.)

ated over a 10-nm^2 area for 100 s using a beam current of 100 pA at 100 keV. Heide (1984) found that the total mass loss is directly proportional to electron exposure. Thus, at temperatures between 9 and 90 K and at 100 keV, the removal rate corresponds to 8 nm/s at 1 A/cm^2. These are values for a single surface of microcrystalline ice; values for amorphous ice are lower. Above 90 K, the mass loss increases exponentially with temperature. Although the damage is primarily confined to the specimen surface, these findings have serious consequences for the analysis of frozen-hydrated sections. However, if the organic sample is totally embedded in ice from the onset of irradiation, little or no damage occurs. This finding puts severe restraints on the accuracy of microanalysis performed on small areas of the sample. Talmon (1984) considers that the radiation-induced etching is not limited to frozen-hydrated specimens only. The thin layers of ice which must inevitably form on any specimen cooled in an electron beam instrument to *reduce* radiation damage, may actually *enhance* the damage at the ice–organic interface.

Chandler (1983) confirms these general findings, although the lowest beam current studied was 1 nA and all the studies were carried out at room temperature. Chlorine was the most unstable element followed by potassium and sodium. Bulk samples and thick sections were more vulnerable than thin sections, frozen-dried material more at risk than resin-embedded samples. This latter finding is contrary to the results of Zierold (1984) who found that mass loss from frozen-dried sections is negligible even at high electron exposures. Coating samples with carbon also reduces mass loss.

All the evidence would suggest that as far as frozen-hydrated bulk samples and thick sections are concerned, one should experience minimal losses from samples maintained at 100–120 K with beam currents of 1–3 nA and analysis times of 100 s.

Dubochet and colleagues (Dubochet *et al.*, 1982a,b; Lepault *et al.*, 1984) have carried out extensive investigations on the effects of radiation damage on frozen sections and frozen aqueous suspensions, and they consider that low temperatures (~100 K) do not prevent damage, but rather only delay its expression. The bubbling phenomenon which a number of workers have observed in irradiated frozen mixtures of aqueous and organic materials, is believed to be due to an accumulation of trapped volatile fragments. In pure ice, much higher electron doses are required to produce the same effect. Dubochet *et al.* (1982a,b) consider that water is more beam resistant than many organic samples. It would appear that the physical state of the water may have an effect on the resistance to radiation damage. Talmon (1982a) refers to work on glass ceramics and organic liquids which show that the vitreous state is more sensitive to radiation than the crystalline state. It remains to be seen whether vitreous water is more (or less) radiation sensitive than crystal-line water. Lepault *et al.* (1984) could find little difference in beam sensitivity of samples embedded in sucrose (presumably vitrified) and samples suspended in water. Dubochet *et al.* (1982a,b) demonstrated that one of the deleterious effects of radiation damage is the devitrification of vitrified water and that the electron dose needed for the transformation increases as the temperature is lowered. The question as to whether cooling to 4 K further reduces radiation damage remains open. In the few examples of pure organic crystals which have been examined, there appears to be a reduction in damage. The cryoprotection factor afforded by low temperature is varied. The reduction can be more than an order of magnitude in some cases (Dubochet *et al.,* 1981); in other cases the extreme-low-temperature protective effect is little better than can be achieved at 100 K (Glaeser, 1971; Siegel, 1972). Jeng and Chiu (1984) have found that the cryoprotection factor for a protein crystal embedded in ice is 5 at 125 K and below.

If it can be shown that there is a significant improvement to the radiation resistance of frozen-hydrated biological material at liquid helium temperatures, then there is every chance one may be able to achieve resolutions of 1–2 nm in thin, unstained aperiodic organic structures (Fernandez-Moran, 1982).

This is a challenging goal for cryomicroscopy and its fulfillment is probably going to require the use of low electron dose techniques on fully vitrified specimens maintained at a few degrees above absolute zero.

9.9. Conclusion

The conclusion must by now be self-evident. For the past 50 years, specimen preparation, dehydration, and beam damage have all conspired to prevent microscopists from obtaining sub-nanometer resolution of aperiodic organic objects. The simple expediency of cooling the sample, and keeping it at low temperatures in spite of all the attendant problems, offers the only hope we have of studying and analyzing the ultrastructure of organic materials.

References

Abrahams, J., and Etz, E. S. (1979). *Science* **206,** 718.

Adrian, M., Dubochet, J., Lepault, J., and McDowall, A. (1984). *Nature* **308,** 32.

Allen, T. D. (1983). *Sem 1983* **IV,** 1963.

Anderson, C. A., and Hinthorne, J. R. (1973). *Anal. Chem.* **45,** 1421.

Anderson, R., and Ramsey, J. N. (1979). In *Introduction to Analytical Electron Microscopy,* ed. J. J. Hren, J. I. Goldstein, and D. C. Joy, Plenum Press, New York, p. 575.

Angell, C. A. (1982). In *Water: A Comprehensive Treatise,* Vol. 7, ed. F. Franks, Plenum Press, New York.

Aoki, M., and Tavassoli, M. (1981). *J. Histochem. Cytochem.* **29,** 682.

Arbruster, B. L., Carlemalm, E., Chiovet R., Garavito, R. M., Hobot, J. A., Kellenberger, E., and Villiger, W. (1982). *J. Microsc.* **126,** 77.

Bachhuber, K., and Frösch, D. (1983). *J. Microsc,* **130,** 1.

Bachmann, L., and Schmitt, (1971). *Proc. Natl. Acad. Sci. USA* **68,** 2149.

Bachmann, L., and Talmon, Y. (1984). *Ultramicroscopy* **14,** 211.

Baggett, M. C., and Glassman, L. H. (1974). *SEM 74* 199.

Bald, W. B. (1983). *J. Microsc.* **131,** 11.

Bald, W. B. (1984). *J. Microsc.* **134,** 261.

Balk, L. J., and Kultscher, N. (1983). In *Microscopy of Semiconducting Materials 1983,* ed. A. G. Cullis, S. M. Davidson, and G. R. Booker, Institute of Physics, London, p. 387.

Balk, L. J., Feuerbaum, H. P., Kubalek, E., and Menzel, E. (1976). *Sem 1976* **I,** 615.

Banbury, J. R., and Nixon, W. C. (1967). *J. Sci. Instrum.* **44,** 889.

Barnard, T. (1982). *J. Microsc.* **126,** 317.

Barnard, T., and Hall, T. A. (1984). *Cryobiology* **21,** 559.

Bauer, V. M., And Butler, W. O. (1983). *Scanning* **5,** 145.

Beall, P. (1983). *Cryobiology* **20,** 324.

Becker, R. P., and DeBruyn, P. P. H. (1976). *SEM 1976* **II,** 172.

Becker, R. P., and Geoffrey, J. S. (1981). *SEM 1981* **IV,** 195.

Becker, R. P., and Sogard, M. (1979). *SEM 1979* **II,** 835.

Beckett, A., Porter, R., and Read, N. D. (1982). *J. Microsc.* **125,** 193.

Beckett, A., Read, N. D., and Porter, R. (1984). *J. Microsc.* **136,** 87.

Behnke, O., Jensen, J. T., and Deurs, B. V. (1984). *Eur. J. Cell Biol.* **35,** 200.

Bendayan, M., and Zollinger, M. (1983). *J. Histochem. Cytochem.* **31,** 101.

Benninghoven, A. (1973). *Surf. Sci.* **35,** 512.

435

Benninghoven, A. (1979). In *Secondary Ion Mass Spectrometry SIMS II*, ed. A. Benninghoven, C. A. Evans, Jr., R. A. Powell, R. Shimizu, and H. A. Storms, Springer-Verlag, Berlin, p. 116.

Berger, M. J., and Seltzer, S. M. (1964). National Research Council Publication 1133, Washington, D.C., p. 205.

Bethe, H. (1930). *Ann. Phys. (Leipzig)* **5**, 325.

Bethe, H. (1933). In *Handbook of Physics*, Vol. 24, Springer-Verlag, Berlin, p. 273.

Bethe, H., and Fermi, E. (1932). *Zeits. Phys.* **27**, 296.

Biddlecombe, W. H., McEvan-Jenkinson, D., McWilliams, S. A., Nicholson, W. A. P., Elder, H. Y., and Demster, S. W. (1982). *J. Microsc.* **126**, 63.

Blackmore, S., Barnes, S. H., and Claugher, D. (1984). *J. Ultrastruct. Res.* **86**, 215.

Blaschke, R. (1980). *Proc. R. Microsc. Soc.* **15**, 280.

Booker, G. R. (1969). In *Modern Diffraction and Imaging Techniques in Materials Science*, ed. S. Amelinckx, R. Gevers, G. Remant, and J. van Landuyt, North-Holland, Amsterdam, p. 597.

Boone, T. (1984). *Ultramicroscopy* **14**, 359.

Boyde, A. (1980). *Electron Microscopy 1980* **2**, 768.

Boyde, A., and Maconnachie, E. (1979). *Scanning* **2**, 149.

Boyde, A., and Tamarin, A. (1984). *Scanning* **6**, 30.

Boyde, A., Bailey, E., Jones, S. J., and Tamarin, A. (1977). *SEM 1977* **I**, 507.

Bresse, J. F., and Lafeuille, D. (1971). *Inst. Phys. Conf. Ser.* **10**, 220.

Broers, A. N., and Spiller, E. (1980). *SEM 1980* **I**, 201.

Brown, J. D., von Rosenstiel, A. P., and Krisch, T. (1980). In *Microbeam Analysis 1980*, San Francisco Press, San Francisco, p. 241.

Brügeller, P., and Mayer, E. (1980). *Nature* **288**, 569.

Bryce, M. R., and Murphy, L. C. (1984). *Nature* **309**, 119.

Bulger, R. E., Beeuwkes, R., and Saubermann, A. J. (1981). *J. Cell Biol.* **88**, 274.

Bullock, G. R. (1984). *J. Microsc.* **133**, 1.

Bullock, G. R., and Petrusz, P., eds (1981, 1983). *Techniques in Immunochemistry* Vol. I (1981), Vol. II (1983), Academic Press, New York.

Campbell, G. J., and Roach, M. R. (1981). *Scanning* **4**, 188.

Cargill, G. S. (1980). *Nature* **286**, 691.

Carlemalm, E., and Kellenberger, E. (1982). *EMBO J.* **1**, 63.

Carlemalm, E., Garavito, R. M., and Villiger, W. (1982a). *J. Microsc,* **126**, 123.

Carlemalm, E., Acetarin, J. D., Villiger, W., Colliez, C., and Kellenberger, E. (1982b). *J Ultrastruct. Res.* **80**, 339.

Carr, K. E., Hayes, T. L., McKoon, M., and Sprague, M. (1983). *J. Microsc,* **132**, 209.

Castleman, K. R. (1979). *Digital Image Processing*, Prentice–Hall, Englewood Cliffs, N.J.

Celotta, R. J., and Pierce, D. T. (1982). In *Microbeam Analysis 1982*, San Francisco Press, San Francisco, p. 469.

Chandler, J. A. (1983). *SEM 1983* **IV**, 2001.

Chang, C. C. Y., and Alexander, J. V. (1981). *Biol. Cell.* **40**, 99.

Chang, J. J., McDowall, A. W., Lepault, J., Freeman, R., Walter, C. A., and Dubochet, J. (1983). *J. Microsc.* **132**, 109.

Cheng, G., Hodges, G. M., and Trejdosiewicz, L. K. (1985). *J. Microsc.* **137**, 9.

Chew, E. C., Riches, D. J., Tam, P. P. L., Tsao, G. S. W., Lam, T. K., and Hou-Chan, H. J. (1983). In *Proc. 41st EMSA Meet.* p. 630.

Chi, J. Y., and Gatos, H. C. (1978). *J. Appl. Phys.* **50**, 3433.

Chiu, W., Cohen, H. A., Grant, R. A., and Jeng, T. W. (1983). In *Proc. 41st EMSA Meet.* p. 428.

Christian, J. W. (1956). *J. Inst. Met.* **84**, 349.

Clark, J., Echlin, P., Moreton, R. B., Saubermann, A. J., and Taylor, P. J. (1976). *SEM 1976* 83.

Clay, C. S., and Peace, G. W. (1981). *J. Microsc.* **123**, 25.

Coates, D. G. (1967). *Philos. Mag.* **16**, 1179.

Coetzee, J., and van der Merwe, C. F. (1984). *J. Microsc.* **135**, 147.

Coetzee, J., and van der Merwe, C. F. (1985). *J. Microsc,* **137**, 129.

Colquhoun, W. R. (1984). *J. Ultrastruct. Res.* **87**, 97.

Coons, A. H., Creech, H. J., and Jones, R. N. (1941). *Proc. Exp. Biol. N.Y.* **47**, 200.

Craik, D. J., and Tebble, R. S. (1965). *Ferromagnetism and Ferromagnetic Domains,* North-Holland, Amsterdam.

Crawford, C. K., (1980). *SEM 1980* **IV**, 11.

Dhalen, H., Scheie, P., Myklebust, R. L., and Saetersdal, T. (1983). *J. Microsc.* **131**, 35.

Danscher, G. (1984). *Histochemistry* **81**, 331.

Davidson, D. L. (1976). *J. Phys. E* **9**, 341.

Davidson, D. L. (1977). In *Proc. 10th SEM Symp.* p. 431.

Davidson, S. M. (1977). *J. Microsc.* **110**, 177.

Davidson, S. M. (1983). In *Microscopy of Semiconducting Materials 1983,* ed. A. G. Cullis, S. M. Davidson, and G. R. Booker, Institute of Physics, London, p. 415.

Davidson, S. M., and Vaidya, A. W. (1977). *Inst. Phys. Conf. Ser.* **33a**, 287.

Davies, G. (1983). *SEM 1983* **III**, 1163.

DeHarven, E. (1983). In *Proc. 41st EMSA Meet.* p. 484.

Dhamelincourt, P. (1982). In *Microbeam Analysis 1982,* San Francisco Press, San Francisco, p. 261.

Diller, K. R. (1982). *J. Microsc.* **126**, 9.

Donolato, C. (1978). *Optik (Stuttgart)* **52**, 19.

Dorsey, J. R. (1969). *Adv. Electron. Electron Phys. Suppl.* **6**, 291.

Downing, K. H. (1983). *Ultramicroscopy 11,* 229.

Downing, K. H. (1984). *Ultramicroscopy* **13**, 35.

Draenert, Y., and Draenert, K. (1982). *SEM 1982* **IV**, 1799.

Dubochet, J., and McDowall, A. W. (1981). *J. Microsc.* **124**, RP3.

Dubochet, J., Knapek, E., and Dietrich, I. (1981). *Ultramicroscopy* **6**, 77.

Dubochet, J., Lepault, J., Freeman, R., Berriman, J. A., and Homo, J. C. (1982a). *J. Microsc.* **128**, 219.

Dubochet, J., (1982b). *Ultramicroscopy* **10**, 55.

Dubochet, J., Adrian, M., and Vogel, R. H. (1983a). *Cryoletters* **4**, 223.

Dubochet, J., McDowall, A. W., Menge, B., Schmid, E. N., and Lickfield, K. G. (1983b). *J. Bacteriol.* **155**, 381.

Duncumb, P. (1957). In *X-Ray Microscopy and Microradiography,* ed. V. E. Cosslett, A. Engström, and H. H. Pattee, Academic Press, New York, P. 435.

Duncumb, P., and Reed, S. J. B. (1968). In *Quantitative Electron Probe Microanalysis,* ed. K. F. J. Heinrich, National Bureau of Standards Special Publication 298, Washington D.C., p. 133.

Echlin, P. (1978). *J. Microsc,* **112**, 47.

Echlin, P. (1981). *SEM 1981* **I**, 79.

Echlin, P. (1982). In *Proc. 40th EMSA Meet.* p. 380.

Echlin, P., and Kaye, G. (1979). *SEM 1979* **II**, 21.

Echlin, P., and Taylor, S. E. (1986). *J. Microsc.,* in press.

Echlin, P., Skaer, H., Gardiner, B. O. C., Franks, F., and Asquith, M. H. (1977). *J. Microsc.* **110**, 239.

Echlin, P., Pawley, J. B., and Hayes, T. L. (1979). *SEM 1979* **III**, 69.

Echlin, P. Broers, A. N., and Gee, W. (1980a). *SEM 1980* **I**, 163.

Echlin, P., Lai, C. E., Hayes, T. L., and Hook, G. (1980b). *SEM 1980* **II**, 383.

Echlin, P., Lai, C. E., and Hayes, T. L. (1981). *SEM 1981* **II**, 489.

Echlin, P., Chapman, B., Stoter, L., Gee, W., and Burgess, A. (1982a). *SEM 1982* **I**, 29.

Echlin, P., Lai, C. E., and Hayes, T. L. (1982b). *J. Microsc.* **126**, 285.

Echlin, P., Chapman, B., and Gee, W. (1985). *J. Microsc.* **137**, 155.

Edelman, L. (1979). *Mikroskopie* **35**, 31.

Eden, M. E. (1985). Personal communication.

Egerton, R. F. (1982). *J. Microsc.* **126**, 95.

Elder, H. Y., Gray, C. C., Jardine, A. G., Chapman, J. N., and Biddlecombe, W. H. (1982). *J. Microsc.* **126**, 45.

Escaig, J. (1982). *J. Microsc.* **126**, 221.

Eskelinen, S., and Saukko, P. (1983). *J. Microsc.* **130**, 63.

Espevik, T., and Elasgeler, A. (1984). *J. Microsc.* **134**, 203.

Estable-Puig, R. F. and J. F., Slobodrian, M. L. L., Pusteria, A., Estable, A. B., and Leblance-Laberge, L. (1975). In *Proc. 2nd Annu. Meet. EMS Canada* p. 40.

Etz, E. S. (1979). *SEM 1979* **I**, 67.

Etz, E. S., Newbury, D. E., Dunn, P. J., and Grice, J. (1985). In *Microbeam Analysis 1985,* San Francisco Press, San Francisco, p. 60.

Eusemann, R., Rose, H., and Dubochet, J. (1982). *J. Microsc.* **128**, 239.

Eveling, D. W., and McCall, R. D. (1983). *J. Microsc.* **129**, 113.

Everhart, T. E. (1958). Ph.D thesis, University of Cambridge.

Evers, P., Robinson, K., and Maistry, L. (1983). *SEM 1983* 333.

Falk, R. H. (1980). *SEM 1980* **II**, 79.

Falls, A. H., Davis, H. T., Scriven, L. E., and Talmon, Y. (1982). *Biochim. Biophys. Acta* **693**, 364.

Falls, A. H., Wellinghoff, S. T., Talmon, Y., and Thomas, E. L. (1983). *J. Mater. Sci.* **18**, 2752.

Fathers, D. J., and Jakubovics, J. P. (1976). *Phys. Status Solidi A* **36**, K13.

Fathers, D. J., and Rez, P. (1979). *SEM 1979* **I**, 55.

Fathers, D. J., Jakubovics, J. P., Joy, D. C., Newbury, D. E., and Yakowitz, H. (1973a). *Phys. Status. Solidi. A* **20**, 535.

Fathers, D. J., Joy, D. C. and Jakubovics, J. P. (1973b). *SEM 1973* 259.

Fathers, D. J., Jakubovics, J. P., Joy, D. C., Newbury, D.E., and Yakowitz, H. (1974). *Phys. Status Solidi A* **22**, 609.

Fernandez-Moran, H. (1982) In *Proc. Eur. Congr EM, Hamburg,* 751.

Ferrel, C. (1956). *Phys. Rev.* **101**, 554.

Ficca, J. F. (1968). In *Trans. 3rd Natl. Conf. Electron Probe Microanalysis* Society of America, Paper 15.

Fiori, C. E., and Newbury, D. E. (1981). In *Analytical Electron Microscopy 1981,* San Francisco Press, San Francisco, p. 17.

Fiori, C. E., Yakowitz, H., and Newbury, D. E. (1974a). *SEM 1974* 167.

Fiori, C. E., Newbury, D. E., Yakowitz, H., and Heinrich, K. F. J. (1974b). In *Proc. MAS 1974* Carlton University, Paper 5.

Fiori, C. E., Myklebust, R. L., Heinrich, K. F. J., and Yakowitz, H. (1976). *Anal. Chem.* **48**(1), 172.

Fiori, C. E., Gorlen, K. E., and Gibson, C. G. (1981). In *Proc. EMSA* Atlanta.

Fiori, C. E., Swyt, C. R., and Gorlen, K. E. (1984). In *Microbeam Analysis 1984,* San Francisco Press, San Francisco, p. 57.

Fisher, K. A. (1982). *J. Microsc.* **126**, 1.

Fletcher, N. H. (1970). *The Chemical Physics of Ice,* Cambridge University Press, London.

Fletcher N. H. (1971). *Rep. Prog. Phys.* **34**, 913.

Fletcher, R. A., Chabay, I., Weitz, D. A., and Chung, J. C. (1984). *Chem. Phys. Lett.* **104**, 615.

Flood, P. R. (1980). *SEM 1980* **I**, 183.

Foley, J. D., and Van Dam, A. (1982). *Fundamentals of Interactive Computer Graphics,* Addison–Wesley, Reading, Mass.

Fotino, M., and Giddings, T. H. (1983). In *Proc. 41st EMSA Meet.* p. 588.

Franks, F. (1980). *SEM 1980* **II**, 349.

Franks, F. (1985). *Biophysics and Biochemistry at Low Temperatures,* Cambridge University Press, London.

Franks, F., and Skaer, H. (1976). *Nature* **262**, 323.

Franks, F., Asquith, M.H., Hammond, C. C., Skaer, H., and Echlin, P. (1977). *J. Microsc.* **110**, 223.

Franks, F., Mathias, S. F., Galfre, P., Webster, S., and Brown, D. (1983). *Cryobiology* **20**, 298.

Franks, J., Clay, C. S., and Peace, G. W. (1980). *SEM 1980* **I**, 155.

Frederik, P. M. (1982). *SEM 1982* **II**, 709.

Frederik, P. M., and Busing, W. M. (1980). *Electron Microscopy 1980* **2**, 712.

Frederik, P. M., and Busing, W. M. (1981). *J. Microsc.* **122**, 217.

Frederik, P. M., Busing, W. M., and Persson, A. (1982). *J. Microsc.* **125**, 167.

Frederik, P. M., Busing, W. M., and Persson, A. (1984). *SEM 1984* **I**, 433.

Fryer, J. R., McNee, C., and Holland, F. M. (1984). *Ultramicroscopy* **14**, 357.

Fujioka, H., Nakamae, K., and Ura, K. (1981). *SEM 1981* **I**, 323.

Furman, B. K., and Evans, C. A., Jr. (1981). In *Microbeam Analysis 1981,* San Francisco Press, San Francisco, p. 336.

Gamliel, H., and Pollicak, A. (1983). *SEM 1983* **II**, 929.

Gamliel, H., Gurfel, D., Leizerowitz, R., and Polliack, A. (1983). *J. Microsc.* **131**, 87.

Garruto, R. M., Fukatsu, R., Yanagihara, R., Gajdusek, D. C., Hook, G., and Fiori, C. E. (1984). *Proc Natl. Acad. Sci. USA* **81**, 1875.

Gibson, J. M., and McDonald, M. L. (1984). *Ultramicroscopy* **12**, 219.

Glaeser, R. M. (1971). *J. Ultrastruct. Res.* **36**, 466.

Glaeser, R. M., and Taylor, K. A. (1979). *J. Microsc.* **112**, 127.

Glaeser, R. M., Chiu, W., and Grano, D. (1979). *J. Ultrastruct. Res.* **66**, 235.

Goldmark, P. C., and Holywood, J. J. (1951). *Proc. IRE* **39**(10), 1314.

Goldstein, J. I., Costley, J. L., Lorimer, G. W., and Reed, S. J. B. (1977). *SEM 1977* **I**, 315.

Goldstein, J. I., Newbury, D.E., Echlin, P., Joy, D.C., Fiore, C., and Lifshin, E. (1981). *Scanning Electron Microscopy and X-Ray Microanalysis,* Plenum Press, New York.

Gonda, M. A., Benton, C. V., Massey, R. J., and Schultz, A. M. (1981). *SEM 1981* **II**, 45.

Gonzalez, R. C., and Wintz, P. (1977). *Digital Image Processing,* Addison–Wesley, Reading, Mass.

Goodman, S. L., Hodges, G. M., and Livingston, D. C. (1980). *SEM 1980* **II**, 133.

Goodman, S. L., Hodges, G. M., Trejdosiewicz, L. K., and Livingston, D. C. (1981). *J. Microsc.* **123**, 201.

Gopinath, A., Gopinathan, K. G., and Thomas, P. R. (1978). *SEM 1978* **I**, 375.

Gopinathan, K. G., Thomas, P. R., Gopinath, A., and Owens, A. R. (1976). *Electron. Lett.* **12**, 501.

Gorlen, K. E., Barden, L. K., Del Priore, J. S., Kochhar, A. K., Fiori, C. E., Gibson, C. G., and Leapman, R. D. (1982). in *Proc. DECUS.*

Gorlen, K. E., Barden, L. K., Del Priore, J. S., Fiori, C. E., Gibson, C. G., and Leapman, R. D. (1984). *Rev. Sci. Instrum.* **55**(6), 912.

Grasenick, F., Jakopic, E., and Waltinger, H. (1972). *Naturwissenschaften* **59**, 362.

Grocki, K., and Dermietzel, R. (1984). *J. Microsc.* **133**, 95.

Gupta, B. F., and Hall, T. A. (1981). In *Proc 38th EMSA Meet.* p. 654.

Haggis, G. H. (1982). *SEM 1982* **II**, 751.

Haggis, G. H. (1983). *J. Microsc.* **132**, 185.

Haggis, G. H. (1985). *J. Microsc.* in press.

Haggis, G. H., Schweitzer, I., Hall, R., and Bladon, T. (1983). *J. Microsc.* **132**, 185.

Hall, T. A., and Gupta, B. F. (1982). *J. Microsc.* **126**, 333.

Hardy, W. R., Behera, S. K., and Cavan, D. (1975). *J. Phys. E* **18**, 789.

Hartman, A. L., and Nakane, P. K. (1981). *SEM 1981* **II**, 44.

Harvey, D. M. R. (1982). *J. Microsc.* **127**, 209.

Hawes, C. R., and Horne, J. C. (1985). *J. Microsc.* **137**, 35.

Hax, W. M. A., and Lichtenegger, S. (1982). *J. Microsc.* **126**, 275.

Hayat, M. A. (1982). *Fixation for Electron Microscopy.* Academic Press, New York.

Heath, I. B. (1984). *J. Microsc.* **135**, 75.

Heide, H. G. (1965). *Lab Invest.* **14**, 396.

Heide, H. G. (1982a). *Ultramicroscopy* **10**, 125.

Heide, H. G. (1982b). *Ultramicroscopy* **7**, 299.

Heide, H. G. (1984). *Ultramicroscopy* **14**, 271.

Heinrich, K. F. J. (1962). *Rev. Sci. Instrum.* **33**, 884.

Heinrich, K. F. J. (1966). In *X-ray Optics and Microanalysis,* ed. R. Castaing, P. Deschamps, and J. Philibert, Hermann, Paris, p. 159.

Heinrich, K. F. J. (1981). *Electron Beam X-Ray Microanalysis,* Van Nostrand–Reinhold, Princeton, N.J.

Heinrich, K. F. J., and Fiori, C. E (1984). In *Microbeam Analysis 1984,* San Francisco Press, San Francisco, p. 175.

Heinrich, K. F. J., Fiori, C. E., and Yakowitz, H. (1970). *Science* **167**, 1129.

Hembree, G. G., Jensen, S. W., and Marchiando, J. F. (1981). In *Microbeam Analysis 1981,* San Francisco Press, San Francisco, p. 123.

Henglein, A. (1984). *Ultramicroscopy* **14**, 195.

Henoc, J., and Maurice, F. (1976). In *Use of Monte Carlo Calculations in Electron Probe Microanalysis and Scanning Electron Microscopy,* ed. K. F. J. Heinrich, D. E. Newbury, and H. Yakowitz, National Bureau of Standards Special Publication 460, Washington, D.C., p. 61.

Herman, E. M., Aloia, K. A. P., Thompson, W. W., and Shannon, L. M. (1984). *Eur. J. Cell Biol.* **35**, 1.

Heuser, J. E., Reese, T. S., Dennis, M. J., Jan, Y., Jan, L., and Evans, L. (1979). *J Cell Biol.* **81**, 275.

Hillenkamp, F., Kaufmann, R., Nitsche, R., and Unsold, E. (1975). *Appl. Phys.* **8**, 341.

Hirsch, P. B., and Humphreys, C. J. (1970). In *Proc. 3rd SEM Symp.* p. 449.

Hirsch, P. B., Howie, A., Nicholson, R. B., Pashley, D. W., and Whelan, M. J. (1965). *Electron Microscopy of Thin Crystals,* Butterworths, London.

Hirsch, P. B., Howie, A., Nicholson, R. B., Pashley, D. W., and Whelan, M. (1978). *Electron Microscopy of Thin Crystals,* 2nd ed., Krieger, New York.

Hirschfeld, T. (1982). In *Microbeam Analysis 1982,* San Francisco Press, San Francisco, p. 247.

Hobbs, P. V. (1974). *Ice Physics,* Oxford University Press (Clarendon), London.

Holt, D. B. (1974). In *Quantitative Scanning Electron Microscopy,* ed. D. B. Holt, M. D. Muir, P. R. Grant, and I. M. Boswarva, Academic Press, New York, p. 213.

Holt, D. B., and Datta, S. (1980). *SEM 1980* **I**, 259.

Hook, G., Lai, C., Bastacky, J., and Hayes, T. L. (1980). *SEM 1980* **IV**, 27.

Horisberger, M. (1983). *Trends Biol. Sci.* **Nov.**, 395.

Hoyer, L. C., Lee, J. C., and Bucana, C. (1979). *SEM 1979* **III**, 629.

Hren, J. J., Goldstein, J. I., and Joy, D. C., eds. (1979). *Introduction to Analytical Electron Microscopy,* Plenum Press, New York.

Hsu, K. C. (1981). *SEM 1981* **IV**, 17.

Huebener, R.P., and Seifert, H. (1984). *SEM 1984* **III**, 1053.

Humbel, B., Marti, T., and Muller, M. (1983). *BEDO* **16**, 585.

Hunziker, E. B., Herrmann, W., Schenk, R. K., Mueller, M., and Moor, H. (1984). *J. Cell Biol.* **98**, 267.

Ikuta, T., and Shimizu, R. (1974). *Phys. Status Solidi A* **23**, 605.

Ikuta, T., and Shimizu, R. (1976). *J. Phys. E* 721.

Ingersol, R. M., and Derouin, G. E. (1969). *Rev. Sci. Instrum.* **40**, 637.

Inove, T., (1983). *SEM 1983* **I**, 227.

Isaacson, M., Ohtsuki, M., and Utlaut, M. (1979). In *Introduction to Analytical Electron Microscopy,* ed. J. J. Hren, J. I. Goldstein, and D. C. Joy, Plenum Press, New York, p. 343.

Jaffe, J. S., and Glaeser, R. M. (1984). *Ultramicroscopy* **13**, 373.

Jaklevic, J., and Goulding, F. S. (1972). *IEEE Trans. Nucl. Sci.* **19**(3), 392.

Jeng, T. W., and Chiu, W. (1984). *J. Microsc,* **136**, 35.

Jeszka, J. K., Ulanski, J., and Kryszewski, M. (1981). *Nature* **289**, 390.

Johansen, B. V., and Namork, E. (1984). *J. Microsc.* **133**, 83.

Johansen, B. V., Namork, E., and Bukholm, G. (1983). *J. Microsc.* **132**, 67.

Johnson, D. F. (1984). In *Analysis of Organic and Biological Surfaces,* ed. P. Echlin, Plenum Press, New York, P. 529.

Jones, A. V., and Leonard, K. R. (1978). *Nature* **271**, 659.

Jones, A., and Smith, K. (1978). *SEM 78* **I**, 13.

Jones, A., and Unitt, B. (1980). *SEM 80* **I**, 113.

Jones, D. B. (1981). *SEM 1981* **II**, 77.

Jones, G. J. (1984). *J. Microsc,* **136**, 349.

Jones, M. P., Gavrilovic, J., and Beaven, C. H. J. (1966). *Trans. Inst. Min. Metall. Sect. B* **75**, B 274.

Joy, D. C. (1982). *Ultramicroscopy* **8**, 301.

Joy, D. C. (1985). *J. Microsc.* in press.

Joy, D. C., and Jakubovics, J. P. (1968). *Philos. Mag.* **17**, 61.

Joy, D. C., and Jakubovics, J. P. (1969). *J. Phys. D* **2**, 1367.

Joy, D. C., and Maruszewski, C. M. (1975). *J. Mater. Sci.* **10**, 178.

Joy, D. C., Newbury, D. E., and Hazzledine, P. M. (1972). In *Proc. 4th SEM Symp.* p. 97.

Joy, D. C., Leamy, H. J. Ferris, S. D. Yakowitz, H. and Newbury, D. E. (1976). *Appl. Phys. Lett.* **28**, 466.

Joy, D. C., Newbury, D. E., and Davidson, D. L. (1982). *J. Appl Phys.* **53**, R81.

Kalab, M. (1981). *SEM 1981* **III**, 453.

Kanaya, K., and Okayama, S. (1972). *J. Phys. D* **5**, 43.

Kanaya, K., Muranaka, Y., and Fujita, H. (1982). *SEM 1982* **IV**, 1379.

Kanaya, W., Moujou, D., and Adachi, K. (1974). *Micron* **5**, 51.

Karp, R. D., Silcox, J. C., and Somlyo, A. V. (1982). *J. Microsc.* **126**, 157.

Katoh, M., and Matsumoto, M. (1979). *J. Electron Microsc.* **28**, 51.

Kaufmann, R., Hillenkamp, F., Wechsung, R., Heinen, H. J., and Schurman, M. (1979). *SEM 1979* **II**, 279.

Kellogg, G. L., and Tsong, T. T. (1980). *J. Appl. Phys.* **51**, 1184.

Kemmenoe, B. H., and Bullock, G. R. (1983). *J. Microsc.* **132**, 153.

Kimerling, L. C., Leamy, H. J., and Patel, J. R. (1977). *Appl. Phys. Lett.* **30**, 217.

Kirkpatrick, P., and Weidmann, L. (1945). *Phys. Rev.* **67**, 321.

Kittel, C. (1966). *An Introduction to Solid State Physics,* Wiley, New York.

Knapek, E. (1982). *Ultramicroscopy* **10**, 71.

Knapek, E., and Dubochet, J. (1980). *J. Mol. Biol.* **141**, 147.

Knight, C. A., DeVries, A. L., and Oolman, L. D. (1984). *Nature* **308**, 295.

Knoll, G., Oebel, G., and Plattner, H. (1982). *Protoplasma* **111**, 161.

Knoll, M. (1941). *Naturwissenschaften* **29**, 335.

Koller, T., Beer, M., Muller, M., and Muhlethaler, K. (1973). In *Principles and Techniques of Electron Microscopy,* ed. M. A. Hayat, Van Nostrand–Reinhold, Princeton, N.J., p. 55.

Kotorman, L. (1980). *SEM 1980* **IV,** 77.

Kourosh, S., and Diller, K. R. (1984). *J. Microsc.* **136,** 39.

Krog, J. O., Zachariassen, K. E., Larsen, B., and Smidsrod, O. (1979). *Nature* **282,** 300.

Kubotsu, A., and Veda, M. (1980). *J. Electron Microsc.* **29,** 45.

Kumon, H., Ohno, K., Matsumura, Y., Ohmori, H., and Tanaka, T. (1983). *J. Electron Microsc.* **32,** 20.

Kuzurian, A. M., and Leighton, S. B. (1983). *SEM 1983* **IV,** 1877.

Kyser, D. F., and Murata, K. (1974). *IBM J. Res. Dev.* **18,** 352.

Lai, C. E., and Hayes, T. L. (1980). In *Proc. 38th EMSA Meet.* p. 800.

Lametschwandtner, A., Miodonski, A., and Simonsberger, P. (1980). *Mikroskopie* **36,** 270.

Lamvik, M. K., Kopf, D. A., and Robertson, J. D. (1983). *Nature* **301,** 332.

Lander, J. J., Schreiber, H., Buck, T. M., Matthews, J. R. (1963). *Appl. Phys. Lett.* **3,** 206.

Leamy, H. J. (1982). *J. Appl. Phys.* **53,** R51.

Leamy, H. J., Kimerling, L. C., and Ferris, S. D. (1976) *SEM 1976* **I,** 529.

Leamy, H. J., Kimerling, L. C., and Ferris, S. D. (1978). *SEM 1978* **I,** 717.

Leapman, R. D., Fiori, C. E., Gorlen, K. E., Gibson, C. G., and Swyt, C. R. (1983). In *Proc. EMSA* p. 10. Reprinted in *Ultramicroscopy* **12,** 281 (1984).

Legge, G. J. F. (1980). In *Microbeam Analysis 1980,* San Francisco Press, San Francisco, p. 70.

Lepault, J., and Pitt, T. (1984). *EMBO J.* **3,** 101.

Lepault, J., Freeman, R., and Dubochet, J. (1983a). *J. Microsc.* **132,** RP3.

Lepault, L. (1984). In *Proc. 41st EMSA Meet.* p. 426.

Lepault, L., Booy, F. F., and Dubochet, J. (1983b). *J. Microsc.* **129,** 89.

Leunissen, J. L. M. (1982). In *Proc Annu. Meet. NVEN,* Wageningen.

Leunissen, J. L. M., Elbers, P. F., Bijvert, J. J. M., and Verkleij, A. J. (1984). *Ultramicroscopy* **12,** 345.

Levi-Setti, R. (1983). *SEM 1983* **I,** 1.

Linton, R. W., Framer, M. E., Ingram, P., Sommer, J. R., and Shelburne, J. D. (1984). *J. Microsc.* **134,** 101.

Llinas, R., Spitzer, R., Hillman, D., and Chujo, M. (1979). *SEM 79* **II,** 367.

Luftig, R. B., and McMillan, P. N. (1981). *Int. Rev. Cytol. Suppl.* **12,** 309.

McCarthy, D. A., Pell, B. K., Molburn, C. M., Moore, S. R., Perry, J. A., Goddard, D. H., and Kirk, A. P. (1985). *J. Microsc.* **137,** 57.

McCully, (1985). *J. Microsc.* in press.

McDowall, A. W., Chang, J. J., Freeman, R., Lepault, J., Walter, C. A., and Dubochet, J. (1983). *J. Microsc.* **131,** 1.

McDowall, A. W., Hoffman, W., Lepault, J., Adrian, M., and Dubochet, J. (1994). *J. Mol. Biol.* in press.

MacKenzie, A. (1977). *Philos. Trans. R. Soc. London Ser. B* **278,** 167.

Madden, M. C., and Hren, J. J. (1985). *J. Microsc.* **139,** 1.

Marchese-Ragona, S. P. (1984). *J. Microsc.* **134,** 169.

Marshall, A. T. (1974). *Micron* **5,** 275.

Marshall, A. T. (1981). *SEM 1981* **II,** 327.

Marshall, A. T. (1982a). *SEM 1982* **I,** 243.

Marshall, A. T. (1982b). *Micron* **13,** 315.

Marshall, A. T., and Carde, D. (1984). *J. Microsc.* **134,** 113.

Marshall, A. T., and Zercher, (1982). *Philips Electron Optics Bulletin* No. 117, p. 16.

Maruyama, *J. Electron Microsc.* **31,** 253.

Maruyama, K., and Okuda, M. (1985). *J. Microsc.* in press.

Mathias, S. F., Franks, F., and Trafford, K. (1984). *Cryobiology* **21,** 123.

Maugel, T. K., Bonar, D. B., Creegan, W. J., and Small, E. G. (1980). *SEM 1980* **II,** 57.

Mayer, E., and Brügeller, P. (1982). *Nature* **298**, 715.

Menzel, E., and Kubalek, E. (1979). *SEM 1979* **I**, 297.

Menzel, E., and Kubalek, E. (1981). *SEM 1981* **I**, 305.

Miller, K. R., Prescott, C. S., Jacobs, T. L., and Lassignal, N. L. (1983). *J. Ultrastruct. Res.* **82**, 123.

Milligan, R. A., Brisson, A., and Unwin, P. N. T. (1984). *Ultramicroscopy* **13**, 1.

Millikin, B. E., and Weiss, R. L. (1984). *J. Cell Sci.* **68**, 211.

Moik, J. G. (1980). NASA Publication SP-431, Washington, D.C.

Molday, R. S., and Mayer, P. (1980). *Histochem. J.* **12**, 273.

Moller, C. (1931). *Z. Phys.* **70**, 786.

Moor, H., Bellin, G., Sandri, C., and Akert, K. (1980). *Cell Tissue Res.* **209**, 201.

Morin, P., Pitaval, M., Besnard, D., and Fontaine, G. (1979). *Philos. Mag.* **40**, 511.

Morrison, J. C., and Buskirk, E. M. (1984). *SEM 1984* **II**, 857.

Mott, N. F., and Massey, H. S. W. (1965). *The Theory of Atomic Collisions,* Oxford University Press, London.

Muller, E. W., Panitz, J. A., and McLane, S. B. (1968). *Rev. Sci. Instrum.* **39**, 83.

Munger, B. L. (1977). *SEM 1977* **I**, 481.

Murakami, T., and Jones, A. L. (1980). *SEM 1980* **I**, 221.

Murakami, T., Kubotsu, A., Ohtsuka, A., Akita, S., Yamamoto, K., and Jones, A. L. (1982). *SEM 1982* **I**, 459.

Murakami, T., Iida, N., Taguchi, T., Ohtani, O., Kikuta, A., Ohtsuka, A. and Iroshima, T. (1983). *SEM 1983* 235.

Muranaka, Y., Hojou, K., and Kanaya, K. (1982). In *Proc. 10th Int. Cong. EM* **3**, 459.

Murata, K., Kyser, D. F., and Ting, C. M. (1981). *J. Appl. Phys.* **52**, 4396.

Murphey, J. A. (1978) *SEM 1978* **II**, 175.

Murphey, J. A. (1980). *SEM 1980* **I**, 209.

Murphey, J. A. (1982). *SEM 1982* **II**, 657.

Myklebust, R. L. (1984). *J. de Physique* **45**, 2.

Myklebust, R. L. (1984). *J. Phys. (Paris)* **45**(C2), 41.

Myklebust, R. L., Yakowitz, H., and Heinrich, K. F. J. In *Proc. 8th Conf. Electron Probe Analysis* paper 26.

Nagele, R. G., Roisen, F. J., and Lee, H. (1983). *J. Microsc.* **129**, 179.

Nagele, R. G., Doane, K. J., Lee, H., Wilson, F. J., and Roisen, F. J. (1984). *J. Microsc.* **133**, 177.

Nagele, R. G., Kosciuk, M. C., Spero, D. A., and Lee, H. (1985). *J. Microsc.* in press.

Nagy, Z. I. (1983). *SEM 1983* **III**, 1255.

Narlen, A. N., Venkatesh, C. G., and Rice, S. A. (1976). *J. Chem. Phys.* **64**, 1106.

Neugebauer, D. C., and Zingsheim, H. P. (1979). *J. Microsc.* **117**, 313.

Newbury, D. E. (1974). In *Proc. 7th SEM Symp.* p. 1047.

Newbury, D. E. (1979). *SEM 1979* **II**, 1.

Newbury, D. E., and Myklebust, R. L. (1984). In *Electron Beam Interactions with Solids for Microscopy, Microanalysis, and Microlithography,* ed. D. F. Kyser, H. Niedrig, D. E. Newbury, and R. Shimizu, SEM, Inc., Chicago, p. 153.

Newbury, D. E., Yakowitz, H., and Myklebust, R. L. (1973). *Appl. Phys. Lett.* **23**, 488.

Newbury, D. E., Yakowitz, H., and Yew, N. (1974). *Appl. Phys. Lett.* **24**, 98.

Newbury, D. E., Yakowitz, H. and Myklebust, R. L. (1976). In *Use of Monte Carlo Calculations in Electron Probe Microanalysis and Scanning Electron Microscopy,* ed. K. F. J. Heinrich, D. E. Newbury, and H. Yakowitz, National Bureau of Standards Special Publication 460, Washington, D. C., p. 151.

Newbury, D. E., Myklebust, R. L., Heinrich, K. F. J., and Small, J. A. (1980). In *Characterization of Particles,* ed. K. F. J. Heinrich, National Bureau of Standards Special Publication 533, Washington, D.C., p. 39.

Niedermeyer, W. (1982). *J. Microsc.* **125**, 307.

Nisonoff, A., Hopper, J. E., and Spring. S. B. (1975). *The Antibody Molecule,* Academic Press, New York.

Nobiling, R., et al. (1977). Nucl. Instrum. Methods **157**, 49.

Nockolds, C. E., Moran, K., Dobson, E., and Phillips, A. (1982). *SEM 1982* **III**, 907.

Nordestgaard, B. G., and Rostgaard J. (1985). *J. Microsc.* **137**, 189.

Nowell, J. A. (1983). In *Proc. 41st EMSA Meet.* p. 504.

Nowell, J. A., and Pawley, J. B. (1980). *SEM 1980* **II**, 1.

Ohtani, O., Gannon, B., Ohtsuka, A., and Murakami, T. (1982). *SEM 1982* **I**, 427.

Okagaki, T., Clark, B., and Fisch, R. O. (1980). *SEM 1980* **III**, 413.

Ostrow, M. Postulka, E., Menzel, E., and Kubalek, E. (1983). In *Microscopy of Semiconducting Materials 1983,* ed. A. G. Cullis, S. M. Davidson, and G. R. Booker, Institute of Physics, London, p. 421

Ourmazd, A., and Booker, G. R. (1979). *Phys. Status Solidi A* **55**, 771.

Panitz, J. A. (1974). *J. Vac. Sci. Technol.* **11**, 206.

Panitz, J. A. (1982a). *J. Microsc.* **125**, 3.

Panitz, J. A. (1982b). *J. Phys. E* **15**, 1281.

Parks, J. E., Schmitt, H. W., Hurst, G. S., and Fairbank, W. M., Jr. (1983). *Thin Solid Films* **108**, 69.

Parsons, D., Belloto, D. J., Schulz, W. W., Buja, M., and Hagler, H. K. (1984). *EMSA Bull.* **14**, 49.

Pashley, D.W., Stowell, M. J., Jacobs, M. H., and Law, T. J. (1964). *Philos. Mag.* **10**, 127.

Pawley, J. B., and Fisher, G. L. (1977). *J. Microsc.* **110**(2), 87.

Pawley, J. B., and Norton, J. T. (1978). *J. Microsc.* **112**, 169.

Perlov, G., Talmon, Y., And Falls, A. H. (1983). *Ultramicroscopy* **11**, 283.

Pesheck, P. S., Scriven, L. E., and Davis, H. T. (1981). *SEM 1981* **I**, 515.

Peters, K. R. (1980). *SEM 1980* **I**, 143.

Peters, K. R. (1982a). In *Proc 40th EMSA Meet.* p. 368.

Peters, K. R. (1982b). *SEM 1982* **IV**, 1359.

Peters, K. R. (1984a). *J. Microsc.* **133**, 17.

Peters, K. R. (1984b). In *Proc. 2nd Pfefferkorn Conference* p. 221.

Peters, K. R., Palade, G. E., Schneider, B. G., and Papermaster, D. S. (1983). *J. Cell Biol.* **96**, 265.

Petroff, P. M., and Lang, D. V. (1977). *Appl. Phys. Lett.* **31**, 60.

Petroff, P. M., Land, D. V., Strudel, J. L., and Logan, R. A. (1978). *SEM 1978* **I**, 325.

Pfefferkorn, G., Brocker, W., and Hastenrath, M. (1980). *SEM 1980* **I**, 251.

Philibert, J., and Tixier, R. (1968). In *Quantitative Electron Probe Microanalysis,* ed. K. F. J. Heinrich, National Bureau of Standards Special Publication 298, Washington, D.C., p. 13.

Philibert, J., and Tixier, R. (1969). *Micron* **1**, 174.

Phillips, T. E., and Boyne, A. F. (1984). *J. Electron Microsc. Techn.* **1**, 9.

Pierce, D. T., and Celotta, R. J. (1981). *Adv. Electron. and Electron Phys.* **56**, 219.

Pinto de Silva, P., and Kan, F. K. W. (1984). *J. Cell Biol.* **99**, 1156.

Plattner, H., and Bachmann, L. (1982). *Int. Rev. Cytol.* **79**, 237.

Plows, G. S., and Nixon, W. C. (1968). *J. Phys. E* **1**, 595.

Possin, G. E., and Kirkpatrick, C. G. (1976). *J. Appl. Phys.* **50**, 4033.

Powell, C. J. (1976). *Rev. Mod. Phys.* **48**, 33.

Pratt, W. K. (1978). *Digital Image Processing,* Wiley–Interscience, New York.

Pscheid, P., Schuld, C., and Plattner, H. (1981). *J. Microsc.* **121**, 149.

Pulker, H. K. (1980). in *Proc. 7th Eur. Congr. EM* **2**, 788.

Pun, T., and Ellis, J. R. (1985). *Signal Processing* in press.

Rash, J. E., and Hudson, C. S., eds. (1979). *Freeze-fracture: Methods, Artifacts, and Interpretations,* Raven Press, New York.

Rasmussen, D. H. (1982). *J. Microsc.* **128,** 167.

Ratliff, F. (1972). *Sci. Am.* **June,** 91.

Rebhun, L. I. (1971). In *Principles and Techniques of Electron Microscopy: Biological Applications,* ed. M. A. Hayet, Vol. 2, Van Nostrand, Princeton, N.J., p. 3.

Rebiai, R., Rest, A. J., and Scurlock, R. G. (1983). *Nature* **305,** 412.

Reimer, L., and Krefting, E.R. (1976). In *Use of Monte Carlo Calculations in Electron Probe Microanalysis and Scanning Electron Microscopy,* ed. K. F. J. Heinrich, D. E. Newbury, and H. Yakowitz, National Bureau of Standards Special Publication 460, Washington, D.C., p. 45.

Revel, J. P., Barnard, T., and Haggis, G. H., eds. (1984). *Proc 2nd Pfefferkorn Conf.,* SEM Inc., Chicago.

Rey, M. E. C. (1984). *J. Microsc.* **136,** 373.

Rigler, M. W., and Patton, (1984). *J. Microsc.* **134,** 335.

Robards, A. W., and Crosby, P. (1979). *SEM 1979* **II,** 325.

Robards, A. W., and Crosby, P. (1979). *SEM 1979* **II,** 325.

Robards, A. W., Wilson, A. J., and Crosby, P. (1981). J. Microsc. **124,** 143.

Rogers, P. A. W., and Gannon, B. J. (1983). *J. Microsc.* **131,** 241.

Romig, A. D., Jr. (1981). In *Microbeam Analysis 1981,* San Francisco Press, San Francisco, p. 249.

Romig, A. D., Jr., Newbury, D. E., and Myklebust, R. L. (1982). In *Microbeam Analysis 1982,* San Francisco Press, San Francisco, p. 88.

Roomans, G. M. (1981). *SEM 1981* **II,** 345.

Rose, A. (1948). In *Advances in Electronics,* ed. A. Marton, Academic Press, New York, p. 131.

Rose, A. (1970). *Image Technology* **June/July,** 13.

Rosencwaig, A., and White, R. M. (1981). *Appl. Phys. Lett.* **38,** 165.

Rosowski, J. R., Hoagland, K. D., Roemer, S. C., and Lee, K. W. (1981). *Scanning* **4,** 181.

Rosowski, J. R., Roemer, S. C., Hoagland, K. D., and Roth, W. A. (1984). *SEM 1984* **I,** 29.

Ross, G. D., Morrison, G. H., Sacher, R. F., and Staples, R. C. (1983). *J. Microsc.* **129,** 221.

Russ, J. (1980). In *Eighth International Congress on X-ray Optics and Microanalysis,* ed. D. R. Beaman, R. E. Ogilvie, And D. B. Wittry, Pendell, Midland, Mich., p. 91.

Russel, P. E., and Herrington, C. R. (1982). In *Microbeam Analysis 1982,* San Francisco Press, San Francisco, p. 449.

Sargent, J. A. (1983). *J. Microsc.* **129,** 103.

Saubermann, A. J., and Echlin, P. (1975). *J. Microsc.* **105,** 155.

Saubermann, A. J., Riley, W. D., and Beeuwkes, R. (1977). *J. Microsc.* **111,** 39.

Saubermann, A. J., Beeuwkes, R., and Peters, P. D. (1981a). *J. Cell Biol.* **88,** 268.

Saubermann, A. J., Echlin, P., Peters, P. D., and Beeuwkes, R. (1981b). *J. Cell Biol.* **88,** 257.

Saxton, W. (1978). *Computer Techniques for Image Processing in Electron Microscopy,* Academic Press, New York.

Schamber, F. H. (1977). In *X-Ray Fluorescence Analysis of Environmental Samples,* ed. T. G. Dzubay, Ann Arbor Science, Ann Arbor, Mich., p. 241.

Scheiwe, M. W., and Korber, C. (1982). *J. Microsc.* **126.** 29.

Schmidt, D. G., and van Hooydonk, A. C. M. (1980). *SEM 1980,* **111,** 653.

Schulson, E. M. (1971). *Phys. Status Solidi B* **46,** 95.

Scott, R. M., and Ramsey J. N. (1982). In *Microbeam Analysis 1982,* San Francisco press, San Francisco, p. 239.

Schimizu, R., and Ikuta, T. (1984). *Appl Phys. Lett.* **44,** 811.

Schimizu, R., Ikuta, T., Yamamoto, T., Kinoshita, M., and Murayama, T. (1974). *Phys. Status Solidi A* **26**, K87.

Schimizu, R., Ikuta, T., Kinoshita, M., Murayama, T., Nishizawa, H., and Yamamoto, T. (1976). *Jpn. J. Appl Phys.* **15**, 967.

Shennawy, I. E. E., Gee, D. J., and Aparicio, S. R. (1983). *J. Microsc.* **132**, 243.

Siegel, G. (1972). *Z. Naturforsch.* **27**, 325.

Silyn-Roberts, H. (1983). *J. Microsc.* **130**, 111.

Simionescu, N., and Simionescu, M. (1976). *J. Cell Biol.* **70**, 608.

Sitte, H. (1982). In *Proc. Int. Cong. EM, Hamburg* **1**, 9.

Sjostrand, F. (1982). *J. Microsc.* **128**, 279.

Skaer, H. (1982). *J. Microsc.* **125**, 137.

Skaer, H., Franks, F., Asquith, M. H., and Echlin, P. (1977). *J. Microsc.* **110**, 257.

Skaer, H., Franks, F., and Echlin, P. (1978). *Cryobiology* **15**, 589.

Slayter, H. S. (1980). *SEM 1980* **I**, 171.

Steinbrecht, R. A., and Zierold, K. (1984). *J. Microsc,* **136**, 69.

Sleytr, R. B., and Robards, A. W. (1982). *J. Microsc.* **126**, 101.

Smith, G. D. W., Delargy, K. M., Barnard, S. J., Williams, P. R., Reed, A. J. G., and VanderSande, J. B. (1981). In *Analytical Electron Microscopy 1981,* San Francisco Press, San Francisco, p. 76.

Soligo, D., Lampen, N., and DeHarven, E. (1981). *SEM 1981* **II**, 95.

Soligo, D., Pozzoli, E., Nava, M. T., Polli, N., and DeHarven, E. (1983). *SEM 1983* **IV**, 1795.

Sommerfeld, A. (1931). *Ann. Phys. (Leipzig)* **11**, 257.

Spencer, J. P., Humphreys, C. J., and Hirsch, P. B. (1972). *Philos. Mag.* **26**, 193.

Spicer, S. S., Schulte, B. A., and Shelburne, J. D. (1983). *SEM 1983* **IV**, 1827.

Statham, P. J. (1976a). *X-Ray Spectrom.* **5**, 154.

Statham, P. J. (1976b). *X-Ray Spectrom.* **5**, 16.

Statham, P. J. and Jones, M. (1980). *Scanning* **3**(3), 168.

Steinbach, W. R., Lohrstorfer, C. F., and Etz, E. S. (1982). In *Microbeam Analysis 1982,* San Francisco Press, San Francisco, p. 279.

Steinbrecht, R. A. (1982). *J. Microsc.* **125**, 187.

Stewart, M., and Lepault, J. (1985). *J. Microsc.* in press.

Stickler, R., Hughes, C. W., and Booker, G. R. (1971). *SEM 1971* 473.

Strahm, M., and Butler, J. (1979). In *37th Annv. Proc. EMSA* p. 598.

Strahm, M., and Butler, J. (1981). *Rev. Sci. Instrum.* **52**(6), 840.

Streitwolf, H. W. (1959). *Ann. Phys. (Leipzig)* **3**, 183.

Sumner, A. T. (1982). *SEM 1982* **I**, 261.

Sumner, A. T. (1984). *SEM 1984* **II**, 905.

Sybers, H. D., Myre, C. D., and Myre, M. V. (1983). *SEM 1983* **II**, 769.

Sze, S. M. (1969). *Physics of Semiconductor Devices,* Wiley, New York.

Takahashi, K., and Tavassoli, M. (1983). *J. Microsc.* **132**, 219.

Takata, K., and Hirano, H. (1984). *Histochemistry* **81**, 435.

Talmon, Y. (1982a). In *Proc Int. Cong. EM Hamburg* **1**, 25.

Talmon, Y. (1982b). *J. Microsc.* **125**, 227.

Talmon, Y. (1984). *Ultramicroscopy* **14**, 305.

Talmon, Y., and Thomas, E. L. (1978). *J. Microsc.* **113**, 69.

Tanaka, K. (1981). *SEM 1981* **II**, 1.

Tanaka, K., and Mitsushima, A. (1984). *J. Microsc.* **133**, 213.

Taub, I-R., and Eiben, K. (1968). *J. Chem. Phys.* **49**, 2499.

Taylor, K. A., Milligan, R. A., Raeburn, C., and Unwin, P. N. T. (1984). *Ultramicroscopy* **13**, 185.

Taylor, P. G., and Burgess, A. (1977). *J. Microsc.* **111,** 51.

Trejdosiewicz, L. K., Smolira, M. A., Hodges, G. M., Goodman, S. L., and Livingston, D.C. (1981). *J. Microsc.* **123,** 227.

Tsuji, T. (1983). *J. Microsc.* **131,** 115.

Tsuji, T., and Karasek, M. A. (1985). *J. Microsc.* **137,** 75.

Ulrich, R. G., and McClung, K. J. (1983). *J. Ultrastruct. Res.* **82,** 327.

Umrath, W. (1983). *Mikroskopie* **40,** 9.

Unguris, J., Hembree, G., Pierce, D. T., and Celotta, R. J. (1985). *J. Microsc.* **139,** RP 1.

van Essen, C. G., and Verhoven, J. D. (1974). *J. Phys. E* **7,** 768.

van Essen, C. G., Schulson, E. M., and Donaghay, R. H. (1970). *Nature* **225,** 847.

van Essen, C. G., Schulson, E. M., and Donaghay, R. H. (1971). *J. Mater. Sci.* **6,** 213.

Van Harreveld, A., and Cowell, J. (1964). *Anat. Rec.* **149,** 381.

Volbert, B., and Reimer, L. (1980). *SEm 1980* **IV,** 1.

Walther, P., Kriz, S., Muller, M., Ariano, B. H., Brodbeck, U., Ott, P., and Scweingruber, M. E. (1984). *SEM 1984* **III,** 1257.

Walz, D. A., Penner, J., and Barnhart, M. I. (1984). *SEM 1984* **I,** 303.

Walzthony, D., Eppenberger, H. M., and Wallimann, T. (1984). *Eur. J. Cell Biol.* **35,** 216.

Warner, R. R. (1984). *J. Microsc.* **135,** 203.

Watson, L. P., McKee, A. E., and Merell, B. R. (1980). *SEM 1980* **II,** 45.

Weibull, C., Carlemalm, E., Villiger, W., Kellenberger, E., Fakan, J., Gautier, A., and Larsson, C. (1980). *J. Ultrastruct. Res.* **73,** 233.

Weibull, C., Villiger, W., and Carlemalm, E. (1984). *J. Microsc.* **134,** 213.

Weiss, R. L. (1980). *SEM 1980* **IV,** 123.

*Wells, O. C. (1974) *Scanning Electron Microscopy,* McGraw–Hill, New York, p. 172.

Wells, O. C. (1976). In *Use of Monte Carlo Calculations in Electron Probe Microanalysis and Scanning Electron Microscopy,* ed. K. F. J. Heinrich, D. E. Newbury, and H. Yakowitz, National Bureau of Standards Special Publication 460, Washington, D.C., p. 139.

Wells, O. C. (1983). *J. Microsc.* **131,** RP5.

Wells, O. C., and Savoy, R. J. (1981). *IEEE Trans. Magn.* **17,** 1253.

Welter, L. M., and McKee, A. N. (1972). *SEM 1972* 161.

Wendt-Gallitelli, M. F., and Woeburg, H. (1981). *SEm 1981* **II,** 455.

Westphal, C., and Frösch, D. (1985). *J. Microsc.* **137,** 17.

Wharlon, D. A., and Rowland, J. J. (1984). *J. Microsc.* **134,** 299.

White, G. K., and Woods, S. B. (1955). *Can. J. Phys.* **33,** 58.

Wildhaber, I., Gross, H., and Moor, H. (1982). *J. Ultrastruct. Res.* **80,** 367.

Williams, D. B. (1984). *Practical Analytical Electron Microscopy in Materials Science,* Philips, Mahwah, N.J.

Williams, D. B., Newbury, D. E., Goldstein, J. I., and Fiori, C. E. (1984). *J. Microsc.* **136,** 209.

Williams, E. J. (1933). *Proc. Roy. Soc. A.* **139,** 163.

Williamson, F. A. (1984). *J. Microsc.* **134,** 125.

Willison, J. H. M., and Rowe, A. J. (1980). In *Practical Methods in Electron Microscopy,* Vol. 8, ed. A. M. Glauert, North-Holland, Amsterdam.

Wilson, A. J., and Robards, A. W. (1982). *J. Microsc.* **125,** 287.

Wilson, D. C., Ambrose, W. W., Crenshaw, M. A., and Hanker, J. S. (1979). In *Proc. 37th EMSA Meet.* p. 360.

Witcomb, M. J. (1985). *J. Microsc.* in press.

Wittry, D. B. (1980). In *European Congress on Electron Microscopy, Leiden* **3,** 14.

Wolfgang, E. (1983). In *Microscopy of Semiconducting Materials 1983,* ed. A. G. Cullis, S. M. Davidson, and G. R. Booker, Institute of Physics, London, p. 407.

Wolf-Ingo, F., Worret, M. D., Cunningham, D. E., and Nordquist, R. E. (1982). In *Proc. 10th Int. EM Congr.* **3,** 253.

Wollweber, L., Strake, R., and Gothe, U. (1981). *J. Microsc.* **121,** 185.

Wouters, C. H., Messeling, S., Daems, W. T., and Ploem, J. S. (1984). *J. Microsc.* **136,** 315.

Wroblewski, R., and Wroblewski, J. (1984). *Histochemistry* **81,** 469.

Yakowitz, H., and Heinrich, K. F. J. (1969). *J. Res. Natl. Bur. Stand. Sect. A* **73,** 113.

Yakowitz, H., Newbury, D. E., and Myklebust, R. L. (1975). *SEm 1975* 94.

Yamada, N., Nagano, M., Murakami, S., Ikeuchi, M., Oho, E., Baba, N., Kanaya, K., and Osumi, M. (1983). *J. Electron Microsc.* **32,** 321.

Yamamoto, T., Nishizawa, H., and Tsuno, K. (1975). *J. Phys. D* **8,** 79.

Zeitler, E. (1982). *Ultramicroscopy* **10,** 1.

Zierold, K. (1982a). *Ultramicroscopy* **10,** 45.

Zierold, K. (1982b). *J. Microsc.* **125,** 149.

Zierold, K. (1982c). *SEM 1982* **III,** 1205.

Zierold, K. (1983). *SEM 1983* **II,** 809.

Zierold, K. (1984). *Ultramicroscopy* **14,** 201.

Zingsheim, H. P. (1984). *J. Microsc.* **133,** 307.

Zubin, J., and Wiggens, J. (1980). *Rev. Sci. Instrum.* **51,** 123.

Index

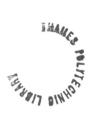